AMERICAN STUDIES – A MONOGRAPH SER[IES]

Volume 292

Edited on behalf
of the German Association
for American Studies by
ALFRED HORNUNG
ANKE ORTLEPP
HEIKE PAUL

MITA BANERJEE

Medical Humanities in American Studies

Life Writing, Narrative Medicine, and the Power of Autobiography

Universitätsverlag
WINTER
Heidelberg

Bibliografische Information der Deutschen Nationalbibliothek

Die Deutsche Nationalbibliothek verzeichnet diese Publikation in der Deutschen Nationalbibliografie; detaillierte bibliografische Daten sind im Internet über *http://dnb.d-nb.de* abrufbar.

UMSCHLAGBILD

© Kong Ho: *20th Anniversary of Americans with Disabilities Act* used with permission

ISBN 978-3-8253-6906-4

Imprimé en Allemagne · Printed in Germany
Umschlaggestaltung: Klaus Brecht GmbH, Heidelberg
Druck: Memminger MedienCentrum, 87700 Memmingen

Gedruckt auf umweltfreundlichem, chlorfrei gebleichtem und alterungsbeständigem Papier

Den Verlag erreichen Sie im Internet unter:
www.winter-verlag.de

Table of Contents

Acknowledgments..vii

Preface..ix

1 Introduction..1

2 Temporalities in Life Writing:
Tito Mukhopadhyay's *Beyond the Silence*.............43

3 Bollywood Film and the Borders of Disability:
Shah Rukh Khan Meets the American President…65

4 "An Anthropologist on Mars":
Temple Grandin's *Thinking in Pictures*…………103

5 "Living Autobiographically" in Modern Dance:
Concepts of Aging in Mikhail Baryshnikov's
"HeartBeat: mb" Performance…………………...131

6 "Like a Hole in the Head": Comedy and
Parkinson's Disease in Michael J. Fox's
Autobiographies *Always Looking Up*
and *Lucky Man*……………………………..…..161

7 Writing the Citizen: Growing Up with Down
Syndrome in *Raising Henry* and *Count Us In*……203

8 *Blue Hawaii*? Adam Horowitz's Film *Nuclear Savage* and Collective Life Writing in the Pacific.....271

9 Trauma, Repatriation, and Representation: Life Writing as an Alternative Form of Knowledge Production.....307

10 Sustainability and Indigenous Life Writing Performances: "Dancing Earth" and *The Cherokee Word for Water*.....337

11 Conclusion.....359

Works Cited.....373

Acknowledgments

This book owes its existence to two research projects I have been involved in: the Research Training Group "Life Sciences, Life Writing: Boundary Experiences of Human Life between Biomedical Explanation and Lived Experience" and the Research Group "Un/Doing Difference," both funded by the German Reseach Foundation. I have learned and benefitted immensely from conversations with my colleages in the "Life Sciences, Life Writing" program, especially Norbert Paul, Thomas Efferth, Manfred Beutel, Ralf Dahm, Thomas Lemke, Tilmann Habermas, Michael Simon, Ilhan Ilkilic, Susanne Michl, Michael Simon, and Claudia Buir. I continue to be indebted to Alfred Hornung for inspiration and support, in matters of life writing and much beyond. My colleagues from the "Un/Doing Difference" group have made me see human differentiation with different eyes. I am grateful to Stefan Hirschauer, Damaris Nübling, Oliver Scheiding, Herbert Kalthoff, Matthias Krings, Carola Lentz and Tobias Boll. For discussions about narrative medicine and beyond, I am deeply grateful to Rita Charon, Maura Spiegel, Deepu Gowda, Craig Irvine, Siri Hustvedt and Danielle Spencer. Without my wonderful team at Mainz, this book would never have been written. I am deeply grateful to Rebecca Schäfer for her meticulous reading of this manuscript, to Nina Heydt for helping me with the bibliography, and to Pia Wiegmink for the formatting of this manuscript. For their support and inspiration, I am indebted to Sonja Georgi, Julia Velten and Christine Plicht. My friends have listened carefully to many of the ideas discussed in this book and were there to remind me to stop working. Renata Kiworr-Ruppenthal and Mechthild Dreyer were there when I needed them most. Marion Stülten and Eva Boesenberg made me feel as if they were right here in Mainz, not in Munich and Berlin. My parents have supported me with their unbelievable patience even when the chips were down. Without my daughter Soraya, with her whirlwind personality and her wisdom well beyond her years, life would be unthinkable. Finally, I am deeply indebted to my husband, Detlef Krejci, for seeing me through; for being my harshest critic and my best friend, and for much more than I will ever be able to say.

Preface

Developments in biomedicine have changed the ways in which we conceptualize what it means to be human: From developments in brain research to reproductive technologies, our ways of being in the world and of coming into the world have changed more fundamentally than we would ever have been able to imagine. Yet, in tandem with these developments in biomedicine, we are now faced with forms of decision-making more complex than we could ever have imagined. Nothing, it would seem, is completely outside our reach, and yet, the choices make our being in the world at once easier and much more difficult. Genetic research may now have found a gene which may be involved in the development of Alzheimer's disease, detecting this gene may be possible even in childhood: "Individuals carrying a particular variant of the apolipoprotein E gene, probably have a higher risk of falling ill with Alzheimer's Disease later in life. Now scientists have found that even in young children, this allele can be related to changes in brain development and cognitive performance" ("Alzheimerdemenz: Belastendes Erbe" 10; my trans.).

Yet, how will the knowledge of having such a genetic predisposition affect the lives of the people whose future thus seems almost mapped out? Under what circumstances do we want to know what our genetic future may hold, and under what conditions would we prefer not to know? And by what compass do we gauge our route in this labyrinth of decision-making made possible by advances in biomedicine? One of the assumptions from which this book proceeds is that in this labyrinth of complex choices, it is to forms of life writing (biographies, autobiographies, blogs, patient narratives) that we may turn for orientation. What these life writing narratives reveal, then, is what course a life has taken *after* a certain decision was made, a decision made possible by advances in biomedicine. This, I propose in this book, is the need for bringing together, for creating a dialogue between, life writing and life sciences: The life sciences may provide us with a way of creating, of enhancing, and of prolonging life; yet, life writing asks, how do we live with these choices? How does the possibility of being able to make these choices change our lives themselves?

Developments in modern biomedicine thus confront us with decisions which we may often feel ill-equipped to make, decisions so existential to our lives or the lives of our loved ones that they seem impossible to make. Such decision-making and the conditions under which they are made, has been the subject of bioethics. Bioethics, in turn, has a strong narrative component. To the extent that the humanities engage with developments in modern medicine, conversely, they too have narratives to offer. If there is a narrative turn in medicine and bioethics, then, there has also been, at the same historical moment, a material turn in the humanities. Drawing on the work of Antonio Damasio[1], among many others, John Paul Eakin has cautioned that the humanities have separated the body from the mind, and the mind from the brain, for too long; that the necessity of overcoming the Cartesian dualism affects not only the life sciences but the humanities as well.

This book thus proceeds from a threefold assumption. First, it argues that overcoming the Cartesian split between body and mind may also require the emergence of a dialogue between life sciences and the humanities. Second, it locates in life writing as a genre a potential link between life sciences and the humanities, precisely because forms of life writing may describe the consequences, on the level of lived experience,[2] of biomedical decisions taken. Third, it locates in the history of the present moment a convergence between life sciences and the humanities, where each of these fields, after a century of separate developments, may be newly attuned to what the other has to offer. As Wolf Singer has recently argued,

> The creative process is the same for science and art. In science, the cognitive process begins with generating hypotheses. [These hypotheses] are first conceived through intuition, often based on criteria of aesthetic consistency which cannot be rationalized. Apparently, scientists are looking for similar criteria as artists: for coherence and closure. Many things in science are dominated by aesthetics. . . . The artist proceeds in a very similar manner; only the material which he handles is different. The artist, too, creates an image of the world as he interprets it, thus re-

[1] I am indebted to Alfred Hornung for this line of argument.

[2] I am grateful to Norbert Paul for this idea.

> maining within a particular descriptive system, he creates new realities, new interpretations [.] The scientist does the same when he creates a model for what can be experienced. Of course, the assumption and the craftsmanship are different, but the underlying processes, it seems to me, are highly similar for science and for art. (80; my trans.)

If indeed, as Singer argues, both the artist and the scientist develop models of the world, then it would seem more urgent than ever at the beginning of the twenty-first century to create a dialogue between these perspectives. Each in its turn may point to the shortcomings of the other. What is so intriguing about Singer's acknowledgment of the "scientific" work of the artist, then, is the absence of a hierarchy between life sciences and art: If indeed there is to be a dialogue between the two, both must meet on par.

Yet art, it may be argued, is different from life writing; in order to be art, it involves the aestheticization of lived experience. At the same time, life writing research has stressed the constructedness of life writing; any autobiography, life writing researchers have argued, also involves a degree of fictionality, of a construction of the self. It is for this reason that I argue that Singer's vision for abolishing the clear-cut distinction, even opposition, between the life sciences and the humanities may involve the inclusion not only of art, but also of forms of life writing.

At the same time, humanities researchers may feel that entering such a dialogue on Singer's terms may be a form of selling out; in order to maintain or regain their self-confidence at a time when many have declared the humanities obsolete, why should the humanities need the recognition of brain scientists like Singer? I believe that such fear of selling out may be unnecessary; even as the humanities must of course generate their self-confidence from within themselves, the willingness of the life sciences to engage with the intrinsic logic of the humanities – vastly different from their own – may nonetheless be beneficial.

Finally, I believe that the terrain whose surface this book can merely scratch is expanding by the minute: Because of the speed at which new developments in the life sciences occur, new ethical dilemmas, new forms of decision-making arise every second of our lives. It seems imperative, then, that the humanities enter into this dialogue, providing their own compasses and cues for decision-making in the era of biomedicine. Art, in its turn, has long taken on this challenge. If indeed art (literature, poetry, painting, photography, film) can be conceived as a form of theory in practice, then, art has long functioned as a compass in the labyrinth of biomedical and bioethical decision-making. To the extent that the humanities include such art forms into their canon, then – from "crip poetry" (Bartlett 16) to ballet –, they, too, enter into the dialogue.

Art, then, may be useful not just in the training of future doctors, but also in guiding us through the ever more complex processes of medical decision-making. To explore these processes, then, does not concern bioethics alone, but it must also centrally concern the humanities. Even as the examples I draw from in this book are taken from (transnational) American culture, my argument about the reach and relevance of the humanities may also be applicable to other disciplines within the humanities as well.

Life writing and life writing research thus converges with, for instance, the sociology of medicine in asking how biomedical developments are understood in the public sphere, how they are translated into social realities. Yet, life writing and art also comment in their own language, on these developments, gauging their desirability; they do not only describe but seek to intervene. In so doing, they also inquire into the reach – the *Deutungsmacht* – which developments in the life sciences have over our lives and the ways we defined them. As Michael Hagner puts it, "Here, too, scientists must be careful not to assume a perspective which is all too organ-centered, drawing conclusions about invariable characteristics of people solely on the basis of characteristics of the brain or its activity patterns" (33; my trans.). This necessity, of course, has been stressed by both brain researchers and geneticists; the field of epigenetics and research into gene expression has stressed the need for multifactorial approaches. What is at stake, then, is not (only) what brain research finds out about the workings of the human mind, but what the consequences (social, cultural, economic) of such findings are. It may be art and forms of life writing, then, which may help us deal with such consequences.

I believe that the discussion around the development of new drugs counteracting some of the effects of Down Syndrome and a photographic exhibit portraying persons with Down Syndrome may serve as an example to describe a canvas of disciplinary and artistic responses. New developments in biomedicine, as in Alberto Costa's work with neurotransmitters such as the receptor NMDA, make possible the development of new drugs targeting neurotransmitters, hence making it possible to counteract learning difficulties; photographic exhibits such as Sigga Ella's "First and Foremost I Am" (2014) stress that regardless of such drugs, we as a society must strive to include all differences, whatever they may be; and Hille Haker, drawing on bioethical debates and coming from the field of theological ethics, stresses that the argument that such drugs, once they have been developed, be *withheld* from persons with Down Syndrome is itself highly problematic. As Haker observes,

> For some, those concerned are only impaired because they lack sufficient social support. From this perspective, not the people living with Down Syndrome have to change, but society has to change in order to provide a place and possibility of belonging for all people. Others see disability as a physical, psychological or cognitive impairment, which is rooted in biological causes, which in principle can be researched and treated. Often, these positions seem mutually exclusive. But this is not the case: In fact, what discussions should revolve around/focus on is the compatibility of social and medical arguments. (77; my trans.)

Medical support, Haker suggests, is a form of social support as well. As Haker goes on to say, "Possibly, those who oppose medical research, end up preventing the individual possibilities of experience for which they are in fact fighting. For medical support is also a form of social aid" (77; my trans.).

The photographs are inseparable, then, from a specific moment in the history of science: a moment in which it now seems possible to make some of the symptoms of Down Syndrome invisible. Whether or not the persons concerned should take the pill or not, at first glance, seems to be a bioethical decision; it is a process of decision-making, however, which art – in this case, photography – has also begun to enter. It is in this sense, then, that the photographs engage in a form of life writing; they make visible the lives behind the "condition," lives which can never be fully captured by a given diagnosis. If the life sciences offer to us a new choice – the possibility of making the symptoms of Down Syndrome invisible – then, the photographs help us navigate the process of decision-making.

The effects of these drugs on the quality of life, but also the ensuing biography of the individual, however, can also be explored through forms of life writing. Thus, in her autobiography *Thinking in Pictures* (1995), Temple Grandin stresses that she has come to be a "believer in biochemistry" (123). As Grandin recalls about her life as a young scientist,

> I went to every doctor in town, but they found no physical cause for the headache that accompanied my anxiety. . . . Medical science was failing me, and I just took each day at a time and tried to get through it. . . . It was then that I turned to biochemistry to help me with the anxiety disorder I had lived with my whole adult life. . . . Six months prior to my eye surgery, I had read an article titled "The Promise of Biological Psychiatry" in the February 1981 issue of *Psychology Today*. (*Thinking in Pictures* 124-25)

What is so striking about this account is that Grandin's experience, and the stance she decides to take, anticipates current debates, at the beginning of the twenty-first century, about the difference, and possible points of intersection, between behavioral psychology and biological psychology (Flor 2016). Faced with the fact that behavioral psychology was unable to help her deal with her panic attacks, Grandin proceeds to do research; her solution, then, anticipates a development – a balance or fusion between behavioral therapy and neuropsychiatry – which has only taken hold at the beginning of the twenty-first century. It is in this sense, then, that it would be highly reductionist to reduce Grandin's narrative to the level of a patient account; it is also an account of the history of science, and it is a book written by a woman who earned a degree in psychology before going on to do her PhD in animal science.

My claim throughout this book is that such accounts are much more than *Betroffenenperspektiven* or patient accounts. In fact, one of the goals of this study is to inquire into the perspectival complexity which has been hidden or obfuscated by the term "*Betroffenenperspektive*." Recent studies in aging research, as in longevity studies and centenarian studies, have drawn attention to the need for extended interviews, for supplementing quantitative through qualitative analyses. In this revision, then, life writing narratives may prove powerful documents for upsetting the dichotomy, and the erstwhile hierarchy, between medical experts and laymen and -women.

What does this mean for our methodological practice? It means that we may come to contextualize cultural texts (literature, art, life writing) not just in historical terms, but also in terms of this history of science. Cultural texts respond to and are shaped not just by historical conditions and legal parameters, but also by new developments in the life sciences. If our lives are reshaped by new developments in the life sciences, then life writing can no longer be separated from life science research.

New developments in the field of biomedicine, this book sets out to argue, make an interdisciplinary canvas of approaches more urgent and more relevant than ever before. It is in this context and out of this sense of urgency that new fields have emerged such as medical humanities and narrative medicine. It is these fields and their "reverse relevance" for a potential redefinition of the humanities that the following chapters set out to explore.

1 Introduction

1.1 Life Sciences and Life Writing

This study begins with a simple question: If the humanities have "exported" some of their methodologies in order to create the field of "medical humanities," what happens to the humanities in the process? My aim in the following chapters is to inquire whether this export of techniques of literary and cultural analysis has any bearing or effect on the field in which these methodologies originate. In other words, are the humanities to remain the same regardless of this "exporting" of some of their methodologies to other fields such as medicine, or is there a sense in which they, too, may benefit from this export? What would happen, then, if the humanities were to set out to "re-import" the very field they had once exported? The central premise of this book is that the emergence of fields such as medical humanities and narrative medicine may have created a space in which a dialogue between the life sciences and the humanities can emerge. This dialogue, in turn, may profoundly alter or at least affect both the humanities and the life sciences. The fields of medical humanities and narrative medicine can hence be read as disciplinary "contact zones" (Pratt 33) between the humanities and the life sciences, and they may have repercussions for the fields which they originally set out to fuse.

This book starts out from a simple premise: that there is a need for a critical and sustained dialogue between the life sciences as a field of both practice and knowledge production, and the genre of life writing as it conveys a deeply personalized experience of human fallibility, vulnerability and ephemerality. It argues that the emergence of medical humanities as a field, as well as approaches such as narrative medicine, have both challenged and enriched the humanities. Conversely, the humanities, through medical humanities and by being asked to be of service to medical practice, have themselves been infused with a new sense of their own relevance, a relevance that may also be deeply ambivalent and often problematic. This book argues that to resist such forms of utilitarianism, to dismiss the question of relevance in and of itself, may also be a dead end for the humanities. What may matter, beyond such mutual suspicion, may be a careful analysis of the agendas of the humanities and of medical humanities, respectively.

Yet, it is also crucial to note that the humanities, particularly in and through the field of life writing research, have been tremendously enriched by new materials which they may previously have construed as rather marginal to their own endeavor. This book suggests that the inclusion of autobiographies such as Tito Mukhopadhyay's *Beyond the Silence*, Michael J. Fox's *Lucky Man* and Jason Kingsley's and Mitchell Levitz's co-written autobiography *Count Us In* may provide a challenge and stimulus for American Studies research in particular, since they force us to reconsider notions of authorship and of collaborative life writing, as well as to rethink the relationship between race, class, gender and sexuality on the one hand and disability on the other.

The agenda for this book is hence threefold. First, it explores the genre of life writing as a textual continuum in which traditional autobiography, biography and a host of other textual forms related to the course – and the meaning – of human life intersect with other forms of testimony and the idea of "bearing witness." Second, the following chapters explore the intersection between life sciences and life writing by arguing that life writing as a genre is particularly suited for opening up the humanities to other forms of research. This openness towards interdisciplinary cooperation which I locate, with Alfred Hornung, in life writing research is based on two aspects inherent in life writing as a genre. First, life writing research starts out from a highly open and extensive form of textuality; at its most extreme, it conflates the oral and the written, "reading," for instance, dance performances as forms of life writing. According to Hornung,

> Auto/biographical narratives display an ever-increasing range of media in which lives or parts of lives are presented: print media, performance, film and video, radio and tapes, or the Internet. Many autobiographies combine different media for intermedial effects, such as the inclusion of photography into texts, voice and music on the radio or tapes, sound and images in filmic auto/biography, or music and dance in self-performances. Autobiographical multi-media performances dissolve the boundaries between genres and technologies of signification. (xii)

Second, the relationship of life writing to the depiction of "life itself" (Rose 40) lends itself in a particular manner to a cooperation with the life sciences.[1] As Hornung goes on to suggest, there are many ways in which "autobiographical narratives mediate between different disciplines of the humanities, the social and natural sciences, and medicine" (xii). Arguably, the life sciences, too, create narratives of human life even if the status of these narratives has been conceived of in vastly different terms, resulting in the fact that these narratives have been said to have supra-narrative status.

The very title of this book may thus, in fact, be a paradox: What would it mean to bring (medical) humanities back to the humanities, as a sort of re-import in both methodological and institutional terms? My point is that medical humanities can be said to instrumentalize, to utilize the humanities as an import or sideline – if a significant sideline – to the training of medical doctors. According to the definition of medical humanities issued by the League of European Research Universities (LERU),

> [the] "medical humanities" include an interdisciplinary field of humanities, social science and the arts, and provide insight into the human condition, suffering, personhood, our responsibility towards each other as well as how social conditions and social institutions influence health and wellbeing and the effects of medical care. They also offer a historical perspective on medical practice. Attention to literature and the arts help to develop and nurture skills of observation, analysis, empathy, and self-reflection – skills that are essential for a humane medical care. (7)

[1] It may be argued in terms of a cautionary note that there is a danger of life writing research going imperial here if life writing research claims for itself all these forms and genres traditionally located in other disciplines as, for instance, performance studies. Even as I acknowledge the risk of any approach going imperial by universalizing itself and, in the process, swallowing up all other disciplines, I would conceive of the link between life writing and other fields within the humanities in terms of complementarity rather than mutual exclusiveness. Thus, a dance performance can be explored both through the lens of life writing research and performance studies.

In this context, the humanities are inflected in a particular way. First, a variety of artistic media and genres are grouped together, and used in the didactics of medicine owing to their ability to "help to develop and nurture skills of observation, analysis, empathy and self-reflection." Here, the reception, the "reading" of "literature and the arts" is itself seen as a practice conducive to a more humane medical practice; the skills gained from the reading of literature, for instance, can be transferred, this approach holds, to medical practice. What this definition does not address, on the other hand, is the idea of creative writing or of drawing, the practice of self-reflection through creative expression which other methodologies, such as narrative medicine as well as the Swiss concept of "Menschenmedizin" have addressed (Hess and Hess-Cabalzar, *Menschenmedizin*).

What has been stressed in medical humanities approaches, then, is the advantage of "importing" the humanities into medicine, especially the didactics of medicine. In this study, then, I am interested in what may be the other side of this process. What happens if these differently inflected humanities are in their turn imported back, or "re-imported" into the humanities? What if we were to consider not the role of "medical humanities" for the practice or medicine, but for the practice of the humanities? In particular, the reinfusion of the humanities with medical humanities may lead us to reconsider some of the categories which the history of literary theory may have caused us to jettison, or to consider these categories in a different light. This may be true, above all, of the category of experience, as I will elaborate in the chapters that follow. What may be at stake here, then, is the difference between material and metaphor. In a given narrative, metaphors may be used to convey a certain illness, disability, or form of physical change; this metaphor can then be discussed, within the field of medicine or medical training, in a medical classroom and can thus serve to enhance processes of empathy on the part of doctors or medical students, with the patient in the (autobiographical or fictional) patient narrative. In so doing, as the LERU definition of medical humanities has suggested, the study of this literary or autobiographical narrative can help change the face of medicine. What, then, if this same narrative were to be reimported into a humanities classroom or re-inserted into a humanities research context? I believe that at its most fruitful, it would carry with it notions about the practice, both social and material, of medicine; in this reimported form, then, the metaphor could be read not only for its narrative but also its "practical" potential. There is, I am well aware, the danger of reductionism here; the humanities, in a line of reasoning that has by now become familiar, are reduced to the "use value" they may have for other disciplines, particularly the social sciences or, in this case, medicine. Yet, I believe that there may be qualities inherent in the concept of "application" or "applicability" which go beyond a reductionist utilitarianism. At the heart of the reimport of medical humanities into the humanities, or into fields such as American Studies specifically, there is a dialogue between the humanities and the practice of medicine. It is this dialogue with which this book will be concerned.

The key point, then, and the telos of medical humanities may be in medical practitioners and humanities scholars reading the same texts, and reading them in dialogue with each other and with each other's readings of these texts.[2] For this may be a pitfall inherent in the logic of utilitarianism. If illness narratives (autobiographies, paintings, music, poetry) are taken from the realm of the humanities to be used in medical classrooms, these narratives are often decontextualized: they become case studies of particular illnesses and they are used, of course, not for the purpose of eliciting aspects about literary theory or the history of autobiography (as I will argue in my discussion of Tito Mukhopadhyay's *The Mind Tree* in Chapter 2), but they are used as patient narratives and are hence reduced to the dimension of illness, even as they broaden the scope of the complexity of illness experience and its connection to the individual life of the patient. What would it mean for the same text to be read within and outside this context of case history and illness narrative? What if, for instance, Michael J. Fox's *Lucky Man* was to be read as an actor's autobiography and not a story about Parkinson's Disease at all? My aim in this study is to explore the potential of such alternate contextualizations of one and the same text. What emerges from this idea, then, is to inquire not just into the logic of a particular text but also and especially into the framework which we read it in. To reimport medical humanities (back) into the humanities may thus open up one more layer of meaning, and it may cause us to reconsider the question of relevance in a different light. What medical

[2] I am indebted to Alfred Hornung for this point.

humanities as a field may imply is also a note of caution, a call on the humanities not to shy away, automatically and on principle, from some degree of utilitarianism. Yet, what is needed, I believe, is to carefully discuss the terms on which the "import" of the humanities into medicine takes place: What would it mean, molecular biologist Ralf Dahm has asked, to know that Monet's style of painting did not simply change because his eyesight was affected by illness but that in changing his painting style, he also changed the history of modern art (324)? What would it mean, in other words, to read Monet's account of his illness not only as an illness narrative and a form of coping with a lack of capability, but also in terms of the history of art? As Dahm writes,

> For artists whose eye conditions were not diagnosed precisely, it is difficult to judge in retrospect if or how their vision, their individual perception and thus their way of painting were affected by possible changes in their visual apparatus. For some painters, however, we can say with certainty that they were suffering from eye conditions. Their symptoms were documented by physicians, friends or by themselves. On this basis, it is possible to assess with relative reliability the impact of a change in vision on particular works of art. [Two] artists in particular form the basis of this article, artists whose eye diseases became manifest in their work: Claude Degas, who, in his last years, developed severe cataracts, and Edgar Degas, who suffered from macular degeneration. (324; my trans.)

To be sure, it could be argued that if illness narrative (or here, illness painting) has a place in medical classrooms, art history does not. Yet, there may be a key dimension in insisting both on the narrative as "case study" and on the context which, in the humanities, this narrative is accompanied by. In this larger framework, "coping" would take on an entirely different meaning: in "coping" with his illness, Monet changed the course which modern painting would take, revealing the complex interrelation between life writing (his change in painting style as a response to the changed capability of his body, or specifically his eyes), and artistic creation. In this interrelation, Monet the painter is not just Monet the patient, just as Tito Mukhopadhyay, I will argue in Chapter 2, is a literary author and not just an autistic writer. To insist on the relevance of art history also for medical humanities in "reading" Monet's painting, then, would be not to insist on or exaggerate the detailed knowledge and minute details of the humanities, to simply resist their "use value" for medical training, but to put Monet's "patient narrative" into a different perspective in which the painter's experience may be different from the patient's. I believe that it is only through this importing not just of the narrative but of its context that medical humanities can live up to their full potential. At the same time, and conversely, of course, the humanities may need to include not just Monet the painter – dismissing any reference to his illness or failing eyesight – but also Monet the patient. Only by so doing, do they stop reducing identity to the ideational aspects of a person's life, disregarding or dismissing the mooring of this identity in a material body as either inconsequential or trivial.

At the same time, the concept of "life writing" as I am using it in discussing the intersection between life writing and life sciences may require some explanation. The texts discussed in the first part of this book, from Chapters 2 to 7 – texts such as Tito Mukhopadhyay's *Beyond the Silence* (2000), or Michael J. Fox's *Lucky Man* (2002) – closely correspond to life writing in the form of written autobiographies by a single author. While some of these autobiographies already strain the limits of the concept of autobiography as such – Mukhopadhyay includes poems into his autobiographical account, Temple Grandin's *Thinking in Pictures* (1995) can also be read as a scientific discussion of the discipline of animal studies –, they can nevertheless still be subsumed under the label of "autobiography." The texts discussed in the second part of this study, on the other hand, point to an understanding of "life writing" which, paradoxically, goes beyond the written document. Rather, these texts define life writing, as Marlene Kadar has done in *Tracing the Autobiographical*, in the sense of testimony, or of performance. Moreover, they are forms of life writing not by an individual, but rather by a collective, a collective often haunted by trauma and histories of oppression. The second part of this book also addresses the question of what Alondra Nelson has called "medical discrimination." If the life sciences have disregarded the human rights of entire communities, such as the rights of the Marshall Islanders subjected to radiation through nuclear testing in the Pacific, how can this infringement of human rights also be accounted for by definitions of ethnic communities ingrained in the social spheres in which life scientists are located? In this sense, Chapters 8 through 10 address the relationship between collective trauma, communal forms of life writing, indigenous rights and environmental justice. By the same token, I am also interested in the question of whether these narratives – documentary films such as Adam Horowitz's film *Nuclear Savage* (2011), for instance – are commonly included into discussions of medical humanities. To the extent that these narratives are not included into medical humanities discussions, but are rather subsumed under indigenous rights discussions, I would argue, we risk perpetuating the practices of medical racism which caused illness and death in the first place. One of the issues that this study tries to address, then, is whether there has been implicit in the concept of medical humanities a certain "color-blindness," the idea that illness narratives convey, first and foremost, the experience of illness, regardless of the social, cultural or racial location of the speaking subject. Conversely, especially the texts discussed in the second part of this book stress the fact that these locations are by no means secondary to the experience of illness, but are in fact central to it. At the same time, this second part of my study is hence concerned not only with the intersection between medical racism and collective trauma, but also with forms of healing and reconciliation.

At the same time, the concept of life writing, especially as it can be seen as being in conversation with the life sciences, questions the very dichotomy between biography and autobiography.[3] This is a difference to which I will return in many of the chapters that follow. While the conflation of the two terms, as Thomas Couser has powerfully argued, can be problematic in many different ways, they may nevertheless be powerful in calling for, for instance, the rights of individuals who as yet may not have full access to channels in which they can represent themselves. As Couser writes in *Vulnerable Subjects: Ethics and Life Writing* (2004), "I am especially concerned here with the representation of subjects who are vulnerable to misrepresentation or betrayal because of some disadvantaged condition, particularly certain kinds of disability" (7).

[3] As Couser puts it, "all autobiography is also in part biography" (Couser, *Vulnerable Subjects* 6).

1.2 Medical Humanities and American Studies

If medical humanities and the re-importation of medical humanities into the humanities is one of the aspects which this book sets out to explore, the notion of "American Studies" is the second one. What does it mean to reintroduce medical humanities not just to the humanities but to American Studies specifically? What is "American" about medical humanities? Or, on yet another level, what do American Studies have to offer to medical humanities? If indeed medical humanities are re-imported into American Studies, what is the specific ground which American Studies as a discipline would provide for this re-importation? In this context, I am interested in two aspects in particular. First, American Studies since their inception have always been a particularly interdisciplinary field. For this very reason, they may provide a particularly fertile ground for the inclusion of life writing research, which is itself interdisciplinary as it combines oral and written accounts, dialogues between historical records and autobiographical narratives, witness accounts and testimonies. It is the idea of "bearing witness" which informs many of the narratives I will discuss in the chapters that follow. In this context, one aspect which I will try to explore is the relationship between medical humanities on the one hand and life writing research on the other. Seen from the perspective of the humanities, much might indeed be gained from the exploration of this link: If medical humanities often dismiss or fail to take into account the specific genres from which a particular narrative is drawn, life writing research may provide an entry point from which to reconsider the notion of genre. Like the category of patient narrative, life writing research is concerned with the notion of lived experience, yet, unlike the majority of medical humanities research perhaps, it is nonetheless concerned with the question of genre, a concern which is, of course, linked to its location within the humanities. The fruitfulness of life writing research, then, is that it is at the same time aware of genre conventions and cultural, historical and political context *and* does not shy away from transcending this context. So what does life writing research have to offer to medical humanities, if the question of genre recedes into the background and if a particular narrative is read as an account of a specific illness, such as Michael J. Fox's account of his Parkinson's Disease? Nonetheless, life writing research can fruitfully complement medical humanities research by reintroducing the notion of genre. What does it mean, as Shapiro has asked, to take into account the expectations, the moorings and the trappings of a particular genre when it comes to telling a particular story? In what way is this story itself inflected by genre conventions? To read life writing into medical humanities and vice versa may hence itself be a crucial endeavor, perhaps, which will be key to the developments of both these fields of research, and of practice.

Yet, what is the role of American Studies in this context? If American Studies has been interdisciplinary from the beginning, it has also been transnational if less explicitly so. There is a profound interconnection, in the texts I will discuss, between what Shelley Fisher Fishkin has called the "transnational turn" of American Studies ("Crossroads in Cultures") and the cultural contexts from which these life writing narratives are drawn. In fact, each of them inflects the idea of "Americanness" differently. Tito Mukhopadhyay describes, in *The Mind Tree*, the fact that with his mother he has migrated from India to the U.S., his mother opening a school for autistic children in California. Yet, his narrative resists an emplotment and a teleology where the U.S. is always-already more enlightened than India when it comes to disability: instead, he is careful to describe his Indian doctor's key influence on his development. Nonetheless, there is a sense in which a certain teleology – the telos of medical humanities as an American telos –, may nonetheless undergird Tito Mukhopadhyay's narrative. What is at stake, then, is what may be termed the "history of the possible." All of the writers discussed in the chapters that follow speak, to some extent, from a U.S.-American location; it is the U.S. as a cultural, political, social, historical and juridical context which provides the framework for these authors' engagement of illness and disability. Yet, the point which they leave open, because they leave it unaddressed, is whether such engagement is possible only in the U.S.; there is clearly a danger here of American exceptionalism in the field of either disability studies or medical humanities. To what extent, then, do medical humanities accounts take their American location into account? Yet, the field of medical humanities as it has been institutionalized and anchored in medical training has by no means been confined to the U.S., and has flourished particularly in the Netherlands and in the UK. What may be needed for an American exceptionalism to be avoided, then, may be taking into account the location of medical humanities research and of life writing narratives. Yet, as has been argued, for instance, in the arenas of ethnic studies and diasporic studies, the U.S. may provide a framework for other, newly emerging fields to draw upon. If, in some contexts, the U.S. can draw on a longer-standing debate on disability studies, it would seem pointless not to use this debate as a potential blueprint or starting point for European discussions of disability. Yet, what may be considered on a different if somewhat related level is the role of the U.S. in the context of knowledge production and the dissemination of knowledge.

I am thus interested in the way in which "Americanness" is configured in different narratives: in the account of an Indian writer and poet with autism who has migrated from Chennai to Los Angeles; in a Bollywood film which chronicles the life of a Muslim man with Asperger's in the wake of the 9/11 attacks; in the performance of a Russian dancer who in the U.S. transformed his classical ballet into a particular kind of modern dance – complete with elements drawn from bioengineering technology – or in the life of a Canadian actor who became a naturalized American citizen and used his citizenship in a campaign to gain political support for stem cell research.

On a different level, this book is also concerned with the concept of autobiography, and the relationship of autobiography (or life writing more broadly conceived) to forms of disability and civic inclusion. A call for such inclusion, arguably, has been central to autobiography from the very beginning. Thus, slave narratives as autobiographies, beginning with Olaudah Equiano's *The Interesting Narrative of Olaudah Equiano or Gustavus Vassa, Written by Himself* (1789) testified not only to the authorship, but also to the humanity of the black subject.[4] It is this concept of autobiography, in turn, that I would like to restore to the framework of medical humanities. Even as medical humanities have centrally referred to the concept of lived experience as patient experience, emphasizing the role of the patient in and for medical treatment, the conceptualization of patient perspective may perhaps benefit from more careful framing. Moreover, a stressing of the concept of the autobiographical, as I will argue especially with regard to Jason Kingsley and Mitchell

[4] See, for instance, Jeffrey Gunn, "Literacy and the Humanizing Project in Olaudah Equiano's *The Interesting Narrative* and Ottobah Cugoano's *Thoughts and Sentiments.*"

Levitz's account in *Count Us In* (1994), may also take into account those aspects of the life writing narrative that have nothing to do with illness in the first place.

In the chapters that follow, one narrative seems to require additional explanation: In a study otherwise concerned with life writing texts, I have chosen to include a narrative which is not literary, but filmic; and I have included a filmic narrative which is not autobiographical in the first place. Perhaps counterintuitively, then, I have included a Bollywood film titled *My Name Is Khan* to explore the ways in which autism may have come to be "mainstreamed" through popular culture, in a film which engages both "Indian" and "American" cultural imaginaries. While this feature film can easily be included in the framework of medical humanities, it cannot be seen as "life writing" in the sense proper. At the same time, many of the autobiographical narratives included here also explore the question of inclusion; there may hence be a continuity between *My Name is Khan* (2010) and for, instance, the Indian American autobiography *The Mind Tree* (2003) by Tito Mukhopadhyay. In investigating the role and potential relevance of medical humanities for American Studies, I am thus also interested in the difference, but also the continuity between life writing narratives and other genres which are similarly concerned with (the meaning of) "disability."

1.3 The Problem of Didacticism

One of the issues which are central in this context, then, may be that of didacticism. From the perspective of medical training, the use of life writing research and illness narratives clearly has a didactic purpose. These texts, it could be argued, need to be deprived of some of their aesthetic qualities in order to be read as patient narratives in the first place. What matters, then, is the question of perspective: These narratives about certain illnesses are read with regard to the patient's coping with his or her experience, and the patient's experience of a certain illness. It is hence the level of both experience and patient psychology which is important to medical humanities as it "imports" the humanities. The aesthetic qualities of a certain text, by the same token, must necessarily be disregarded as excess, as surplus; they cannot really be dealt with through the methodological toolbox of medical humanities. The question why a certain illness should be expressed in a particular genre –

the choice of poetry over a novel, for instance – seems to be of secondary importance for medical humanities. From a humanities perspective, on the other hand, this choice of genre would in itself be significant: The minute a given topic is treated in a particular genre – such as, for instance, the discussion of organ transplantation in a dystopia such as Ishiguro's *Never Let Me Go* (2005)[5] –, this will shape, even if it does not determine, the expression of patient experience and of narrative illness. Arguably, of course, *Never Let Me Go* is not an illness narrative; yet, it may nonetheless serve to draw attention to the power which genre may exert over the narrative that it contains.

Yet, crucially, the idea of didacticism may not only apply to the teaching of cultural, filmic, literary or poetic texts in a medical humanities framework, but also to the writing and reading of illness narratives themselves. It may also be pertinent, in other words, to the humanities as they come to deal with experiences of illness, partly in response to the emergence of medical humanities within the framework of medicine and of medical training. What is at stake here may in fact be the idea of the "activist" component in literary texts, and in the humanities practice of reading such texts. This question of didacticism has been addressed in recent literary criticism especially with regard to the emergence of ecocriticism as a discipline, and the related emergence of what Graham Huggan and Helen Tiffin have termed "postcolonial ecocriticism". In their recent study *Postcolonial Ecocriticism* (2010), Graham Huggan and Helen Tiffin explicitly address the question of genre, and its relationship to the didacticism of a given text. They use Indian writer and activist Arundhati Roy as a case in point. While Roy's debut novel *The God of Small Things* (1997) earned her the Booker Prize in 1997, she subsequently turned away from fiction toward activist non-fiction, and embraced ecocritical concerns. In tandem with this move away from fiction-writing towards more overtly didactic forms such as the essay, Roy's style and her tone became an overtly activist one: every sentence, its author implied, needed to be taken at face value. There was little difference, then, between the essay and the political pamphlet; in fact, Roy's activism seemed to take pride in this lack of difference. Writing for the (ecological) cause, she implied, had to be direct, and it had to be

[5] I am indebted to Ruth Steinberg for this point.

didactic, exhorting its readership (the Indian government, local Indian communities, the global community) to change its ways. Yet, as Huggan and Tiffin go on to ask, what does such overt didacticism mean for the reading of such texts? What would it mean for literary criticism to take a given text "at face value"? Such a reading, Huggan and Tiffin note, is a deliberate disregard of the "constructedness" of a text, to which the question of genre no longer seems to apply. As Huggan and Tiffin observe, "If Roy's message is crystal clear, unashamedly partisan in its intentions, her text remains a curiously unresolved mixture: part hard-headed investigative report, part sentimental political fable; part historically situated postcolonial allegory, part universal Green manifesto and call to arms" (48). It is this dismissal of the aesthetic, then, which Huggan and Tiffin go on to resist, pointing instead to the fact that an overtly didactic text is no less "constructed" than a more explicitly literary one.

What, then, would this mean for medical humanities? In my reading of texts such as Michael J. Fox's *Lucky Man* (2002) or *Always Looking Up* (2009), I am struggling with the temptation of reducing autobiography to political activism: Surely, Fox's is a straightforward call for inclusion; it is an activist call for the implementation of stem cell research, and for a turnaround in the way we treat persons with disabilities. What, however, is the difference between Michael J. Fox writing in his autobiography that even simple acts such as brushing one's teeth may be difficult for a patient with Parkinson's Disease (PD) like himself, and Michael J. Fox *staging* such difficulty in a TV interview? What, in other words, is the difference between Michael J. Fox's "having" PD and his playing a PD patient in TV series such as *The Good Wife* (2009-2016)? Crucially, what may be at stake here is the very difference between Mikhail Baryshnikov's staging his own aging process and the simple "fact" of *being* older. What Baryshnikov does in his "HeartBeat: mb" performance (1998) is to interrogate, through the staging of processes of physical change related to aging, the meaning of such physical change. Staging is hence crucially different from simply expressing this change: If the body indeed is the dancer's medium, Baryshnikov's performance estranges the medium from itself, and draws our attention not to what the medium expresses but the qualities of the medium itself. Similarly, the process of physical change is no less present, even if it is differently visible, in Michael J. Fox's account of living with Parkinson's Disease: Like that of the dancer, the actor's body, too, is his medium; it is this medium, as Michael J. Fox puts it with characteristic self-irony, which has been sabotaging him for the last two decades. It is this sabotage, then, that Fox draws attention to, but he does so in a manner which is itself constructed, and makes no secret of such constructedness.

What, on the other hand, would we lose if we took these narratives or performances not as constructions, but as straightforward expressions of patient "truths"? From a pragmatic standpoint which may at first sound absurd, we would deprive the humanities of their material, and would rob literary studies of the literary aspect of their work. What is at stake here is the question of whether "coping" is the right word to be applied to these narratives expressing illness or aging. The point is not so much how we "cope" (on a psychological level), but how we make sense of and ascribe meaning to changes in the human body. If indeed illness or age are social and not only biological categories, then the question is not how individuals affected with physical change "deal with" such alteration, but what meaning they themselves ascribe to the way in which their bodies have changed. It is in the ascription of such meaning, then, that the aesthetic is far from obsolete: it is part and parcel of writing about illness and aging. What such a reading restores to the "patient" or subject whose narrative we are reading, then, is precisely the idea and the concept of authorship. It is by becoming the author of his own illness, then, that Michael J. Fox stops being a patient, or becomes a patient differently conceived. The staging of the physical change of his body, then, is implicitly connected to the idea of authorship: What Baryshnikov does on stage in his "HeartBeat: mb" performance, Michael J. Fox does in the interview. Moreover, it is here that the concept of "haunting" recurs: For to view the interview simply as a patient narrative, simply as an expression of illness experience, would deprive the patient, paradoxically, of his individuality. What is at stake here is not just anyone having PD, but Michael J. Fox struggling with his own diagnosis. The point to be derived from this idea, however, is not that Fox is different from, let alone superior to other PD patients. Rather, he writes in his autobiography how much he himself draws solace from finding himself to be part of a patient community. Yet, what both the concepts of staging and of haunting imply is that each experience of illness is inscribed on the body of a particular individual: the moment of illness must be seen to be haunted by this previous performance, here that of Michael J. Fox the actor. To the extent that we take the haunting seriously, then, marks the extent to which we will be able to "honor" the patient's story, as Rita Charon has put it in the context of narrative medicine (*Narrative Medicine* 3). The challenge for medical practice, then, may consist in taking seriously this haunting; it may consist in insisting on viewing, paying attention to and taking into account the individual's previous performances. When we see Michael J. Fox in the doctor's chair, then, we also see the actor from *Back to the Future* (1985). The key issue to be addressed here is that this haunting will be clear, even self-evident for Michael J. Fox the megastar, but will not be seen as relevant to those patients who happen not to be famous. If the concept of haunting is taken seriously, however, each patient's previous performances need to be considered, whether or not he is in fact a "performer" in Michael J. Fox's sense. It is in drawing attention to such haunting, then, that the genre of autobiography may be particularly important: For Fox, just like Kingsley and Levitz, chooses to write an autobiography, not a patient narrative. Even if this autobiography can be read as a patient narrative, it is nonetheless part of a different genre, a genre which has to be taken seriously if we are to live up to the true potential of both medical humanities and of the humanities "reimporting" medical humanities. It is in this sense that it is by no means coincidental that the autobiography of Michael J. Fox should have many of the same sections which can be found in the collaborative autobiography of Jason Kingsley and Mitchell Levitz. Each of these narratives, it must be stressed, performs a *life*, not an illness.

As I am arguing throughout this study, "illness autobiographies" can be seen to "hijack" the form of illness narrative and patient account and sabotage them from within. In the very concept of "illness autobiography," the two terms contained in this definition are continually in a tension with each other: In fact, the concept of "autobiography" may sabotage the very notion of illness, since autobiography is about writing a person's *life*, not his or her illness. It is in this sense that I argue in each of the chapters that the illness or disability autobiography can be seen as a Trojan horse sabotaging the framework it is being read in: If indeed, these autobiographies are being read in the framework of medical humanities, they sabotage this framework by being more than medical (narratives), by being, precisely, autobiographies in the fullest sense of the term. Life writing, these texts emphasize, can never be reduced to just one facet of the life that is being written. In this vein, Tito Mukhopadhyay's autobiography, even as it describes his life with autism, is also a postcolonial autobiography, and the story of a life that, through the author's move from India to the U.S., has become transnational. Similarly, the autobiography which Jason Kingsley has co-authored with his friend Mitchell Levitz, a text to which I will return in Chapter 7, can be read as much as a narrative of a young man with Down Syndrome as it can be read as a portfolio of a young man entering the job market, or a narrative of initiation as Kingsley is growing up and begins dating. This idea of the Trojan horse of illness autobiography, I am arguing throughout this book, is what the humanities can bring to medical humanities: Crucially, it could be argued that medical humanities so far have imported the narratives themselves (importing them as illness accounts or patient narratives), without simultaneously importing the humanities framework of interpreting these narratives. Rather, the narratives are being used by medical humanities for the didactics of medicine. What would happen, however, if the tension between the interpretative framework and the text itself were taken into account? It is this sense of illness autobiographies containing a "full" account of a person's life that is also at the heart of Rita Charon's idea of narrative medicine, and of "honoring the stories of illness" (*Narrative Medicine* 3). Charon writes, "Along with their growing scientific expertise, doctors need the expertise to listen to their patients, to understand as best as they can the ordeals of illness, to honor the meanings of their patients' narratives of illness, and to be moved by what they behold so that they can act on their patients' behalf" (*Narrative Medicine* 3).

My insistence on reading these autobiographies not only as illness narratives but as autobiographies in the full sense of this concept, then, is to put Rita Charon's idea of narrative medicine, of "honoring the stories of illness" into the practice of literary analysis. It is in this sense, then, that literary research is not only supplementary to medical practice, but it can re-import the knowledge gained from new interdisciplinary fields such as narrative medicine into literary research. Thus, the very field of narrative medicine, created by Rita Charon, emerged as a field linking literary and medical research, and literary and medical *practice*. According to Charon, "[To be] empathetic and effective in the care of individual patients . . . requires what psychologists and literary scholars call narrative knowledge. . . . If narratives are stories that have a teller, a listener, a time course, a plot, and a point, then narrative knowledge is what we naturally use to make sense of them" (*Narrative Medicine* 9). Here, literature is by no means seen as being merely supplementary to medical practice; rather, narrative medicine deliberately applies some of the key methods of literary analysis – particularly the strategy of close reading – to "reading" stories of illness. As Charon goes on to say, "Medicine can benefit from learning that which literary scholars and psychologists and anthropologists and storytellers have known for some time – that is, what narratives are, how they are built, how they convey their knowledge about the world, what happens when stories are told and listened to, how narratives organize life, and how they let those who live life recognize what it means" (*Narrative Medicine* 9). Reimporting narrative medicine into literary practice, then, is to suggest that we may gain an additional dimension in the reading of autobiographies which is also, but by no means exclusively, about illness.

This, then, may be a difference between medical humanities and narrative medicine. For in its inclusion of what they see as "patient narratives" in different forms, medical humanities run the risk of dismissing a number of aspects which, seen from a literary or cultural studies perspective, would be inseparable from these representations of illness. First, it sees these representations, first and foremost, as representations of illnesses, not as autobiographies in the full sense of this term; second, it tends to dismiss the aesthetic qualities of these representations. Narrative medicine, on the other hand, urges us to "honor the stories of illness" (Charon, *Narrative Medicine* 3), thereby seeing in these narratives their quality as narratives about lives, and not only lives lived with illness. In order to "read" these lives, then, narrative medicine employs the tools of literary analysis. What Charon emphasizes, then, is the idea of "narrative knowledge" (*Narrative Medicine* 11). This idea could not be more central at the intersection between life writing and life sciences. Charon argues not only that knowledge is always, to some extent, conveyed in narrative[6], but that narrative enables a form of knowing that is itself specific. Charon suggests, "Medicine is joining other disciplines

[6] This idea is at the core of Timothy Lenoir's and Hans-Ulrich Gumbrecht's "Writing Science" series.

such as anthropology, history, psychology, social science, law, and even mathematics in recognizing the elemental and irreplaceable nature of narrative knowledge" (*Narrative Medicine* 11). What is at stake here, then, is the role of narrative in fostering interdisciplinary research. As Charon implies in this passage, narrative research – itself a term that can be read in multiple ways – has triggered a plethora of new fields, in which the notion of narrative and the methodology of narrative research have "invaded" fields which had previously been seen as unrelated to narrative, or at least fields in which narrative was seen as subordinate to the methodologies proper. Thus, the field of ethnography was fundamentally changed by the "writing culture" debate spearheaded by the work of James Clifford.[7] Similarly, the field of Critical Race Theory linked literature and the law.[8] Finally, Charon herself mentions her indebtedness to the field of "literature-and-medicine" (*Narrative Medicine* 4), and the work of Stephen Marcus.[9]

1.4 The Haunted Stage

What medical humanities approaches may run the risk of neglecting, then, is the constructedness of stories about illness. Here, too, narrative medicine may seem crucial: For discussions of narrative medicine have stressed the fact that patient narratives are never transparent (Shapiro 68); they are not mimetic but representational of a given illness or condition. Narrative medicine employs the tools of literary studies, cautioning about what has been called, in literary studies, mimetic fallacy. Narrative medicine is keenly aware, then, of the constructed quality of the narrative; it is attuned to its representational aspect (Shapiro 68). This is an issue to which I will return in more detail below.

It is this notion of representation, then, which I would like to relate to the concept of the performative. In this sense, I am also interested in the continuities between literary and theatrical representations. Applying

[7] See, for instance, James Clifford and George E. Marcus, *Writing Culture*.

[8] See, for instance, Crenshaw et al., *Critical Race Theory*.

[9] See, for example, Stephen Marcus' use of Sigmund Freud's theory in *The Other Victorians: A Study of Sexuality and Pornography in Mid-Nineteenth-Century England*.

performance studies to literary analysis, I would argue, can enhance our notion of embodiment, which, arguably, is central to narratives about illness, as well as narratives of aging. It is for this very reason, then, that this book explores the potential of Marvin Carlson's memorable concept, the "haunted stage," to performances of life which emerge in these narratives of life writing. I am interested, then, in the relationship between a written text – which, in many of the instances discussed in this book, is an autobiographical written text – and the performance of life which it chronicles. What applying Carlson's image of the haunted stage, taken from theater studies, to the study of a literary text can do, I believe, is to help us grasp the relationship between the written text – which, in many different ways, reduces the writer's body to a two-dimensional description which unfolds on the written page – and the materiality of the author's body[10] whose illness or disability the text conveys, discusses and grapples with through narrative form. Even more importantly for the purposes of this study, I am interested in how this haunting of the performance of the self by previous performances affects not only the audience – a process of reception that Carlson is most concerned with, but also the "actor" himself. I am interested, throughout these pages, in how the physical body of the past is superimposed on the present-day physicality of the same body. What happens, I ask, in this act of (narrative) superimposition?

Even more importantly, this study both starts out from and seeks to modify sociological interventions taken from the field of citizenship studies, especially from the notion of "biological citizenship."[11] While discussions of biological citizenship, as I will elaborate below, have looked at the ways in which individuals or patient groups call for the inclusion of their own life narratives and lived experiences into discussions of patient rights, social inclusion, and medical practice, I am interested in the aesthetic form through which they can be said to call for

[10] This is not to say, of course, that the author's subjectivity equals that of the narrator in these texts; it is, however, to explore the material dimension of the body of both the author (who, in autobiographical form, often addresses an illness or disability that he or she is confronted with) and the narrator whose physical body is imagined and portrayed in the written account.
[11] I will return to this concept below.

such inclusion. It is here, I believe, that Carlson's approach may provide a valuable tool. I am interested, then, in the ways in which the idea of "haunting" can be said to inform narratives of illness, and of health, and the complex forms of temporality through which both relate to each other. Carlson writes,

> At various periods and in various theatrical cultures, almost every element in production – from the narratives presented to the bodies of the actors – has been reused. And any regular theatregoer is familiar with the experience of a performance calling to mind the ghosts of previous performances. *The Haunted Stage* explores the process by which theater recycles material, and examines how that reuse stimulates the spectator's memory – memory not of broad cultural or historical phenomena but of specific theatre experience. (dust jacket n. pag.)

In Chapter 3, addressing Indian actor Shah Rukh Khan's Bollywood performance of an autistic man in *My Name Is Khan* (2010), I will be using the idea of the actor haunted by his previous performances very much in the sense envisioned by Carlson. Similarly, I will argue in Chapter 5 that Mikhail Baryshnikov, in his "HeartBeat: mb" performance from 1998, deliberately plays with the notion of such haunting. At the same time, however, I believe that there is a sense in which the potential of Carlson's notion of the haunted stage exceeds the haunting of the actor's performance, and can also be applied to our witnessing, as audiences in a different sense, performances of life. In fact, as I will elaborate in Chapter 6, Michael J. Fox is concerned with the superimposition of his performance as an actor in various roles (such as the sitcom *Spin City*) and the body which increasingly interfered with the actor's performance. Just as the actor's performance in a given film was haunted by his previous on-screen appearances, Fox argues that he kept comparing the performance of his body to those performances that his body had previously been capable of. There is a striking similarity here to Mikhail Baryshnikov's "HeartBeat: mb" performance, in which the Russian American dancer deliberately draws the audience's attention to the ways in which his present-day body can no longer "mimic" the moves that the body of his younger self was capable of.

At the same time, perhaps counterintuitively, Carlson's concept of the haunted stage can also be upset in its temporality in these narratives of lived experience. For an audience witnessing Baryshnikov's superimposition of his younger self on his present-day self, there can be a sense of being haunted by their own future: What Baryshnikov depicts, in his middle age, is what a younger audience may in time come to experience as well. It is in this sense and at this point that this (possible) future of being haunted by illness or disability may reflect what Judith Butler, in another context, has termed "precarious life" (*Precarious Life* x).[12] For Butler, catastrophes such as the terrorist attacks of 9/11 remind us of the vulnerability of our lives, a "precariousness" in which our vulnerability to being hurt by physical violence may parallel our susceptibility to illness or disability. Throughout the following chapters, then, I will return to the ways in which Carlson's concept of the haunted stage can be said to emerge in various contexts of life writing.

It is in this context that I am drawing, throughout this study, on Marvin Carlson's memorable metaphor of the "haunted stage." As I will elaborate in the pages that follow, Carlson suggests that a particular actor's performance of a given role will be perceived by his audience not just as a performance in the present, but will carry within it traces of each of the actor's previous performances that the audience has seen. Each performance, Carlson writes, is also shaped by the audience's memory of the performance's "predecessors." I believe that in many of the narratives that will be discussed in this book, there is a sense of "ghosting"; in some instances, however, this "ghosting" may be more straightforward than in others. In Michael J. Fox's narrative, for instance, there is a sense in which he superimposes his younger self – before the onset of Parkinson's Disease –, on the self that is writing. There is hence a complex layering of past and present here; it seems to Fox ironic that his body, always too short for its age, should have spoken of an off-centered relationship between corporeality and temporality, which would later be refigured through Fox's having Young Onset Parkinson's Disease. Similarly, Baryshnikov inscribes into his performance, if implicitly so, the younger self he once was; and the audience comes to measure his appearance in "HeartBeat: mb" against the virtuoso dancer he once was. In all these narratives, however, this ghosting

[12] For a more detail discussion of Butler's concept, see Chapter 3.

by no means only takes shape in terms of decline; rather, it is a complex dialogue between the past and the present.

What Carlson's memorable metaphor can bring to the discussion of "illness" narratives, I believe, is the sense of embodiment, an embodiment with which, I will argue in the chapters that follow, these texts choose to conceal and reveal in a curious strategy of what I call "disembodied embodiment." Moreover, I believe that the metaphor of "ghosting" is powerful in that it erases, for my purposes here, the distinction between health and sickness, between ability and disability: If qualities of health and of sickness are superimposed on one and the same body in an imagination of the past in the present or a prefigurement of the future in the present, what emerges is a fluidity between health and illness which, I believe, is crucial in distinguishing illness and disability from other "differences" such as race or gender, which can usually not affect one and the same body. Illness, as Thomas Couser, following Susan Sonntag, has powerfully argued, affects us all, just as age does; yet, in the prior case, we may choose to make believe that this difference will never affect us or, if it does, it will take us by surprise. "We" may thus be "immune" to racial difference or gender difference if we happen to be members of a group not affected by racial or gender discrimination; age, on the other hand, affects us all, and many of us will come to be affected by disability. As Couser argues, "Because, as Sander Gilman puts it, 'we are all at risk – we will all be ill, will fail, will die,' it would seem that we might all identify with the lives these narratives depict" (*Recovering Bodies* 16). Seen from this perspective, then, we may all in a sense be haunted or affected by life writing narratives about age, illness, or disability.

I believe that it is for this reason that these texts engage the quality of haunting that Carlson has described for the stage in their textual aesthetics; and they engage this metaphor by reminding us of the vulnerability not just of the lives of the authors of these narratives, but a vulnerability which, as human beings, we all share.

What then, is the temporality of this haunting? In the era of biomedicine, I believe, the layering of the past and the present, and the present and the future, takes a very specific shape. To the extent that genetic discourse has inscribed ideas of probability, locating in a particular genetic dispossession the possibility, even probability, of future illness, the present is being "haunted," in a complex upsetting of temporality and of chronology, by the future, or by a future that is now being imagined as likely. This is where my approach would, at the same time, overlap with many discussions about the "reach," both discursive and material, of biomedicine, and where it would, at the same time, seek to transcend these discussions. For I believe that Carlson's intervention, in the realm of theater studies and theater history, is key in articulating, on the level of performance and the reception of this performance by the audience, the ways in which we experience the present. Particularly in the era of genetic prediction and the "technological reproducibility of human life" (Weiß, "Einleitung" 7; my trans.), there is a sense in which health is haunted, again in reverse chronology, by the future of impending illness. What is at stake in the understanding of the temporality of our lives if human beings are understood in public or in policy debate, especially in debate by health insurances, as "future patients"? I believe that these complex, often counterintuitive and often contrary temporalities are more than just inscriptions; they are "theaters" in which we come to experience a temporal period which is asynchronous with the present – the past in the present, the future in the present – as if it were happening already. One of the questions which I would like to ask is how we, as human beings, make sense of such temporalities, of temporalities and probabilities which biomedicine has made more complex than ever. In this attempt at sense-making, it has seemed to me that Marvin Carlson's metaphor of the haunted stage (of the present) and of the present being ghosted by the past (to which I would add the counterintuitive sense of the present being haunted by an impending or probable future) may be useful.

Our lives, however, are more than a theater; they are real in a sense of which our bodies daily remind us of, putting in relief the vulnerability and ephemerality of our lives. At the same time, I believe that this metaphor taken from theater studies can go a long way in explaining the ways in which we live our lives, and in which we experience the present, interwoven as it is with a complex form of temporality – indeed, of temporalities – which have, more than ever, been complicated through biomedicine: through the choices which it has made possible, but also through the decisions which it may force us to make.

This sense of haunting, for the writer or performer himself/herself, can also take the sense of being haunted by the image of a previous self, an image of the difference between ability and disability, between illness and health that Emily Perl Kingsley has addressed in her memorable essay “Welcome to Holland” (1987). In an essay which, as Rachel Adams has argued almost a decade later, was the “road map” to many mothers of children born with Down Syndrome, Perl Kingsley writes that once her son Jason had been born, and had been born *differently* than she had expected, she had to come to terms with this superimposition: The mother she had imagined she would be – the mother of the child she had imagined her son would be – had to reconcile this image to the reality of her present-day life, and the future of a different form of mothering. Rome, Kingsley writes, is different from Holland; and part of coming to terms with the challenge of raising a newborn son who had Down Syndrome was the haunting of Holland by Rome. As Perl Kingsley writes,

> When you’re going to have a baby, it’s like planning a fabulous vacation trip - to Italy. You buy a bunch of guide books and make your wonderful plans. The Coliseum. The Michelangelo David. The gondolas in Venice. You may learn some handy phrases in Italian. It’s all very exciting.
>
> After months of eager anticipation, the day finally arrives. You pack your bags and off you go. Several hours later, the plane lands. The stewardess comes in and says, “Welcome to Holland.”
>
> “Holland?!?” you say. “What do you mean Holland?? I signed up for Italy! I’m supposed to be in Italy. All my life I’ve dreamed of going to Italy.”
>
> But there’s been a change in the flight plan. They’ve landed in Holland and there you must stay.
>
> The important thing is that they haven’t taken you to a horrible, disgusting, filthy place, full of pestilence, famine and disease. It’s just a different place.
>
> So you must go out and buy new guide books. And you must learn a whole new language. And you will meet a whole new group of people you would never have met.
>
> It’s just a different place. It’s slower-paced than Italy, less flashy than Italy. But after you’ve been there for a while and you catch your breath, you look around.... and you begin to notice that Holland has windmills....and Holland has tulips. Holland even has Rembrandts. (n. pag.)

Many of the narratives I will discuss here start with this moment of difference, of the awareness that the present is different from the future one had originally imagined in the past. Kingsley's narrative begins, as does Rachel Adams' memoir, with a sense of grief, of mourning the life she thought she was going to lead. The question both narratives ask, then, is whether the narrative of Holland will always be haunted by the imagination of Rome, or whether, quite to the contrary, Holland will become a narrative in its own right, a narrative which we will cease to compare to the narrative it might have been, and that we once thought it was going to be. I believe that this sense of ghosting, the awareness of the shape, the shaping and reshaping of our lives assumes a particular quality in the era of biomedicine precisely because of what Martin Weiß has called the "Veränderbarkeit," the malleability of our lives through biomedicine and biomedical technologies. As Thomas Lemke has cautioned, current debates, for instance, on the role of genetic screening and genetic prediction particular in the field of human reproduction may be profoundly dissimilar from the history of eugenics, but there may nonetheless be continuities between the two. What may be at stake in both instances, then, is the idea of the malleability of human life, the extent to which we may influence, in the present, the shape that our lives or that of our children will have; and the extent to which we can influence these futures on a corporeal, on a genetic level. As many of the narratives discussed in this book illustrate, there is a curious dichotomy between the idea of a certain "mastery" over our lives suggested to us by biomedicine, and the awareness that these lives are nonetheless shaped by contingency to an extent which is greater than we might otherwise have imagined. The challenge, then, may be to take seriously the extent of such haunting, the awareness of the fact that our perception and experience of the present will be haunted by our past expectations – or imaginary performances – of this present. There is a sense in which the haunting of the present – by the past and the future – as the twenty-first century opens, has become more powerful and more pronounced than ever before. Even if the slogan that "we are our genes" has been severely criticized and its reach has been severely compromised – scientists do not know why in one individual, genetic predispositions lead to illness and an individual with a similar disposition remains healthy – there is nonetheless a sense in which the possibility of such prefigurement seems more palpable than ever.

What my reading of these autobiographies seeks to add to current discussion, then, is an analysis of the "textures"[13] of these narratives, the way in which – as literary narratives – they can choose to disclose or conceal a difference which is physical, and hence visible to the observer. I am drawing on what Toni Morrison has once said, in the context of race and of color-blindness, about the literary text. As Morrison notes in her memorable collection of essays, *Playing in the Dark* (1992), she once wanted to write a book which entirely sidestepped the logics of racial coding.[14] What would it mean, then, to "sidestep" the logics which code (dis)ability? And how would we do so in a literary narrative? The point which I would like to make here is not only that one and the same text, as Thomas Couser has argued, contains chapters which pertain to a particular illness or disability while others go beyond the framework of illness or disability, as in Couser's distinction, but it is at the heart of recontextualizing life writing texts by taking into account multiple frameworks of reference. As Couser has asked, "Under what circumstances does the story of a bodily dysfunction come to represent an entire life?" (*Recovering Bodies* 14). The aim of this study is to explore instances in life writing narratives where these narratives revolve around "bodily dysfunction," but also other instances in which they exceed this focus. As Couser goes on to note, "The relation between bodily dysfunction and personal narrative is a complex one; the former may both impel and impede the latter" (*Recovering Bodies* 5). Taking my cue from Couser, I will explore in the chapters that follow where reading life writing narratives is "impelled and impeded" by what we might term somatic readings; this double bind, moreover, may be located both on the level of the text (in its sabotaging particular strategies of reading, for instance), and in our practices of reading it, as well as the contexts in which we do so.

I am interested, then, in the way in which these narratives – presumably "only" narratives of illness or disability – circulate in multiple frameworks at one and the same time, and in the ways in which they strategically engage, in their narrative, these multiple frameworks. I believe that they do so in playing with the sense of the haunting of

[13] I am indebted to Norbert Paul for this term.

[14] This is an idea which I will discuss in more detail in Chapter 6.

health by illness or disability which I am trying to capture through Marvin Carlson's metaphor of "ghosting." To say, as Couser does, that a "full" autobiography which also touches on the author's illness is much more than a narrative about illness, then, may ultimately reinscribe the dichotomy of health/illness as a framework of reference. My aim, then, is to inquire about the "beyond" of illness narratives, to look at the way in which they strategically engage – through "disembodied embodiment" – our notions of normalcy. I believe that this strategic engagement of the "fullness" of these lives has not yet been adequately addressed either through quality of life research or even through narrative medicine. In none of these frameworks, I argue in Chapter 7, would we be able to account for the fact that the structure which Kingsley and Levitz's collaborative autobiography follows is that of a citizenship test.

Drawing on the work of Richard Schechner and Joseph Roach, Carlson is especially interested in processes of surrogation, an idea which, I would argue, may also have powerful repercussions for medical humanities. Carlson writes,

> Richard Schechner's oft-quoted characterization of performance as "restored behavior" or "twice-behaved behavior" looks in the same direction, as does Joseph Roach's relation of performance to surrogation, the "doomed search for originals by continuously auditioning stand-ins." The physical theatre, as a site of the continuing reinforcement of memory by surrogation, is not surprisingly among the most haunted of human cultural structures. (1-2)

I am interested, then, in the continuity between representation (in this case, autobiographical representation) on the one hand and reception on the other. I am thus using Carlson's seminal ideas of the haunted stage by deliberately going against the grain of his argument to focus less on discontinuities than on continuities between the artistic and the non-artistic, between the representational and the "experiential." Even as I recognize that there may be a fallacy of the real at work in my argument, I am interested nonetheless in the continuity between representation and lived experience. Illness, disability or processes of aging can be said to disrupt life narratives, and hence introduce – in the ways in which they are represented in autobiographies and other forms of life writing – a rereading of one's own life before this disruption. Carlson's idea of the haunted stage is concerned, quite specifically, with theater as a unique art form; it is this uniqueness, I am well aware, that my argument runs the risk of dismissing. According to Carlson,

> This process [of haunting] occurs, of course, not only in the arts but in any human activity involving interpretation, which includes any human activity to which consciousness is brought, but the major feature generally separating a work of art from other activities of the consciousness lies in the particular way it is framed, as an activity or object created to simulate interpretation, that is, to invite an audience to interact with it. (5)

Yet, while I acknowledge the powerful ways in which Carlson's work illuminates the particular qualities of theatre as an art form based on the corporeal presence of the actor, I am interested in what this notion of corporeality may bring to medical humanities and autobiographical narratives concerned with the ways in which the human body may come to change through processes of illness or aging.

This application of Carlson's metaphor of the haunted stage to the realm of medical humanities, however, may involve a different notion of spectatorship. Arguably, if described in Carlson's terms, the spectator or the person re-reading a previous life in the light of the present one is the autobiographer herself. Thus, as I argue in Chapter 6, Michael J. Fox looks back on his life before the onset of Parkinson's Disease in an autobiography whose writing was triggered by his PD diagnosis; he becomes a spectator looking back not only on his previous on-screen performances, but also on his previous "life." In both senses of these lives, I believe, Carlson's idea of "haunting" can be used to illuminate the experience of this superimposition of lives, and of the "interpretive" processes which we may use to make sense of them. To be sure, "interpretive" is by no means meant to be a trivializing of lived experience, quite the contrary. Throughout this study, I am interested in the ways in which narratives add an aesthetic dimension to the idea of "coping," a term commonly used in both medical humanities and psychosomatic research to describe a person's coming to terms with his or her illness.

What I am concerned with, in particular, in an attempt to apply Marvin Carlson's idea of the haunted stage – or as I argue with regard to Michael J. Fox's discussion of his early appearance on *Back to the Future*, the "haunted screen" – is what Carlson calls the "haunted body" (52): I am interested in the way this haunting – quite literally, by a previous performance – may affect not just the body of the actor, but the body of human beings quite generally. We may be haunted, in other words, by the previous performances, on other days or in other periods of our lives, of our older, our former selves. This is always true of autobiographies; in fact, this haunting – the attempt at making sense of these previous performances, to be the interpreter of our previous self's performance – may inform the very project of autobiographical writing itself. What is so intriguing about Carlson's concept, I believe, is precisely its use of the notion of embodiment, a notion which may transform our readings of autobiographies which are concerned not only with the way the author-narrator's identity has evolved over time, but also with the way in which this identity is moored in a particular physical and material "home," the body itself.

As I will elaborate with regard to the Russian ballet dancer Rudolf Nureyev in Chapter 5, Carlson addresses the effect of aging in particular. Referring to Richard Schechner's work in particular and the latter's idea of surrogation, Carlson goes on to note,

> That public . . . looked past the infirmities of his physical body to his "other body, the one that existed outside itself in the fact of his performances of it. Transcending the body of flesh and blood, this other body consisted of actions, gestures, intonations, vocal colors, mannerisms, expressions, customs, protocols, inherited routines, authenticated traditions –"bits."" Unlike the physical body, "the actions of this theatrical body could not be invalidated by age or decrepitude." The power of performance memory, reinforced by the repetition of familiar gestures, intonations, and mannerisms, here proved more powerful than the actual physical appearance of [the aged actor] himself; the ghost had a greater performative visibility than the body it haunted. (58)

What would this passage mean, then, if it were applied to narratives of aging or illness? For our perception of Muhammad Ali, for instance, it means that our seeing the bent body of Ali, the "greatest" boxer of all time, evokes a particular sense of haunting: the incongruence of the present body ghosted by Ali's previous performance – as both a "loudmouth" and a prize-winning boxer – is made all the more tragic because we see in Ali's body bent by Parkinson's Disease, the presence of his former self who had vowed to the world that he would never be swayed. It is here that the previous performance – that of the world champion in heavyweight boxing – will inevitably haunt our reception of Ali's present-day appearance. What this also means, however, is that our vision of Ali will never be reduced to Parkinson's Disease; it will always be informed by his former, younger and healthier body which remains with us, a world audience, as a "ghost." This, at the same time, is the vision of narrative medicine which calls for ways of resisting the reduction of a present-day patient to the narrative – or the diagnosis – of his illness. We have a different image of Ali, the patient affected by PD, then, because we have already witnessed Ali in his former life, that of a world champion. In witnessing his present-day performances, then, we are not, as Carlson puts it, newcomers to this performance; we do not judge or comprehend Ali simply by what we see in the present. To use Carlson's words, the "voice [or body] that might seem to an outsider grown thin with age [or illness]" (58) would continue to carry weight and cadence in our perception because we would see in this performance the performer's previous self, superimposed on the present one.

What narrative medicine seeks to restore, then, is the sense in which this ghosting may resist a person's reduction to narratives of illness even if this person is not a celebrity of public life. What the bringing of performance studies to medical humanities – or to narrative medicine, for that matter, – may yield is precisely to add another dimension to our sense of embodiment.

1.5 Medical Humanities, Narrative Medicine, and Life Writing Research

It is at this point that I would like to return to the intersection between medical humanities, narrative medicine, and life writing research. Over the last decade, medical humanities have emerged as a vibrant, interdisciplinary new field which have sought to explore the notion of medicine and medical practice, but also the concepts of illness and health from a variety of different angles, including cultural studies, sociology, and art history. At the same time, medical humanities have been key to the restructuring of medical training, with "texts" usually taught in the humanities being included in the medical curriculum. As a different but to some extent related approach, narrative medicine has emerged as a method aimed to include narrative into (the practice of) medicine, and to train medical practitioners to listen to, and appreciate the complexity of (patient) narratives. Narrative medicine brings together medical practitioners and literary scholars to explore the common terrain that narrative provides as a bridge between medicine and the humanities. If "medical humanities" are thus a field or research, narrative medicine is a method seeking to change the practice of medicine. It is thus aimed less at changing the humanities than at changing, through the inclusion of the humanities (and literary narratives more specifically) the "face" of medicine. Moreover, narrative medicine is not only a practice of reading, but also of writing; in narrative medicine programs, writing is seen as key to "learning" empathy. As Marini observes quoting Spiro,

> Accomplishing such acts of witnessing allows the physician to proceed to his or her more recognizably clinical narrative tasks: to establish a therapeutic alliance, to generate and proceed through a differential diagnosis . . . to interpret physical findings and laboratory reports correctly, to experience and to convey empathy for the patient's experience and, as a result of all these, to engage the patient in obtaining effective care. (qtd. in Marini 8)

Narrative medicine thus brings together not only medical doctors and literary scholars, but also includes writers as experts in narrative. The involvement of award-winning author Siri Hustvedt in the narrative medicine program at Columbia University is a case in point here.

While narrative medicine is concerned with the concept of narrative (patient narratives in particular, but also the narratives of doctors about their own medical practice), it does not address the relevance of "life writing" in this context. In the humanities, conversely, life writing research has emerged as a field whose potential it may be, as I have argued above, to bridge the gap between the humanities on the one hand and medicine and the natural sciences on the other. Many of the "texts" which have been included into medical humanities, such as patient autobiographies, thus fall within the realm of life writing, even if "life writing" does not figure as a genre in these discussions. Looking at medical humanities and narrative medicine from the perspective of the humanities – and of American Studies in particular –, I am thus interested in the ways in which life writing texts are being read and included in different disciplines. What if, I would like to ask here, one and the same autobiography is being read in a literary and a medical classroom? More than mere parallelism, I am interested in the ways in which these readings may differ, but also the ways in which they may converge. What happens to the humanities, in other words, after the emergence of medical humanities? If the emergence of medical humanities has changed the face of medicine, then, it may also – if counterintuitively – have changed the face of the humanities. It is this process that I am trying to explore in the chapters that follow. At the end of each chapter, I will discuss how that chapter's outlook and the material analyzed in it may contribute to the framework of medical humanities.

One of the key questions which this book seeks to explore is the potential impact of medical humanities, paradoxically, on the humanities. If medical humanities emerged, in the 1980s and 1990s, as a way of bringing narrative into medicine, of enhancing the relevance of patient narratives for medical practice by expanding the fields, genres and formats from which such patient accounts were to be drawn, medical humanities implicitly also emerged as an attempt to bring the humanities (back) into medicine and the practice of medicine. The focus was to some extent on medicine, and here particularly on medical training or the didactics of medicine. As Johanna Shapiro has argued, "Several scholarly trends, such as narrative medicine, patient-centered and relationship-centered care, have long advocated for the value of the patient's voice in the practice of medicine. As theories of textual analysis are applied to the understanding of stories of illness, doctors and scholars have the opportunity to develop more nuanced and multi-faceted appreciation for these accounts" (68). As Shapiro's account of the emergence and the relevance of medical humanities and narrative medicine (particularly with reference to the work of Rita Charon and Sayantani DasGupta) makes clear, the impetus of medical humanities is not of itself novel, as it incorporates and is able to incorporate various other, and previous approaches, such as narrative health and "patient-centered care" (68). Yet, from the perspective of the humanities, my aim is to ask not only what the humanities can do for medicine but also what medicine can do for the humanities. For what would medical humanities mean not just for the humanities as a form of scholarship, but as a form of practice? What would Shapiro's distinction between "doctors and scholars" mean not just for the current practice of medicine, but for the humanities? What is the notion of "practice" in the humanities? I believe that to tie back the (interdisciplinary) field of medical humanities to the current practice of the humanities may have profound implications for this latter field not only in a struggle for relevance: To be sure, it would be short-sighted to reduce the humanities to a sort of utilitarian ethics, to argue that they are "relevant" only insofar as they can prove their use value to fields such as medicine. Yet, what an encounter with medicine via the missing link of medical humanities as a medium of translation may bring to the humanities may be a renewed attention to narrative and the status of narrative in a variety of different contexts: It is here that one of the pitfalls of life writing research as a field of inquiry can lie: For even if there is a continuity between, say, patient narratives and fictional narratives, what distinction nevertheless needs to be made between these two kinds of narrative? Are some narratives more "real" than others? Is the need to listen to some stories more "existential" than the need to listen to others? As Shapiro convincingly argues, neither medical practice nor medical humanities as an emerging field of inquiry may be well-advised to naively assume the innocence or the primacy of narrative. Every narrative, regardless of its context, is always a construction of reality, is always a performance in and of itself. According to Shapiro, "we realize, for example, that a patient's story is rarely "just a story," but is rather the conscious and unconscious representation and performance of intricate personal motives and dominant meta-narrative influences. Overall, this complexifying of narrative is beneficial as it reduces readers' and listeners' naïve assumptions about reliability and authenticity" (68). There is an interesting link here to the field of life writing research as it has been used in the context of human rights narratives. The connecting link between human rights activism and stories of illness or disability may be located precisely in the idea of the experimental. Arguably, through the prevalence of post-structuralism and the paramount of *textuality* as it has come to be applied to all texts, the notion of lived experience may itself have become suspect to the humanities. To focus on the experiential, it may seem, is only one step away from the trap of mimetic fallacy. To focus on lived experience as a truth in and of itself is to fall prey to the fiction of authenticity, to "naïve assumptions about reliability and authenticity," as Shapiro puts it (68). And yet, some fields within the humanities such as Ethnic Studies or Minority Studies have stressed the mooring of cultural practice in social and cultural experience. In these fields, the author has never been quite dead since writing was said to emanate from a particular cultural and historical location. At this juncture, human rights research or rather, the life writing research which has been done, especially by Sidonie Smith and Kay Schaeffer, with regard to human rights activism, has stressed life writing as a field which fruitfully links an awareness of the textual nature of human rights narratives with the notion of lived experience. Life writing research can be located, then, half-way between the textual and the "actual," even if, of course, the latter is never accessible to us in unmediated fashion. Nonetheless, life writing research is crucial in stressing the fact that there may in fact be a sliding scale of "textuality," there may be different degrees of textualization. Illness, as Michael J. Fox has suggested, is not a performance, but an experience ("Michael J. Fox on George Stroumboulopoulos"). There is a sense here, however, in which there is something about the notion of illness which causes us to shy away from the textual. As Shapiro goes on to say, "the readers of such [illness] narratives, whether they are physicians trying to educate themselves about the patient experience, or rather patients attempting to make sense of their own encounter with illness, tend to assume that these accounts represent objective truth – 'what really happened'" (68). There is, of course, a subjective dimension to this experience as "objective truth," a dimension which exposes objectivity as a myth in the first place. Yet, I believe that there is a sense in which life writing accounts differ from fiction in the urgency they convey, particularly, as Schaeffer and Smith point out, when it comes to breaches in the integrity of human life as in human rights violations. These breaches in the integrity of human life, incidentally, may cut to the heart of the matter, and to the blind spot of mimetic fallacy as a notion to the extent that it runs the risk of disregarding the experiential notion of human life. In this regard, it may be useful to recall Martha Nussbaum's critique of Judith Butler's work. Hate speech, Nussbaum noted in her critique of what she saw as Butler's poststructuralist politics, may be more than a textual move. To be sure, Butler has long made clear that her focus on the deconstructive potential of parody by no means meant a retreat from the "actual," from the everyday life of politics and the vulnerability of human subjects. In particular after 9/11, it is the physical vulnerability of human subjects which has been paramount in Butler's notion of "precarious life." Thus, life writing research has been instrumental in stressing the fact that the breach of the integrity of human life is not just ideational, but physical and material. It is the materiality, the biological condition of human life that medical humanities can bring to the humanities with renewed force.

Thus, there is a sense in which from the perspective of literary history *and* the history of medicine, the developments in both fields may be particularly conducive to a focus on interdisciplinary research between medicine and the humanities: For the humanities, life writing research has meant a renewed attention paid to the material dimension of human life and the relevance of the body to any notion of human "identity." According to Couser,

> although our selves and our lives are fundamentally somatic, the body has not until recently figured prominently in life writing. Traditional biographers usually treat illness as an interruption of the life that is their proper concern, except when it threatens life or ends it. And although autobiographers are better situated than biographers to report on the somatic lives of their subjects, traditionally they too have seemed disinclined to do so. (*Recovering Bodies* 5)

The humanities may thus recently have been marked by a "somatic turn," just as medicine may have taken a more narrative direction. For different branches of medicine, there has been an increasing need for individualized medicine, and for integrating the patient's perspective into medical practice. This shift, many clinicians argued, also involved a different sense of "positivism" in clinical practice. As Shapiro notes,

> In the post-Flexnerian era, physicians increasingly viewed the patient's story with a certain skepticism and discomfort because of its subjectivity and perceived unreliability. Instead, they came to depend more on impartial data obtained from various technological manipulations of the Foucauldian clinical gaze (CT scans and MRI imagery, lab values, stress tests, etc.), as well as their own positivist scientific expertise. Various scholarly trends have reintroduced the importance of the patient's story to the field of medicine. The thrust of narrative medicine scholarship, for example, has been to move the patient's voice from a position of relative marginalization to one reinvested with a measure of authority. (68)

There is, of course, the danger of a false dichotomy here: one telos of medical research would need to be not, of course, a discarding of laboratory medicine but rather the integration of laboratory medicine *and* patient narratives. To speak only of Foucauldianism here perhaps, would be to sidestep the complexity inherent in such a dialogue. Yet, a perspective focusing on or stressing the need for a constructive dialogue between life sciences and life writing would highlight the fact that these perspectives are by no means mutually exclusive. In fact, they are short-sighted only if they assume from the very beginning such mutual exclusivity and hence the ubiquity and universal applicability of their own specific approach. As Marini has emphasized in her recent discussion of narrative medicine, then, effective health-care can be ensured only through a fusion between Evidence-Based Medicine (EBM) and narrative medicine. According to her, "Narrative medicine is democratic . . . : It is able to connect patients and health-care providers and link evidence-based medicine and medicine based on narrative, as well as clinical science and human science" (Marini 8).

I believe that the greatest risk that the humanities may run in incorporating or reimporting medical humanities is that paradoxically, they, too, will reduce stories of illness to being just that, stories of illness. To the extent that they read these texts as autobiographical texts in the sense proper, comprising stories of illness but also of the unfolding of a life completely unrelated to illness, the humanities, too, will be able to do what Rita Charon calls "honoring the stories of illness" (*Narrative Medicine* 3). In fact, this is where my reading of autobiography converges with Charon's account of narrative medicine: To Charon, each patient narrative is also an autobiography; it contains the sum total of a patient's life, not only aspects about his or her illness. It is in this sense, then, that I would like to call for a re-reading of life writing narrative in the framework of medical humanities but also and especially in a sense unrelated to this framework. To re-import medical humanities, then, is at the same time to look beyond medical humanities, and to incorporate into the practice of life writing research what Rita Charon calls "honoring the stories of illness," or, perhaps, honoring the stories as the stories they are, and as the life writing narratives they are meant to be. It is in this sense that I see a convergence between Charon's concept of "narrative medicine" on the one hand and life writing research on the other.

What, then, are the loose ends of this analysis? First and foremost, even as the concept and genre of life writing can be seen as a liberating and democratizing concept, there seems to be a pitfall here since, as Johanna Shapiro has argued, there is a privileging, if not of the autonomous subject – many of the texts which this study will explore are collaborative autobiographies in varying senses of the term –, then at least of the writing subject (68). As I will argue in many of the chapters, for instance, with reference to Tito Mukhopadhyay's poetic/ autobiographical narrative *The Mind Tree* or Michael Bérubé's *Life As We Know It* (1996), reference is often made that without the right and the faculty to represent themselves, these "disabled" subjects would have remained "vegetables," as Tito Mukhopadhyay puts it in his interview on "Breaking the Silence," a special feature of CBS's documentary program *60 Minutes II* ("60 Minutes"). This idea may in turn be seen as a highly contentious argument. The capability to represent oneself in written form, then, is itself said to be coterminous with the emergence and the recognition of subjectivity. There is no space, then, of subjectivity outside language. Valorization depends, in a way, on the act of being read; subjectivity is not valued as a concept in itself but it is seen as emerging only in the process of recognition, and the recognition by a reader.[15]

1.6 Biological Citizenship

One of the issues which this study seeks to explore, then, is the concept of "biological citizenship" (Lemke 127; my trans.). All of the texts and performances discussed in this book can be seen as being in dialogue with the concept of biological citizenship which, many critics argue, is the "frontier" of the twenty-first century. Yet, as Thomas Lemke has argued, it may be more productive for us not to understand "biological citizenship" as a given, which, for my purposes here, would then be seen to be exemplified by particular life writing texts, but biological citizenship may rather constitute a definitional force-field which, as the twentieth century opens, is still open to discussion. What is at stake in these debates, then, is the way in which the concept of the biological constitution of our lives and our bodies has come to be understood as the basis of the rights and duties associated with the holding of citizenship. Following Nikolas Rose, Lemke and Wehling cite a number of models

[15] I am indebted to Katja Sarkowsky and Mary Kempering for this point. The discussions at the conference "Autobiography and the Production of Knowledge" (University of Münster, March 2015) were invaluable in the reshaping of my argument.

which have characterized contemporary debates on biological citizenship. They begin by saying that the concept of "biological citizenship" not only coincides with what Kymlicka had earlier called the "return of the citizen" (Lemke and Wehling 72; my trans.), but that it may also constitute one of the key concepts of the future: "It does not seem to be an exaggeration to call this term a 'key concept' of the future . . ." (Lemke and Wehling 74; my trans.). Biological citizenship, as it has, for instance, been addressed in the work of Nikolas Rose, can also be related to the concept of "genetic citizenship," which has been explored by Rayna Rapp and which I will discuss in more detail in Chapter 7. What is crucial for my purposes here is that the concept of "biological citizenship" can be said to break down the barrier between medical experts on the one hand and, on the other hand, patient groups as lay persons whose perspective would have little bearing on medical opinion. According to Lemke and Wehling, the concept of biological citizenship sets out to break down the barrier between these two realms:

> [the] boundaries between lay people and experts, between active researchers and passive beneficiaries are being undermined. Even if Heath, Rapp and Taussig mention the danger of "genetification" inherent in biomedical practices and quotidian discourse, their depiction of genetic citizenship stresses, above all, its political advantages and its implications for critiques of power. If we follow these authors, new developments in genetics lead to "new forms of democratic participation, they dissolve the boundary between state and society, between private and public interest." (79; my trans.)

It may thus be highly remarkable, or perhaps not surprising at all, that virtually all of the texts discussed in this book correspond to one or more of the parameters outlined by Lemke and Wehling. What this implies is that "biological citizenship" has already crystallized as a discourse on the relationship between biology and citizenship, in which life writing texts can be said to intervene, but by which they are also shaped. In the chapters that follow, I will relate each of the narratives to the parameters of biological citizenship outlined above; and I will investigate what may be some of the shortcomings of this association.

At the same time, this book is thus interested in the relationship between autobiographical writing on the one hand and the discourse of citizenship on the other. In what way, and through what formal and aesthetic means, can autobiographical texts inscribe (biological) citizenship, and on what levels? Yet, conversely, to what extent can all of the texts discussed in this study be subsumed under the category of citizenship discourse? It may be misleading to see these different autobiographical (and sometimes also biographical) narratives only as interventions into the current debate on biological citizenship. For these texts are not (only) political interventions but they are, first and foremost, literary texts (and, in the case of Baryshnikov's work, artistic performances). Through this aestheticism, moreover, they elicit particular responses; responses in which political activism – the call, for instance, for the civic inclusion of disabled individuals – is inseparable from the aesthetic form in which it is framed, and which may have profound consequences for its impact and its social, cultural and political reception. It is this aesthetic specificity, I believe, which distinguishes, say, an activist call for biological citizenship on a website, from the life writing narratives which are the topic of this book. If Abraham Lincoln famously argued that Harriet Beecher Stowe started the Civil War, what is at stake, then as now, is to investigate the textual (and emotional) politics through which public sentiment (and ultimately, political activism rooted in such sentiment) can be mobilized through particular aesthetic and literary strategies.

The question of citizenship, in turn, is closely connected to social justice debates. It is for this reason that many of the following chapters will return to Martha Nussbaum's seminal study, *Frontiers of Justice: Disability, Nationality, Species Membership* (2007). Not only, as Nussbaum argues, is disability closely connected to notions of citizenship and the question of who should and should not be allowed to actively participate in a given nation's social, political and civic life, but many of these concerns raise fundamental questions about our notion of humanity itself. The idea of species membership, in the texts I will investigate in this book, is perhaps most explicitly raised in Temple Grandin's complex autobiographical text, *Thinking in Pictures*. In her autobiographical narrative, Grandin claims that owing to her different way of thinking and of perceiving the world, she may be able to empathize, on a different and quite exceptional level, with the cattle whose living conditions she sets out to ameliorate, working for companies such as McDonald's. A similar perspective is also addressed in Dawn Prince-

Hughes' *Songs of the Gorilla Nation: My Journey through Autism* (2004).

Finally, the aim of this study is to ask how these questions of citizenship can be related to the idea of knowledge production. In this context, I am interested in the ways in which life writing narratives can be seen as forms of knowledge production in their own right. To argue that life writing narratives have to be included into medical discourse is thus only one part of the discussion which is currently being held at the nexus of life writing and life science; what may be at stake, beyond the politics of mere inclusion, is the level and the institutional context in which such an inclusion takes place. What, then, would be the life writing equivalent of the ICD-10? What if the knowledge produced in life writing texts, came to be part of the everyday practice of diagnosis and prognosis?

This study sets out to address the juncture between life writing and medical humanities as a juncture fundamental to our understanding of notions of illness, aging, and disability. For the more we insist on reading these texts as autobiographies and not, as Couser once noted, as "pathographies" only, we will refuse to imply that a person can ever be defined by, let alone reduced to, the state of his health or the chronology of age (*Recovering Bodies* x). It is for this reason, I argue in this study, that life writing research may have much to offer to medical humanities, just as conversely, medical humanities may have come to inform the ways in which we read these autobiographies which, among many other things, also address notions of physical change or deviance from whatever it is that we conceive as "normal." It is for this reason that, while the concept of biological citizenship may inform some of the narratives I will discuss in the following chapters, these narratives can never be reduced to notions of citizenship, or to the "biological" qualities of the individuals in whose names they call for civic inclusion. The aesthetics of autobiography, then, exceed any petition or plea, on the political level, for social inclusion. It is this excess of the aesthetic, I believe, where life writing research may productively complicate the framework, often geared towards the didacticism culled from "patient experience," of medical humanities. The following chapters, even as they seek to engage in a dialogue between life writing research and medical humanities, will thus also focus on elements of playfulness, on the junctures in which these autobiographical texts deliberately undo the frameworks they know they will be included in.

It is this "unruliness" of autobiographical narratives, in turn (Charon, *Narrative Medicine* 4), which may provide not only a key link in the space in-between life sciences and the humanities, but also the need for an ongoing discussion between the two. For where medical classrooms would run the risk of reducing a given autobiography to a patient narrative, humanities scholarship and life writing research would stress the multifacetedness of this narrative, as well as its cultural, historical, social and political context. This context, in turn, may be necessary for the medical practitioner to understand all the aspects in the patient's narrative, even those aspects which at first may seem irrelevant to the diagnosis. This need to listen to all the facets in a patient's narrative, then, is stressed in Charon's approach to narrative medicine. The central question in this context is where the difference lies between patient narrative and autobiography. Charon's intervention is crucial in insisting that this question may ultimately unanswerable, that each of these narratives is irreducible in its complexity. It is in their shared attention to the unruliness of autobiographical narratives that life sciences and life writing research may converge; and it is this "unruliness" (Charon, *Narrative Medicine* 4) also, which makes an ongoing dialogue between these two fields not only fruitful, but necessary.

2 Temporalities in Life Writing: Tito Mukhopadhyay's *Beyond the Silence*

I would like to start this chapter[1] with an experiment, the experiment of simply citing a poem:

> Many things can happen in a minute.
> This or that;
> Some of this and some of that;
> All of this
> And none of that;
> Or all of that
> And none of this.
> It depends on which you consider important,
> this or that (Mukhopadhyay, *The Mind Tree* 142)

Across many cultures and ages, it has been argued that if someone wanted to be a good statesman, he had to be a good poet first. Poetry, it was argued, was the aesthetic form in which we wonder about what it means to be human. From the very beginning, this aesthetic form was associated with temporality, or rather, with the suspension of temporality. Not only in Shakespearean sonnets, the poet's aim was to transcend the span of his own mortality; the poem, in its universality and its universal appeal to humanity as an existential condition, was to transcend both space and temporality.

[1] The ideas gathered in this chapter were first presented at the conference "Der Wert der Literatur in den Medical Humanities," ("The Value of Literature for Medical Humanitites") organized by Mariacarla Gadebusch-Bondio, Pascal Berberat and Pascal Fischer of the Institute for History and Ethics of Medicine at TU Munich in 2013. I am grateful for the organizers' invitation and critical comments, which were central to my writing of this chapter.

Yet, what would happen if I were to write that this poem had been written by a boy of nine? My assumption is that at this very moment, we would read the poem differently; and we would now read it as an acceleration of time. A child prodigy - for only a child prodigy would be able to compose such a poem at the age of nine – is by definition ahead of his time; he has accelerated his mental capacity beyond or ahead of his biological age.

As a third step in my experiment, what would happen if I were to add that not only had this poem been written by a boy of only nine years of age, but that it had been written by a nine-year-old boy from India, and that it had originally been written in English? To the context of temporal acceleration, I believe, the context of spatial acceleration would now be added, if I am permitted this mixing of metaphors. It is here that the poet's location takes a yet more specific shape. He is marked not only as a nine-year-old child prodigy, but as a child from a highly educated, presumably high caste, middle-class Indian family. Not only would the child be assumed to have appropriated an aesthetic form far beyond the reach of his fellows in age, but – as an Indian boy poet – he would also, in a postcolonial reading of the poem, be said to have appropriated the form of the English sonnet. When we learn about the poet's name – Tito Mukhopadhyay – our assumptions will be confirmed: it is the name of a Brahmin boy from Bengal.

I have so far imposed on the reading of the poem the lens of age and that of cultural context. Yet, my claim is that all of these readings would come to nil if I were to provide one more piece of information about the poet. What if I were to state that this nine-year old boy from India, Tito Mukhopadhyay, was diagnosed with autism?

From one minute to the next, the entire context in which we read the poem would change, and, I would argue, it would change in a way more radical than in any of my previous readings of either temporal acceleration or postcolonial context. All at once, the poem and the boy poet's writing would be conceived in terms of disability. Into this reading, moreover, the limits of credibility would intrude: Could this poem really have been written by an autistic person? In this very question, the writer of the poem would cease to be a poet and start being a patient: he would be conceived of in terms of the diagnosis which erases both his individuality and his artistic genius: He is what he has been diagnosed to be. The poem, however, is curiously at odds with this diagnosis: If a poem is conceived of as the most sublime form of cultural expression, how can a "disabled" mind produce such a form of art?

2.1 The Limits of Credibility

Crucially enough, the context in which Tito Mukhopadhyay's poem has been framed for publication is one of authentication, of credibility, and of trust. Indeed, the publication of an autistic boy's poetry strains the limits of our credibility; the dust jacket description of the boy's writing says as much. It is a description, which, not accidentally, comes from Oliver Sacks, a neurologist who has become famous for his popular scientific accounts, such as *Awakenings* (1990), in which he looks into the lives behind the cases of specific illnesses. About Tito Mukhopadhyay's *The Mind Tree*, Sacks writes on the book's dust jacket, "This book is fascinating, but it is also shocking, since we have always assumed that autistic persons are incapable of either introspection or of contemplative thinking – let alone was it believed that they possessed poetic fantasy. Tito gives the lie to these assumptions and forces us to reconsider our notions of autism" (n. pag.). It is the engagement of the concept of credibility, I would argue, which accounts for a shift in register. From one minute to the next, our reading of the poem turns from literature to the realm of biomedicine. As Norbert Paul has argued, this realm, first and foremost, is the domain of establishing trust: "In our post-industrial and postmodern societies of knowledge, crises have long been understood as crises of trust. All societies live in and on economies of trust. What far-reaching consequences breaches of trust have for the capital of trust in biomedicine, was evidenced by the scandal around Hwang Woo-suk, who on 17 June 2005 published fabricated evidence on stem cell research" (556). The framing of Tito Mukhopadhyay's poem *not* in terms of artistic merit but in terms of (biomedical) credibility, I believe, is also a narrowing down of the meanings of the poem to a single reading: In this reading of a poem which has been produced by an autistic person, we may no longer look at the poem in its own right, but will, rather, conceive of it in terms of disability. The poem is no longer just a poem; it is a document which belongs into the domain of illness narratives. In this framing, Oliver Sacks, the neurologist, informs us that the poem has really been written by an autistic person, Tito Mukhopadhyay; and it is thus that credibility is established. As a neurologist, we assume that Sacks is qualified to define what an autistic mind can and what it cannot produce. Our marveling at Tito Mukhopadhyay's mental ability is thus all the more pronounced because it is described as standing in contrast to his condition. Precisely because this trustworthiness of Mukhopadhyay's account is emphasized not by a literary critic, but by a neurologist engaging in popular science, the book is framed as the cultural production of disability. The context in which we read the poem is thus not the context of literary studies but that of disability studies; what takes place is a *medicalizing* of literary analysis.

2.2 The Riddle of Perspective

Tito Mukhopadhyay's narrative is troubling to read, first and foremost, because it is riddled by perspective. As the narrative of *Beyond the Silence* opens, the third person perspective and the subjectivity of an I narrator blur into each other, confounding the reader as to who is speaking here: "It is important to mention that a time came when he lost control over these images that formed around him. He got lost in a situation that was unreal or super real" (Mukhopadhyay, *Beyond the Silence* 8). There are, then, two explanations for this superimposition of perspectives which, crucially enough, can also be said to inform the cover photograph. In the photograph, we see a young boy looking at the ocean, and we look at him from behind. The facelessness of the boy may imply the fact that his is a mere case study; the "case" of autism is revealed through Tito Mukhopadhyay's example. The fact that the boy is photographed from behind mirrors the third-person-perspective: his is an autistic body to be inscribed by the medical diagnosis of disability. Yet, another, alternative reason why the boy should have been photographed from behind is that this perspective enables us to look at a young boy contemplating eternity by looking at the sea: As Sacks notes, the boy's prose implies both his ability of artistic creation and of introspection. It is this eternity, then, which we contemplate with him, looking at the ocean through his eyes. The fact that the boy should have been photographed from behind, then, implies two readings of Tito Mukhopadhyay's narrative which are mutually exclusive. We either look at Tito Mukhopadhyay from the perspective of case studies or illness narratives, *or* we look at Tito Mukhopadhyay looking at the world, thus looking at the world with Tito Mukhopadhyay. We are either distinct from him – as Sacks is in reinforcing the able-bodiedness of his own subject position by writing about Mukhopadhyay's disability – or we learn, through Mukhopadhyay's unusual perspective, something about ourselves.

As the narrative progresses, it becomes clear that the reason why Tito Mukhopadhyay should be writing about himself in the third person is *not* that he sees himself as a medical case, looking at himself through the eyes of his doctor, but it is quite simply the fact that Mukhopadhyay is writing about his own life in retrospect. As the narrative progresses, it becomes clear that it is the older Tito Mukhopadhyay – writing this retrospective account of his nine-year-old self at the age of eleven – looking at the younger self from the outside, looking at him from behind: "My story, through the boy in the story" (Mukhopadhyay, *Der Tag* 88; my trans.). In the narrative, the eleven-year-old Mukhopadhyay looks at his nine-year-old self who hears the diagnosis through the ears of his mother listening to the doctor tell her that her son will never be able to lead a self-directed life:

> Time was running out and the parents took the boy to a speech therapist. He was a bit impatient to handle a two years eleven months old boy and declared after ten minutes observation that he was sorry to say that the boy was mentally retarded. I still go back to that moment and find that it was like a lightening striking down upon the family. The mother staggered back into the hotel room, hugged her son and wept bitterly. The boy was sad too but could not show any feeling of pain. (*Beyond the Silence* 10)

What emerges in this passage is an intrusion of temporality. From the very beginning, Tito Mukhopadhyay's life is described as a race with temporality: When he was two, time started running out for his parents; his development stubbornly refused to match the expectations of normalcy. It is when time starts running out, then, that his parents take him to the doctor; and the doctor informs them that not only has their son been unable to keep up with normal child development, but he will always continue to lag behind. From the moment of the diagnosis, his condition is described as being "retarded," as failing to keep time, as falling out of the temporality of the normal.

It is from this diagnosis of an abnormal or retarded temporality that the story of his life, written by himself, unfolds. In this narrative, Tito Mukhopadhyay proceeds to contrast different forms of temporality, continually re-establishing his own reality vis-à-vis other forms of temporality which mark him as belated, as being out of time. It is this temporality of the normal which turns him into what he describes as a social outcast, a person outside the stream of everyday human productivity. In his narrative, Mukhopadhyay writes about what is perceived by others as his own uselessness, and he writes about this uselessness in English verse:

> All the world was a busy place
> And I was an idle kind
> Disqualified in the human race
> A different form of mind (*The Mind Tree* 103)

The diagnosis of autism, however, supplies us with one more explanation for the riddle of perspective in Mukhopadhyay's narrative. For a long time, "pronoun reversal" – in the sense of a confusion of pronouns, as in referring to oneself in the third person – was seen as one of the characteristics of autism as a form of psychological impairment (Lee et al., "I, You, Me"). Yet my point is that it would be too facile to reduce Tito Mukhopadhyay's writing to being a mere effect of his medical condition. As the prerogative and the creative freedom of a writer, the decision for Mukhopadhyay's writing about his younger self in the third person stands squarely in the tradition of autobiographical writing; it is a decision motivated by literary tradition, not by medical diagnosis.

What life writing supplies to the tenets of life science, then, is the excess of individuality which cannot be contained in mere case studies. First and foremost, Tito Mukhopadhyay's life writing gives the lie to the medical diagnosis which prophesied to him – and to his parents – that he would never be able to write. Life writing can hence be seen as corrective to medical diagnosis; the temporality of Mukhopadhyay's life writing clashes with the temporality which has been predicted for him by medical science. Moreover, Mukhopadhyay's life writing lays bare the workings of medical science; his life narrative is a log book which both mirrors *and* refutes his medical file. From the psychologist's office he is sent to the neurologist's, and from there to a psychiatric clinic. Mukhopadhyay's account of the medical sector could not be more devastating; time and again, the trauma that his narrative revolves on is the pronouncing of diagnoses which seem to run counter to his own conception of self. His narrative is thus also a self-diagnosis, a retrospective, self-directed account in which he re-assesses medical diagnoses through the prism of his own experiences: "The boy went to the Institute where the clinical psychologist after studying him, told the parents that they had an 'AUTISTIC' son. "It is a state when the child is so withdrawn that he is unable to understand what is going on around him." "I understand very well," said the spirit in the boy" (Mukhopadhyay, *Beyond the Silence* 22-23).

2.3 Collaborative Life Writing

At the same time, in writing down his life, Tito Mukhopadhyay is writing not only his own life but also that of his mother. The doctor's original diagnosis seems to spell out not only his own, but also his mother's doom. The story is so haunting in its driving home the point that in a number of ways, Mukhopadhyay's life cannot be written without simultaneously writing the life of his mother: His diagnosis, the story makes clear, is also her doom. What the account makes painfully clear is that while we have a globalized system of medical knowledge, this knowledge has to contend with local practices. According to Norbert Paul, "biomedicine has long become a global phenomenon, yet its local instantiation is strongly affected by the particular cultural, social and economic frameworks in which it is placed" (550). The diagnosis of autism, in India, clashes with the religious notion that an autistic person is a person possessed. As Tito Mukhopadhyay's narrative chronicles in painstaking detail, he watches one religious healer after another enter his home in his mother's desperate attempt of clutching at straws:

> The next thing that thc boy found was that his mother was turning very religious. She started to believe in everything that was told to her. . . . A gentleman suggested that mother should separate rice from the grains before dawn. . . . It took her all night to separate the required number of grains. That was a monsoon month and under a pouring sky, the white cloth was placed on the road – so that the boy spoke. (*Beyond the Silence* 11)

Eventually, Mukhopadhyay manages to convey to his mother that he both understands her desperation and is devastated by the fact that his mother, too, may think of his disability as a cursed condition.

But how could Mukhopadhyay have written down his own story in the first place, thus refuting the diagnosis of his doctors in terms of both disability and temporality? One of the most powerful moments in the narrative is that once his mother gave up shelling grains of rice to make her son speak, she proceeded to teach him herself. The power of the narrative lies in the description of two people, a mother and her son, setting out to beat medical diagnosis, *and* to refute a religious system stigmatizing people with autism. What Tito Mukhopadhyay and his mother grapple with is both the realm of the medical and the realm of the social; their goal is to oppose both the medical prognosis and the religious prophecy with another, an alternative kind of temporality; a temporality in which Mukhopadhyay progresses at his own pace. It is by dedicating her life to her son, moreover, that his mother steps out of the temporality of the normal; she gives up her career in chemistry – a career which caused relatives to ascribe to her the reason why her son is autistic in the first place – and dedicates her life to teaching her son to catch up with the temporality of the normal.

And yet, Tito Mukhopadhyay's writing down his own story is collaborative in a sense whose complexity by far exceeds our established notions of collaborative writing: The point which he makes in his story is not only that with the aid of a spelling board, his mother taught him to spell out the words with which he could describe his life. Rather, Mukhopadhyay goes on to describe that he was able to spell out the words on his spelling board only when his mother was holding the board.[2] It is at this point that his mother, through a method not of medi-

[2] The method of "assisted writing" has been a highly controversial one. As Temple Grandin has noted in *Thinking in Pictures*, critics were able to prove that in the majority of cases, the writing subject was not the person holding the board but the person prompting them. It is, however, crucial to note in this context that Grandin herself met Tito Mukhopadhyay and vouches for the authenticity of his writing: "His typing is truly independent and he was not prompted after he typed each short sentence to keep him on task and to prevent him from running across

cal training but of intuition, uses her own body as an extension of her son's. The same notion of physical collaboration is true of the signature moment in which Mukhopadhyay "finds" his own voice:

> Then she did 'it' with all her suddenness. She gave him a push from the back on his chest. The boy was not prepared for the push, and he gave a sound "uh!" as the air pushed out of his mouth due to the reflex action of the push. "There! Your voice is found! Now with each push, you will find it," she told him. Then for the next 10 minutes, they did the voice finding process. (*Beyond the Silence* 81-82)

It is here that Mukhopadhyay contrasts social conventions with his own notion of authenticity. Ultimately, as in the doctor's and the patient's collaborative attempt to come up with the right kind of therapy, Tito Mukhopadhyay's and his mother Soma's attempt at beating the temporality of medical prognosis is a method of trial and error. The *context* in which Mukhopadhyay is able to speak may seem strange to the average onlooker, he is well-aware; but the judgment of such visual incongruence is itself based on the assumption of normalcy. As Mukhopadhyay goes on to say,

> I would tell the people, those who deal with the autistics, "Try to follow the same system, which works best for your subject consistently and universally. At that time, there should not be any 'social customs' that come in the way of the procedure. It may look very 'unnatural' when a person is pushed or urged to speak, but it would be a great help for your subject." No, dear psychologists, you do not make yourselves inhuman by the . . . slight pain [which you inflict]. (*The Mind Tree* 85)

The power of life writing, as much as the power of Tito Mukhopadhyay's poetry interspersed into the writing of his life, is the suspension of physical materiality. In this writing, we imagine Mukhopadhyay, but we do not see or hear him physically. The point is not only that we look at him through his eyes, not our own, it is also that the power of his narrative is such that it suspends our own sensual per-

the room. . . . This convinced me that Tito was not being cued by his mother" (*Thinking in Pictures* 80-81).

ception. In this sensual perception, the narrative makes clear, the judgment of the abnormal resides. It is one thing, in other words, for us to read Tito Mukhopadhyay's description of the fact that even though he has learned to speak, it is often hard to understand him; it would be quite another, however, for us to listen to his words.

It is for this reason, then, that I have chosen in this paper to try to tell you Tito Mukhopadhyay's story, rather than refer to the CBS documentary about Mukhopadhyay's amazing ability to rise above his diagnosis. I am thus concerned in this chapter with the relevance of the genre of life writing and the medium in which a given life is being told for our perception of normalcy. The power of writing about a life – and the solace of reading this life writing – may lie precisely in the suspension of visual and acoustic perception. Tito Mukhopadhyay writes to us about the disability of his body by confronting us in a disembodied form. We witness his body only in his writing. Had we looked at the CBS documentary, on the other hand, we would have seen a boy sitting on his bed, with his body spinning for no apparent reason. It would have been at this very moment, I believe, that our gaze would have taken on the parameters of a medical, a diagnostic gaze; we would have looked at the boy's body not as the body of the author who wrote these poems, but as the body of a severely autistic person. His body would have ceased to be the poet's body and would have become simply the body of an autistic boy spinning on his bed.

2.4 "Frontiers of Justice"

Why, then, should we read Tito Mukhopadhyay's story and the poems that have been incorporated into it? It is here that I would briefly like to take into account the work of American philosopher Martha Nussbaum, reading two of her recent books in conjunction with one another: Nussbaum, in her volume *The Clash Within* (2009), has written about India, as a space of a radical asynchronicity of time, as the simultaneous existence, even clash, of the atavistic and the modern. In another book published two years before *The Clash Within*, a book entitled *Frontiers of Justice* (2007), Nussbaum has addressed the "case" of autism as a frontier to our notions of democracy. What is significant for my purposes here, however, is that Nussbaum, for all her attempts to delineate a universal, a comprehensive theory of justice, has chosen not to refer to autism as an abstract case study, but as a story which, to Nussbaum, is much closer to home. Nussbaum, writes, in *Frontiers of Justice*, about her own nephew, Arthur, who has been diagnosed with autism. Nussbaum starts, in a striking parallel to Tito Mukhopadhyay's life writing, by highlighting her nephew's complex grasp of the relativism of human signification. In this passage, Martha Nussbaum, the philosopher, muses about her ten-year-old nephew's thoughts being ahead of her own (*Frontiers of Justice* x).

I am interested, then, in this shift in register, the moment in which a philosophical account of the nature of modern democracy suddenly changes in genre to write the life of the philosopher's nephew. In Nussbaum's account, Arthur never becomes a case study. We should think about Arthur's life and our ability to include him, Nussbaum reminds us, because this will not only enable him to lead a life in which he can live up to the fullest of his abilities, but because our notions of democracy have to be measured against Arthur's life, and about what life we make possible for him. To return to the cover image of Tito Mukhopadhyay's book, it is by looking at Mukhopadhyay that we may come to look at ourselves.

What, then, would it add to our reading of Tito Mukhopadhyay's story to know that shortly after the completion of his book, he and his mother have moved to California? Mukhopadhyay's has become a transnational narrative, adding to the notion of complex forms of temporality a complex form of spatiality, and hence the idea that the struggle against the stigmatizing of autism, too, needs to be a transnational endeavor.

As in Nussbaum's account, Tito Mukhopadhyay emphasizes that we may have stressed the fact that the autistic person needs help in order to speak over the *content* of what he says. In order for American democracy to live up to the fullest of its potential, Nussbaum writes, it needs to find a way to help people like her nephew participate in the social and the political fabric. Frontiers of Justice, in Nussbaum's words, are constituted by the normalcy of time, a time in which Mukhopadhyay's problem of synchronicity – the curious mixture of the slowing and the acceleration of time – will no longer be out of place. He writes, "One day I dream that we can grow in a matured society where nobody would be 'normal or abnormal' but just human beings, accepting any other human being – ready to grow together" (*The Mind Tree* 90). This passage is remarkable in its deliberate upsetting of the temporality of the normal: what is retarded, Mukhopadhyay implies, is a way of thinking which cannot go beyond the limits of ability. A world which can only conceive of ability and disability in terms of black and white but does not know the nuances of grey, he reminds us, is chronologically lagging behind its own potential.

The story of Tito Mukhopadhyay's life, as it has unfolded since the publication of the book, has progressed remarkably, and it has progressed by coming full circle. Eclipsing for good the dichotomy between an India steeped in superstition and a U.S. as the teleology of medical science, Mukhopadhyay's mother Soma has founded, in Los Angeles, a school for autistic children. In this school, she teaches autistic children the way she has taught and continues to teach her own son. The children's parents have been amazed at the rapid progress which, under Soma's tutelage, their children have been making. As Portia Iversen describes the method's success for her son Dov, "I was like a kid in a candy shop. I didn't know where to start. You know? What's your favorite color? What do you want to be when you grow up? I mean, you know, all the things you ask your child over the years. Every day, there was a whole new set of things I was finding out."

Soma's approach, a CBS television documentary makes clear, is intuitive; and yet, it works. As Michael M. Merzenich, a neuroscientist at the University of California at San Francisco, remarks in an excerpt from "Breaking the Silence," the special feature of CBS's documentary program *60 Minutes II* on autism, "I think it's almost certain that this method can be used with many, many autistic children, and the initial indication from the studies in Los Angeles is that it might apply even to the substantial majority of these children" ("60 Minutes"). It is at this point that we may have come full circle from Oliver Sacks. If Sacks, as a neurobiologist, set out to authenticate Tito Mukhopadhyay's writing, Mukhopadhyay's narrative transcends the authentication of an autistic life by a medical expert. His mother's founding a school for autistic children in Los Angeles, moreover, continues to turn the tables on notions of medical expertise and laypeople's intuition: In this upsetting of *Deutungshoheit*, of the power of interpretation, it is the mother of an autistic son who goes on to teach the neurobiologist about how the temporality of a life lived with autism can in fact refute medical prognosis.

The greatest gift, and the most supreme intuition, then, is Mukhopadhyay's mother Soma's acceleration of time. To the temporality of biomedicine, Soma opposes another temporality, the temporality and accelerated temporality of teaching her son every single waking moment of his life. Tito Mukhopadhyay himself comments on his mother's attempt to accelerate time, to beat the biomedical diagnosis of his own mental "retardation" by speeding up the process of teaching; his comment, however, is not without ambivalence: "He felt she was being a bit cruel as she told him, 'Our one day should be equal to two days'" (*The Mind Tree* 64). Yet, the fact remains that with this method of beating medical prognosis by disbelieving in it, Mukhopadhyay's mother has enabled her son to participate in social life to an extent which has dazzled not only neurobiologists, but also the parents of other autistic children. As the interviewer in the excerpt from the *60 Minutes II* documentary asks him in closing, what would have happened to Mukhopadhyay had his mother not dedicated her life to teaching him? His answer is simple: "I would have been a vegetable." ("60 Minutes")

What remains, then, is the power of writing, and the necessity of including alternative forms of temporality into our own notions not only of normalcy, but also of social justice. In her philosophical treatise, Martha Nussbaum envisions, in a utopian form of temporality, a time when her autistic nephew would be allowed to vote and hence fully participate in American democracy; when the content of what he thinks would be privileged over the way in which he is able to say it. By the same token, Tito Mukhopadhyay may be able to write only when his mother is holding the spelling board, but what he writes is certainly worth reading, and it may be worth reading far beyond the context of disability studies. Whether this form of temporality is a utopian one is for us to decide.

At the heart of Tito Mukhopadhyay's narrative is thus also a refraction of the debate around biological citizenship. What is at stake here on a more abstract level is the idea outlined by Lemke and Wehling in reference to the work of Nikolas Rose and Paul Rabinow, that personal accounts (by individual patients or patient collectives) can also help to abolish the gap between lay experience and expert knowledge (79). Tito Mukhopadhyay's narrative can thus be said to participate in two frameworks simultaneously: First, as I have argued above, it intervenes in the discussion of autobiography; and second, it can be seen to respond to and inscribe its own position into, the debate around biological citizenship. In this latter debate, it is closely aligned with the idea of what Thomas Lemke calls "embodied health." In this sense, a question once asked by W.E.B. Du Bois, "How does it feel to be a problem?"[3] is taken up by these narratives as interventions, by the "patient," into medical discourse. How does it feel, these narratives ask, to be "disabled"? How does it feel to be "autistic," or even more crucially, as Tito Mukhopadhyay's narrative puts it, to be labeled "autistic"?

2.5 Towards an Ethics of Usefulness?

At first sight, there could be no better narrative to testify to the intricate interweaving of life sciences and life writing. Tito Mukhopadhyay's text starts with the inscription of a young boy's life by the life sciences, starting with the medical diagnosis of autism. At this critical juncture, life science seems to have the power to determine a life, by predicting its outcome or rather, the lack of its progress, and a boy's future participation in society. Yet, as the narrative progresses, it becomes clear that Mukhopadhyay's mother Soma sets out to predict the diagnosis and the prognosis of the life sciences, using life writing – in the literal sense of teaching her son to write his own life – as a field in which to refute the predictions of the life sciences. At the end of the *60 Minutes II* documentary excerpt, then, we have come full circle. Precisely because Soma has succeeded in proving the life science prognosis wrong through the successful career of her son, life scientists – such a neurologists in California – now take their cue from life writing. The power of interpretation, of what it means to be autistic, has been successfully redefined by a mother's dedication to change the life of her son.

At the same time, there are a number of loose ends in my argument that I have so far failed to take into account. For what is the emplotment of Tito Mukhopadhyay's narrative, and the emplotment of my analysis so far? Crucially, as Shapiro has argued, any study located in the field of medical humanities needs to be acutely aware of the concept of emplot-

[3] I am indebted to Anirban Halder for this point which he explores in much more detail in his current research project on trauma and life writing.

ment: What story is told, and for what audience? What are the narrative patterns which inform the telling of a particular illness narrative? What genres does this telling preclude by following particular expectations or rather, the expectations of one particular audience instead of another? My analysis in this chapter has, so far, followed the trajectory, and the teleology, also embedded in Tito Mukhopadhyay's own narrative, as well as the documentary *60 Minutes II*. Seen from this angle, Mukhopadhyay's story is in fact a success story: Through the constant care and the dedication of his mother, Mukhopadhyay was able to make a life for himself, even if this life does not quite enable him to live independently of his mother. As the documentary makes clear, he will never be able to lead a life of his own. There is, hence, an ethical aporia which arises from the particular emplotment of Tito Mukhopadhyay's narrative in both his prose as it has been published in *The Mind Tree* and in the *60 Minutes II* documentary. For how could we question the dedication of his mother, how could we question her self-denial as his constant caregiver? If the emplotment which the narrative in both the documentary and Mukhopadhyay's own life writing follows is that of an individual rising above his diagnosis, disproving the prediction of the life sciences through the very act of leading a creative life, there are in fact two protagonists to this narrative. By enabling her son to rise above his circumstances, Mukhopadhyay's mother also tries to rewrite her own life. Yet, as the documentary in particular makes clear, both these forms of life writing are inextricably intertwined, one is impossible without the other. Following Thomas Couser's argument in *Vulnerable Subjects: The Ethics of Life Writing*, we might thus ask about the ethics of such "collaborative life writing" (34). The question of authorship here must be understood in a figurative sense: Tito Mukhopadhyay writes his life both in prose form and in verse; yet, within the lines of his autobiography, his mother's "authorship" of his life is also visible. Moreover, Soma's presence in the above-cited documentary on autism, can clearly be seen as a biography or "heterobiography" (Couser, *Vulnerable Subjects* 35) of her son. It is in this context that Couser's cautionary remarks about the "vulnerable subjects" both of collaborative life writing and of parental autobiography may apply. Couser writes,

> Although issues of literary ethics may arise in any genre, ethical dilemmas seem to be inherent in collaborative life writing in ways that are pe-

> culiar to it. . . . The inherent discrepancy between the partners' contributions may be complicated by an imbalance of power between them. Often, collaborations involve partners whose relation is hierarchized by some difference in race, culture, gender, class, age or (in the case of narratives of illness or disability), somatic, intellectual, or emotional condition that renders them vulnerable to exploitation. (*Vulnerable Subjects* 37)

Crucially, then, it might hence be argued that the story which Tito Mukhopadhyay tells not only to the camera and the reporter on *60 Minutes II*, but also in his essays and his poetry, is in fact told to his mother. Here, his mother has assumed not only the role of his caregiver, but also that of his *doctor* – having developed a form of treatment herself, which then later will be taken up by neurologists at the University of California, San Francisco. In this context, it could be argued that life writing inspires, even informs, the life sciences and not only vice versa. And Mukhopadhyay, as especially the excerpt from the *60 Minutes II* documentary makes clear, wants to be a "good patient" ("60 Minutes"). It is this form of audience expectation – Mukhopadhyay's talking, first and foremost, to his mother – which informs the particular emplotment of his narrative. If through this very enmeshment of his own story with that of his mother, who literally enables him to live the life he has been enabled to live by her constant care, he is a "vulnerable subject" in Couser's terms, what are his possibilities of being not a conformist subject – a subject conforming to the emplotment which his mother has mapped out not just for his narrative but also for his life – but, instead, an unruly subject? How can Mukhopadhyay break out of this emplotment? Analyzed from this perspective, there may, in fact, be fractures in the narrative and in the emplotment and teleology which underlie it. For as Mukhopadhyay's prose makes clear, he is aware that there may be a certain cruelty involved in his mother's constant monitoring of his progress. This unruliness may emerge from a statement I have already quoted above: "He felt she was being a bit cruel as she told him, 'Our one day should be equal to two days'" (Mukhopadhyay, *The Mind Tree* 64). How, then, can we account for this slippage in register, in the tone of constant reverence which his narrative otherwise adopts for his mother? By making Mukhopadhyay overcome, as she sees it, the curse of his own condition, his mother devises a bodily regime for her son's everyday life. As Couser has emphasized, however, it would be both unfair and ultimately short-sighted to fault caregivers like Soma for her own way of coping with her son's diagnosis. What emerges, however, is nonetheless a question of ethics. Crucially, Soma never once "second-guesses" her approach; the idea of power, and of her son's being a "vulnerable subject" for her emplotment of his life, never enters the picture. As the reporter on *60 Minutes II* excerpt asks her:

> INTERVIEWER: What if you slacked off? What would happen do you think?
>
> SOMA: I did not. I cannot even imagine myself doing that. ("60 Minutes")

In the documentary, his mother takes Mukhopadhyay to see the Hollywood Walk of Fame. As they are walking along Hollywood Boulevard, however, she is constantly correcting him. Both enabling and urging her son to "look normal" and to behave normally, his mother hence keeps a constant regime, a pattern of behavior, which he willingly seems to follow. From her perspective, Soma urges her son to rise above the "tics" prompted by his narrative each and every waking moment of his life.

The key question, asked by the reporter in the *60 Minutes II excerpt* is precisely the highly problematic concept of the social "usefulness" of a person with autism, a question whose ethical underpinnings neither Soma herself nor the documentary quite addresses: If it had not been for his mother's constant prompting of Mukhopadhyay, he would have been, in his own words, "a vegetable" ("60 Minutes"). Yet, whose words are these? And whose value judgment of a successful life, a "gelingendes Leben," do they imply? This is a question, the question of social and economic usefulness, which Mukhopadhyay himself has addressed in his poetry. Can the "overcoming" of autism as a diagnosis really be collapsed into the utilitarian logic of social and economic usefulness? Nonetheless, there is a sense in which, quite similarly to the teleology inscribed in Oliver Sacks' *Awakenings* – where the use of L-dopa temporarily rouses patients from the sleep into which they had fallen decades earlier – we cannot but sympathize with these autistic individuals being reintegrated into their parents' lives. As one mother puts it in the *60 Minutes II* documentary excerpt, it was through Soma's rapid prompting method that after years of silence, she was finally able to lead a conversation with her own son ("60 Minutes"). There is a sense here –

and a sense prompted by the teleology of the documentary, in which the end may justify the means: Even if her regime of her son's "tics" required a certain degree of coercion, the documentary implies, does not his success in the end justify this regime of Mukhopadhyay by his mother? What is at stake here is, in fact, the very pitfalls of co-authorship, and of a particular kind of vulnerability and physical and emotional dependency. The point here may be precisely that this mutual inscription of one life on another – the mother's life being intricately bound up with that of her son – cannot quite be unraveled; what may matter instead is our awareness of the complications, the ethical dilemmas, arising from this double inscription.

The question of the economic usefulness of autistic persons, incidentally, has been hotly debated in recent years. Perhaps problematically, companies have responded to the increasing alienation of workers from the workplace and the increasing specialization of labor which is often akin to automatization by deliberately seeking out employees with autism: It is their highly specialized brain, they have argued, which enables employees with autism to focus, for hours on end, on tasks which non-autistic individuals would have difficulties in carrying out, thinking this to be a brainless occupation. As in Soma's reasoning, if with a different twist, there may be a sense of teleology here where autistic individuals are suddenly "useful" for the workplace not despite, but because of their disability. Crucially, however, there are a number of ethical pitfalls in this form of emplotment in which the hiring of disabled individuals takes the shape not of affirmative action hiring practices but, conversely, of staying within a neoliberal doctrine. Seen from this angle, the problem of our postmodern economy is *not* the degree to which it takes the alienation of labor by forcing workers to execute the same highly specialized task for an entire workday, but the idea that the workers stubbornly fail to keep pace with the degree of their own automization. Thus, in a neoliberal variation of the idea that some workers (often unskilled or migrant workers) may be willing to take underpaid or hazardous jobs even if the local workforce refuses to do so, the point here is that autism may in fact be turned into an asset under such neoliberal conditions. The goal is not to rethink the logic of automatization and of increasing specialization of certain tasks, but simply to look for individuals who may do the trick. This neoliberal reasoning is then turned into an altruistic scheme as it benefits not only the company but also the autistic individual who is suddenly able to lead a "productive" life. Seen from Mukhopadhyay's angle, the very fact that his mind has a different shape would now turn him into the most productive of workers.

At the same time, there is yet another issue involved in the idea of co-authoring a life. As both Tito Mukhopadhyay's narrative and the documentary makes clear, his life is so enmeshed with that of his mother as to be virtually inseparable from it. What is at stake in parenting a disabled child, both Tito Mukhopadhyay's narrative and autobiographies such as Kingsley and Levitz's *Count Us In* imply, is the issue of the child's growing independence from his parents. It is in this sense that *Count Us In*, as I will argue in Chapter 7, lays bare an idea which is perhaps "under erasure" (Derrida 1997) in Mukhopadhyay's narrative. As Jason Kingsley's mother Emily Perl Kingsley writes in her introduction to her son's autobiography, and as Jason Kingsley himself reiterates in an open letter to his parents, it is hard for parents to let go, to accept their child's growing independence (Kingsley and Levitz 152). If this is true of all parents, *Count Us In* implies, it may be particularly so for parents with children with disability. The difference between *Count Us In* and the *60 Minutes II* documentary, then, is that it not only elaborates on, but critically interrogates the issue of co-authorship. This, in turn, is an ethical question: If the mother's life is based on taking care of her son, what would be at stake if the son wanted to strive for single authorship? What this implies, also, is the possibility of a productive dialogue between life science and life writing. Tito Mukhopadhyay's book has been discussed as a paradigm case of autism and the ensuing ethical questions in the work of Kern-Stähler and Thiemann (2015). Yet, the question of medical ethics alone may fail to address the complexity of Mukhopadhyay's narrative. Read through Couser's idea of co-authorship in narratives of disability, Mukhopadhyay's text gains a complexity, which a "medical ethics" reading of the same text may not possess. At the same time, a literary analysis – minus the framework of medical analysis – may fail to inquire into the medical-ethical dimension of the notion of co-authorship.

This chapter has tried to address a number of questions which are also at the core of the chapters to come. First, my aim has been to inquire into the intersection between narrative form and the representation of disability and genetic difference.[4] I have argued that written autobiography may be a form of aesthetic disembodiment, which allows us to imagine the subject of difference without visually witnessing this subject's physical difference. Such visuality, I have argued with regard to the difference between Tito Mukhopadhyay's autobiographical writing and his presence on the *60 Minutes II* episode "Breaking the Silence" may lead to a "medialization" of the writing subject. This chapter has thus implicitly engaged with the concept of "medical humanities" in that it has called for taking into account the aesthetic specificity of the genres through which disability or difference are conveyed. One idea that this chapter has not addressed but which would require further research is the question of why narratives on autism have been proliferating in different years, appearing not only in terms of biography and autobiography, but also in popular culture. Autism, we may argue, has been "mainstreamed" through popular culture, being central in TV series such as *Bones* and a host of other detective series, including *Monk*. What is it about autism, then, that fascinates contemporary popular culture? Autism has thus arguably been turned into a paradigm case through which we have come to investigate spectrums of difference. This role of autism as a paradigm case, in turn, may be both fruitful and problematic. While this is not a question to which this study can do justice, we must nevertheless remain vigilant as to what may be termed the "currency" of difference, which comes to inform our understanding of disability or genetic difference. The next two chapters will thus also be concerned with representations of autism as they will trace the presence of autism as a form of difference in both autobiography and popular culture. While the following chapter (Chapter 3) on Bollywood film will address the role of mainstream media for creating potential presences for persons with

[4] One of the central ideas in this context, which will come up time and again throughout these chapters, is the relationship between difference, illness and disability. Some authors discussed in this book refer to severe autism as a form of disability; others, like Temple Grandin, stress the fact that it has genetic causes and may hence be considered a genetic difference. In neither of these understandings of autism as a condition is autism seen as an illness; yet, as Grandin states in *Thinking in Pictures* and as I will elaborate in Chapter 4, autism was originally treated as a psychological or even psychiatric illness.

autism, Chapter 4 discusses Temple Grandin's groundbreaking autobiography *Thinking in Pictures*, which can be seen to turn the tables on the mainstream itself.

3 Bollywood Film and the Borders of Disability: Shah Rukh Khan Meets the American President

The 2010 Bollywood film *My Name Is Khan* can be said to transgress a number of borders. As a film about a man with Asperger syndrome, it addresses the question of disability and can hence be seen as Bollywood's entering into the discussion of medical humanities; as a film about 9/11, it investigates the concept of the U.S. nation space in the wake of global terrorism; and as a film about Hindu-Muslim romance, it explores the possibility of interreligious dialogue within the Indian diasporic community on American soil. Drawing on concepts of life writing as well as Thomas Couser's work on "vulnerable subjects" (*Vulnerable Subjects* xii), this chapter asks what lives can be written and rewritten by Bollywood film.[1] Moreover, taking Martha Nussbaum's recent questions about the "frontiers of justice" into account, it wonders why the American president – from George W. Bush to Barack Obama – should figure so prominently in discussions of the access we provide to disabled communities. For why should Bollywood's fictional protagonist, Rizvan Khan, go on a mission to speak to the president himself?

3.1 Bollywood Meets Medical Humanities

If Bollywood film can long be said to have gone transnational, I believe that *My Name Is Khan* is emphatically transnational in yet another sense: in Bollywood's entering the field of medical humanities. Not incidentally, *My Name Is Khan* is one of the highest grossing Bollywood films on the international market to date. By the same token, Indian

[1] The argument addressed in this chapter were first presented at the MESEA annual conference in Saarbrücken in 2014. I am grateful to Astrid Fellner for inviting me, for her critical ideas, which have shaped the reworking of this chapter.

actor Shah Rukh Khan's award-winning film *My Name Is Khan* could be said to breach three different kinds of borders at one and the same time: As a Bollywood film about a man with Asperger's, it could be said to breach the borders of medical humanities; as an Indian film set in the U.S., it could be said to breach the borders of transnational American Studies; and as a film concerned with the effects of 9/11 on both the U.S. and the rest of the world it could be said to address what Samuel Huntington has infamously and wrongly called "the clash of civilizations." In this chapter, I am interested in the ways in which these multiple borders may be said to overlap, as well as with the ways in which they may in fact collide. For who transcends which borders in *My Name Is Khan*?

My interest in this chapter, then, is in the way in which Shah Rukh Khan's memorable performance in *My Name Is Khan* is "ghosted" in multiple ways even before the film actually opens. I am thus concerned with the ways in which Marvin Carlson's concept of the "haunted stage" can be adapted to film studies; and with the ways in which Shah Rukh Khan's body on Bollywood's filmic screen may be doubly or perhaps triply haunted in both a performative and a cultural sense. This latter sense of haunting is described by Carlson as follows:

> All theatrical cultures have recognized, in some form or another, this ghostly quality, this sense of something coming back in the theatre, and so the relationships between theatre and cultural memory are deep and complex. Just as one might say that every play might be called *Ghosts*, so, with equal justification, one might argue that every play is memory play. . . . It is the repository of cultural memory, but, like the memory of each individual, it is also subject to continual adjustment and modification as the memory is recalled in new circumstances and contexts. The present experience is always ghosted by previous experiences . . . . (2)

What Shah Rukh Khan's performance in *My Name Is Khan* is haunted by, I will suggest in this chapter, is precisely the specter of Hindu-Muslim violence in India, as well as, for an American audience, the more recent history of the racialization of Muslim male bodies in the aftermath of the 9/11 attacks. What interests me here, then, is the cultural dimension of haunting which, in the case of Khan, the actor, and the film, *My Name is Khan*, deliberately addresses two sets of ghosting: both these hauntings, however, center on the sign of the Muslim male body which is seen, in both cases, as transgressing against the sanctity and religious integrity of the nation – the Indian and the U.S. American nation, respectively. This twofold engagement is itself highly significant for Bollywood film: For as Meenakshi Mukherjee and a host of other critics have argued, Bollywood film has often viewed its "exotic" Western settings as a mere backdrop to what is in fact an iconically "Indian" story. In keeping with such an Occidentalist exoticism, Switzerland has often been Bollywood's location of choice, a choice which has made the Alps a topic not just of Tirolian nationalism, but of Indian cinema's aesthetic style. Not only is *My Name Is Khan* not set in the Alps, then, but the change in setting is highly significant for the filmic plot itself. In *My Name Is Khan*, the Alps have been exchanged for the hilliness of San Francisco; Bollywood may still be enamored with mountain peaks, then, but the setting is no longer picturesque but urban, even if the quaint urbanity of San Francisco is not quite the grittiness of LA. The change from the Swiss Alps to San Francisco, however, is significant in one more respect: For while, as Mukherjee has noted, Bollywood has been prone to view the exoticism of Western locations only as a backdrop to its plot of Indian culture reexamining itself, *My Name Is Khan* breaks not only with the alpine tradition, but it similarly disrupts the tradition of Bollywood film not engaging with the cultural politics of its location. Switzerland, then, has been interesting to Bollywood for its haystacks, not the history of its politics. This is not the case, however, for the American backdrop to *My Name Is Khan*. In this film, the San Francisco streetcars – as the American equivalent of the Swiss Alps – can be seen to reach into the film; in more than one sense, the protagonists of *My Name Is Khan* are touched by the American setting which they inhabit. And in the sense of this modification, the film aspires to be not only an Indian, but also in a sense an American film.

The haunting of the body of the film's main actor, Shah Rukh Khan, is thus doubly reconfigured before the film even starts: it is a Muslim body which, the film makes clear, has a racialized history in both an Indian and a U.S. historical context. The concept which the film engages is thus the "out-of-place-ness" of Muslim bodies on both Indian and U.S. American soil. Yet, why should the film choose to heighten this out-of-place-ness by giving its protagonist not only a Muslim, but an autistic cultural difference? As I will argue in this chapter, not only does Bollywood film go transnational in *My Name Is Khan*, but it also goes medical; it engages not only the idea of transnational American Studies but that of medical humanities as well.

To return to the second notion of "ghosting" in Carlson's study, Shah Rukh Khan's performance in *My Name Is Khan* may be ghosted as the "body of the actor" it is: Seen from this perspective, the audience's perception and reception of Khan's performance in this, his more recent movie, will be haunted or informed by his innumerable on-screen performances. As Carlson goes on to say,

> Often these memories have been consciously utilized by the theatre culture, but, even when they are not, they may well continue to operate, affecting reception in powerful and unexpected ways. The most familiar example of this phenomenon is the appearance of an actor, remembered from previous roles, in a new characterization. The recycled body of an actor, already a complex bearer of semiotic messages, will almost inevitably in a new role evoke the ghost or ghosts of previous roles if they have made any impression whatsoever on the audience, a phenomenon that often colors and indeed may dominate the reception process. (8)

Thus, the "ghost" which Shah Rukh Khan can be said to lay to rest through his memorable performance in *My Name Is Khan* is his earlier encounter with disability in a film called *Koi... Mil Gaya* (2003). Incidentally, Bollywood film has been said to be a latecomer to medical humanities which, through this very assertion, is implied to be a Western concept. *Koi... Mil Gaya* can thus be seen as Bollywood's earlier attempt to deal with disability in rather unfortunate terms: For the genre in which a disabled boy suddenly appears in Bollywood film is in fact the Indian version of *E.T. the Extra-Terrestrial* (1982). Significantly for my purposes here, this film, *Koi... Mil Gaya*, too, starred Shah Rukh Khan, yet not as the protagonist, but as the able-bodied friend to a boy who is, after all, trying to talk to aliens in outer space. Even if the film tries to be sympathetic to disability, it is nonetheless dubious in linking this deviance to other forms of non-normalcy from outer space. Thus in *My Name Is Khan*, Shah Rukh Khan the actor can actually be said to return to the filmic scene of the crime when it comes to disability. In *My Name Is Khan*, Shah Rukh Khan the media persona may actually have learned his lesson in turning the tables on our very definition of normalcy. Not only does Khan move from a sympathetic bystander to being the protagonist of disability, but the film proceeds to turn the concept of disability on its head. In *My Name Is Khan*, the only people whom we would have hoped came from outer space are the religious fundamentalists, both Indian and American, who believe that every person named "Khan" is simultaneously also a terrorist.

The film *My Name Is Khan* is thus far from being only a film about disability, it is also a film about religious fundamentalism. It is here, moreover, that the concept of transnationalism and of the film's engaging the concept of transnational American Studies may be the most productive. For the film is transnational not only in its economic success, but also in the way in which it skillfully engages two national histories, that of its Indian and its American audiences, respectively. Crucially, the film skillfully drives home the point that religious fundamentalism may be the skeleton in the closet of both Indian and American audiences. The scene which *My Name Is Khan* creates is of a moment in historical time when both the U.S. and India come face to face with their suspicion that Islam is inseparable from religious violence and global terrorism. It is this fear of Islam which the film conjures up for both Indian and American audiences by asking the same question over and over again: When we hear the name "Khan," whom or rather what do we see?

3.2 Writing Lives

I am interested in the ways in which life writing as both a genre and a concept may be used to highlight the continuity between fiction and historical time. For what *My Name Is Khan* addresses is a Hindu nationalist fear of Islam played out on American soil. Seen from this angle, Bollywood film becomes a canvas on which not only transnationalism, but interreligious debates are being played out. For the specter which *My Name Is Khan* conjures up is precisely the fear, from an Indian nationalist perspective, of interreligious romance. The love plot it centers on is that of a romance between Khan, a Muslim man with Asperger's and Mandira, a Hindu hairdresser who lives in San Francisco. In its defiance of concepts of religious purity and anti-Muslim sentiment, then, the film deliberately taunts an Indian mainstream audience by taking literally the name of its main actor, Shah Rukh Khan.

The history of Bollywood film, of course, adds its own twist to the film's curious charade of the absence and presence of Islamic cultural difference. For as a film industry, Bollywood is also a Hindu film industry, a film industry catering to the Hindu majority in India. Shah Rukh Khan could only have become one of Bollywood's megastars, then, by playing Hindu protagonists on screen. The frontier which *My Name Is Khan* crosses, curiously enough, is thus that it takes, for the first time in Bollywood's filmic history, the name of its megastar at face value. In *My Name Is Khan*, the actor's name is really Khan; Khan the name is thus an ambiguous concept on whose meaning – and disruptive meaning – the film can in fact be said to capitalize. *My Name Is Khan* thus gives the lie to the numerous previous films in which Khan starred with his film partner, Kajol, in ways so successful that it has earned them the nickname "the golden pair." For in these previous blockbusters, the bottom line of Bollywood as Hindu mainstream cinema remained intact: The actor's name may be Khan, these films held, but on screen he can only romance Kajol, the Hindu actress, because his stage or rather, his screen persona is that of a Hindu hero. Not so, however, in *My Name Is Khan*: In this film, Khan gets to marry Mandira aka Kajol as the Muslim man he is or rather, the Muslim character he plays on screen.

Yet, there is a sense in which reality trumps fiction in *My Name Is Khan*. For the banter which the film holds out to a religiously fundamentalist audience is that the interreligious romance which *My Name Is Khan* enacts has long become reality for Shah Rukh Khan himself. I would argue that the film *My Name is Khan* is so memorable and so sophisticated precisely because it engages the multiple ways in which Shah Rukh Khan's persona will be "ghosted" for both Indian and non-Indian audiences. Even before the film opens, Shah Rukh Khan's life, off screen, has breached the very taboos that the film engages. In a country where Hindu fundamentalists rage in their blogs about the defilement of Hindu beauties by Muslim men on Bollywood's celluloid screen, Shah Rukh Khan has made matters worse by romancing a Hindu woman not only in film, but off the screen as well. In what in India is called a "mixed marriage," Shah Rukh Khan married Gauri in a traditional Hindu ceremony. Not only is *My Name Is Khan* ghosted by Shah Rukh Khan's pervious performances, but it is ghosted by his performances in real life as well.

For the cultural climate which the film taunts is that of a Hindu nationalist community which has long become diasporic. It is an audience, what is more, which zealously keeps track of Muslim transgressions against Hindu concepts of propriety. If Bollywood is the film industry of the Indian Hindu mainstream, then, *My Name Is Khan* proceeds to marginalize itself. It is in this transgression, then, that I would like to engage the concept of life writing. In his book *Husband of a Fanatic* (2005), Indian Canadian writer, director and critic Amitava Kumar describes his marriage to a Muslim woman poet, Mona Ahmad Ali. As Kumar vividly describes, this marriage has earned him hate mails from the diasporic Hindu nationalist community, marking him as a traitor to Hinduism overseas. It is in order to meet the man who wrote some of the hate mails, then, that Kumar proceeds to have lunch with a bigot: Mr. Barotia. Crucially, then, Mr. Barotia's criticism of Kumar's transgression and his enshrining of Hindu fundamentalist values hinges on Bollywood film. It is as a fundamentalist viewer of the country's mainstream film industry, then, that Mr. Barotia keeps track of Hindu-Muslim encounters, on the screen and in life. Not surprisingly, in Mr. Barotia's narrative, Shah Rukh Khan the actor does not figure in positive terms. Thus, Khan's relationship to a Hindu woman – both in real life and on screen in *My Name is Khan* – can also be read through Amitava Kumar's account of his own interreligious marriage to Mona Ahmad Ali, a fellow writer and a poet. Crucially, if my chapter tries to engage the intersection between Bollywood film and life writing, it is striking that Amitava Kumar should begin his own account of his marriage to a Hindu woman with a reference to Bollywood film.

Set in his home in Toronto, Kumar's narrative starts out with the perhaps absurd but real-life scenario of himself having lunch with a bigot. He sets out to meet the man on whose website he was listed as one of the enemies of Hindu India, and, over lunch, to talk to him in the hope of making sense of what is after all the politics of hate. In their matter of fact conversation, it is to Bollywood film that the bigot alludes. With his young niece helping out in the kitchen, Mr. Barotia, the bigot, explains:

> The litany was familiar and quickly wearying. Mr. Barotia began with the names of all the male Indian film stars who were Muslim and married to Hindu women. "Sharmila Tagore is now Ayesha Begum and that pimp Aamir Khan is married to a Hindu girl. Her name is Gauri." These women have been forced to convert, he said, and now Muslims were having sex with them, thereby defiling them. . . . He was using a vulgar

> Hindi word for what he was describing, a word common on the streets in India, and he said it so loudly, and so repeatedly, that I was startled and immediately thought of his niece in the kitchen. (Kumar 6)

What is remarkable here is that to Mr. Barotia, the bigot, every Khan may in fact look alike; while the name of actor Aamir Khan's wife is Kiran, Gauri is the name of Shah Rukh Khan's wife, not the wife of Aamir Khan. It is here that Mr. Barotia, without even knowing it, drives home the irony at the heart of the film *My Name Is Khan*: To a religious fundamentalist, all Khans look alike. Moreover, for Hindu fundamentalists like Mr. Barotia, the act of a Muslim actor's romancing a Hindu woman on screen will be made worse by the knowledge that such inter-religious romance for Khan, is not only fiction. Film, is thus ghosted by life writing, and as the nightmare of Hindu fundamentalism, truth is indeed stranger than fiction.

As Kumar writes with bitter irony, for Mr. Barotia, 9/11 is a gift – at least this is how the bigot sees it. As he enthusiastically tells Kumar about the unfolding of his own life in the U.S.:

> Mr. Barotia had told me earlier that he had come to the United States in 1972. For twenty-five years he had worked as a legal secretary in Manhattan. . . . Mr. Barotia said that he had gotten along well with his colleagues and they treated him as "a partner in the firm," and one of them even called him after the attacks of September 11 to say, "Jagdish, we thought you were obsessed with Muslims. But [now we know] you were right." (Kumar 8)

3.3 Romancing Disability

My Name Is Khan is thus remarkable because it breaches two taboos at the same time: it is a film about a Muslim man marrying a Hindu woman; and it is a narrative about a non-disabled woman marrying a man who has Asperger's. Particularly with regard to the latter transcendence of social frontiers, we may ask whether India transcends its distrust of disability on American soil or whether this cultural context could in fact be said to trigger or even inform such transcendence. It is in the U.S., by the same token, where his fear of the color yellow is taken not to be a symptom of his disability – Asperger's – but a symptom of his humanity. As Mandira, an Indian woman from across the street reminds him, everyone is afraid of something:

> *RIZVAN is standing at a pedestrian crossing in San Francisco, trying to cross the street. When he is halfway across, he looks at the yellow stripes and freezes. A streetcar is fast approaching. The driver is shouting for RIZVAN to move. He seems paralyzed, unable to move. Within inches of him, the streetcar comes to a halt. The passengers get out of the streetcar, angry.*
>
> CONDUCTOR [*shouting*]: Hurry, get out of here!
>
> MANDIRA [*unseen, walking towards them from behind*]: Hey, you guys, just leave him alone. Stop it! Stop it, okay? Just go. Go, please.
>
> *The crowd of white Americans disperses. Only an African-American pedestrian is still standing with RIZVAN, looking at him in concern. MANDIRA still remains unseen, speaking with RIZVAN from behind.*
>
> MANDIRA: Are you okay? Hey. Are you scared? It's okay. Look, there's nothing wrong with being scared. Just don't make your fear so large that it stops you from achieving your goal. Okay. All right, bye.
>
> *RIZVAN turns to see MANDIRA walk back to the hairdresser's salon, where she works. He still hasn't seen her face.* (*My Name Is Khan*)

To be afraid of some things, then, lies in the nature of our humanity. Yet, who is transcending which border in this scene? Is the U.S. a country in which Asperger's is no longer out of place, or is it the backdrop of a world in which Mandira, the Indian hairdresser living in San Francisco, can accommodate her fellow Indian's vulnerability? Is it as an Indian woman that Mandira can deal with Khan's condition or has her Americanness taught her to cope with his disability? The point that the movie can be said to make is that it refuses to answer this very question. Where does Indianness end when it comes to disability and where does Americanness begin?

I am interested, then, in the question of the difference which a given genre – here, the genre of Bollywood film, can accommodate: *My Name Is Khan* is Bollywood film, then, minus dance, but not without music; it may be a film about disability, yet without having to feature the aliens. In keeping with the telos of virtually all of Bollywood's movies, there is a wedding, even if this wedding happens not at the end, but half-way through the film. I believe that the film's wedding scene is significant here for a number of reasons. First, it conforms to the standards of Bollywood film and Indian mainstream audiences by giving us features of a traditional Hindu wedding – the hennaed hands, the sharing of sweets; and yet, it features a Muslim protagonist with Asperger's who wears not a *kurta*, but a tuxedo for his wedding. And yet, his Hindu bride makes no secret of his attractiveness, regardless of the cultural provenance of his suit.

In its depiction not only of a Hindu-Muslim intermarriage, but of the intermarriage between a disabled man and a non-disabled woman, the film varies yet another feature of its signature aesthetics. A long-standing feature of any Bollywood film has not only been the scene of a couple embracing on a haystack or being caught in the rain, but also the question of whether under these circumstances, the couple is in fact allowed to kiss. Until the 1990s and due to the censorship of the Hindi film industry, Bollywood invented the trick of the "übertragener Kuss" ("forbidden kiss").

Khan's romance with Mandira, incidentally, could be seen as another, albeit unusual version of the forbidden kiss or *übertragener Kuss*. Even as the morality and the aesthetics of Bollywood film has changed dramatically at least since *Salaam Namaste* (2005), where the Indian female protagonist living in Australia has a child out of wedlock and must thus be assumed to have kissed at least once, *My Name Is Khan* can be said to add another twist to the question of whether or not kissing is appropriate in Bollywood film. With the waning of censorship in the 1990s, kissing has no longer been tabooed on Bollywood screen; yet, it has still been viewed with suspicion by some parts of the audience which saw in Bollywood's signature feature of the "übertragener Kuss" one of Bollywood's major distinctions from Hollywood film. In *My Name Is Khan*, then, Bollywood can be said to have its cake and eat it, too: Because Khan has Asperger's, there can be sex without kissing; and Bollywood film can imagine sex, paradoxically, without even showing it:

> *Khan and Mandira are sitting on their bed.*
>
> MANDIRA: Khan.
>
> KHAN: Yes.

MANDIRA: We can't do this without touching.

KHAN: I know.

MANDIRA: You know?

KHAN: Yes. I have read it in this book. [*showing her the book.*] *Intercourse for Dumbos* by Dr. Richard K. Woomer.

MANDIRA: Okay.

KHAN: Nice pictures. [*giggles*] Mandira, I think we should do it [*looks at his watch*] now.

MANDIRA: One minute, and …

KHAN: No, no, no, not one minute. It will take longer than one minute.

They both laugh. The scene ends. (*My Name Is Khan)*

If Kumar evokes the shocking quality, for a Hindu fundamentalist gaze, of Hindu-Muslim romance, *My Name Is Khan* doubles this shock by letting a disabled Muslim man touch a non-disabled Hindu woman. It is here, too, that the film deliberately defies the limits of appropriateness. To be sure, it may be Shah Rukh Khan's "ghosting" here which helps the film's portrayal of the sexual attractiveness of a man with Asperger's: For who would have thought of Dustin Hofmann as Hollywood's autistic in *Rain Man* (1988) as a love interest?

Yet, it is true for both Hollywood's and Bollywood's enactment of autism as a form of disability that this deviance is being embodied by non-autistic actors: What is at stake here may thus in fact be a new form of minstrelsy, the minstrelsy of disability. What, however, of Khan's performance of disability in *My Name Is Khan*? For all the film's political correctness and its turning of the concept of disability on its head, is there not a sense in which Khan's performance is a minstrelsy of disability on an Indian mainstream screen? To be sure, Khan the actor carefully researched the part, to the extent that he suffered physically from his strife for accuracy:

> Not prone to headaches, Khan ignored them the first few times, and popped pills when the pain continued. When that didn't help either, he decided to see a doctor. . . . The actor suffered from severe migraines and a crick in the back of his neck during the shooting of [the film]. . . . The pain in the neck and the headaches were caused by the expressions

> and posture of Rizwan Khan, [Khan's] character in [the film]. Rizwan, who has Asperger's Syndrome, has a way of jutting his neck out at a particular angle and wears an expression which has his eyebrows raised in every scene. As he would shoot for hours, he'd get severe migraines. Today, he's been seeing a physiotherapist to get rid of the pain in his neck. (Upala KBR n.pag.)

Yet, there is clearly a difference between the mask of disability and its physical presence. If the actor himself had had Asperger's, would he still have been allowed to romance Kajol in the film? This is perhaps the limit of ghosting: Behind the fixed stare and the arched neck, we still see Shah Rukh Khan the megastar, whose physical presence, for audiences across the globe has not quite been repelling. Even if with *My Name Is Khan*, Bollywood courageously squares the domain of medical humanities, it still managed to turn it into a blockbuster, and for such blockbusting, it needs its megastars.

Moreover, there may be one more qualification to this transgressing of both religious boundaries and the notions of normalcy. Within Bollywood's cultural imaginary, Khan's bride, Mandira, would be seen as highly Westernized; her arranged marriage having failed, she is now divorced with a six-year old son. If, as Amitava Kumar and a host of other critics have argued, it is the rape scenario, the image of a Hindu bride being attacked by a Muslim transgressor which has loomed large in the internet forums of Hindu fundamentalist haters of Bollywood film – then Mandira does not qualify for this Hindu-Indian version of the cult of true womanhood. And yet, the fact of transgression – and the transvaluation of an interreligious marriage as positive – remains: The point which the movie makes is that transgression does take place, even if the couple's actual lovemaking is never actually shown. And even if the couple's touching is never shown, it is talked about, for Bollywood's standards, with an unprecedented degree of explicitness. At the same time, it may be argued that the fact that Khan happens to be autistic may serve to appease, for a mainstream Hindu audience, the very specter of the Muslim rapist, a specter also alluded to in Kumar's discussion of Mr. Barotia. In a highly problematic sense, then, the reference to Khan's disability may render his masculinity less threatening to a mainstream Hindu audience.[2]

Yet, one of the questions which I would like to ask in this chapter is what disability has to do with this sudden presencing of Muslim identities on Bollywood's celluloid screen. There is a sense here in which two wrongs may make a right: Why should a full-scale acknowledgment of the complexity of Muslim culture in India be possible only through the mask of disability? And is there anything problematic about conveying disability through the prism of Muslim cultural difference, and vice versa? By the same token, what happens when the difference or disability of Asperger syndrome is mapped onto a Muslim body, even if the body is that of Shah Rukh Khan, the Bollywood megastar?

3.4 *My Name Is Khan* and the Politics of 9/11

Half-way into the film, Rizvan Khan thus realizes that he has fulfilled his late mother's wish and has indeed made a life for himself, a life often deemed impossible for people with Asperger's. And yet, what the film drives home is that Rizvan's life in the U.S. is fraught not only by his mental condition, but as the life of a Muslim man in the U.S.. The borders which *My Name Is Khan* engages by being not only a film about autism, but also a film about 9/11 and the U.S. in the wake of the terrorist attacks, are the multiple ways in which our own bodies are precarious ones. Khan's life becomes "precarious" in Judith Butler's terms not only because he is a man with Asperger's, but also because he is an Indian Muslim. In fact, one of the feats of the film consists in juxtaposing these two forms of precariousness. As Butler writes at the outset of her study, the sense of precariousness is true of *all* lives: "That we can be injured, that others can be injured, that we are subject to death at the whim of another, are all reasons for both fear and grief. . . . One insight that injury affords is that there are others out there on whom my life depends, people I do not know and may never know. This fundamental dependency on anonymous others is not a condition that I can will away" (*Precarious Life* xii). I am interested, then, in a threefold meaning of

[2] I am indebted to Katrin Horn for this aspect.

precariousness which, I suggest, may also shed light on the role of medical humanities for American Studies. For as Thomas Couser has argued in his study, *Vulnerable Subjects*, American Studies seems particularly well-equipped for dealing with difference. In its explorations of the dimensions and specific experience of subjects who have been vulnerable in terms of race, class and gender, it has already paved the way, arguably, for dealing with the difference of disability. Yet, the key question which I would like to ask with both Judith Butler and the film *My Name Is Khan* is whether there is a difference in or among these differences. As Couser has noted, one of the major obstacles faced by persons with disability is their inability to write their own lives. To the extent that we are storied individuals in John Paul Eakin's sense, then, this inability to write one's own life can at once result in a loss of agency, of the power to make one's voice heard and one's subjectivity recognized by others. There may be a difference, then, in a marginalized ethnic writer not being able to publish his or her story in the context of a culturally biased publication industry, then, and an obstacle which is much more fundamental to the telling of this story. What concerns me here, however, is not the attempt to balance one difference against another in a one-upmanship of difference: Rather, it is to argue that we may want to be particularly careful in *differentiating difference*. For my purposes here, then, it may be crucial to distinguish among forms of precariousness even as we acknowledge the continuities between them. All human lives, Butler notes, are subject to being hurt; yet, as she goes on to observe in the wake of 9/11, some bodies – bodies singled out as male Muslim bodies – have been particularly vulnerable to the disruption of their physical and psychological integrity. And yet, there is a sense in which the above quote also resonates in a particular way with the difference of disability: the "fundamental dependency on anonymous others" (*Precarious Life* xii), which Butler writes about, may be particularly true for people with disability.

My Name Is Khan is thus a film not only about autism but also about 9/11. What the film revolves around is the historical moment starting from which the phrase "my name is Khan" could never again be an innocent, a neutral sentence stating a person's name. Yet, it has been argued by some critics that this assumption of 9/11 as a singular turning point in the perception of Islam in the "Western" imagination is actually misleading. The assumption is true in the sense that the events of 9/11 seemed unprecedented; it is not true in the sense that the 9/11 attacks triggered or reactivated anti-Muslim sentiment which had been there in the social unconscious to begin with. Similarly, the movie makes clear, as does Amitava Kumar's life writing, that the events of 9/11 struck a chord of hostility not only in U.S. mainstream cultures, but in India as well. And yet, as both Butler and *My Name is Khan* emphasize, there is a sense in which 9/11 seemed to mark a new chapter not only in American history, but in world history as well.

For as the film opens, Rizvan's mother tells her son, in their home in Mumbai, about the idiocy of Hindu Muslim violence:

> [*subtitle*] Hindu-Muslim Riots 1983
>
> *Burning debris on the street, in a Muslim neighborhood.*
>
> MAN [*in the street, to his friends*]: Each one of them should be shot dead mercilessly. Didn't even spare our women. Dogs! Rogues! Idiots! Are you guys with me? Rogues. All of them. [*RIZVAN is watching the men from the balcony; as he turns back inside, he is repeating, in a monotonous voice, what he has heard.*]
>
> RIZVAN [*repeating, in Hindi*]: Each of them should be shot dead mercilessly.
>
> MOTHER: I had told you not to step outside. Now, come on. Let's eat.
>
> RIZVAN [*repeating*]: Rogues. All of them. Each of them should be shot dead mercilessly. Rogues. All of them.
>
> MOTHER: What did you say?
>
> RIZVAN: Rogues. All of them.
>
> MOTHER [*agitated*]: Where did you hear that?
>
> RIZVAN [*keeps repeating*]: Each one of them …
>
> MOTHER [*shouting*]: Shut up!
>
> RIZVAN: Rogues. All of them.
>
> MOTHER [*slapping him*]: Shut up, Rizu. Come with me. Come. [*showing him a piece of paper*]. Look at this. [*She starts drawing stick figures*]. This is you, Rizvan. Who?
>
> RIZVAN: Rizvan.

> MOTHER: Yes. [*Drawing another stick man.*] And this is the person who has a stick in his hand. And he is beating you.
>
> RIZVAN: It's bad … Beating is bad.
>
> MOTHER: Yes, it's bad. [*keeps drawing*] Now, this is you again, Rizvan. And this is the person who has a lollipop. And he gives it to you.
>
> RIZVAN: Lollipop is sweet. It's a good thing.
>
> MOTHER: Good boy.
>
> RIZVAN: Good boy.
>
> MOTHER: Now tell me, which one of these is a Hindu and which one, a Muslim?
>
> RIZVAN: Both look alike.
>
> MOTHER [*stroking his head*]: Good. Remember one thing, son. There are only two kinds of people in this world. Good people who do good deeds. And bad people who do bad. That's the only difference in human beings. There's no other difference. Understand? What did you understand? Tell me.
>
> RIZVAN: Good people. Bad people. No other difference. (*My Name Is Khan)*

The politics of stick figures, then, encapsulates the message of the film. His mother's instinctive understanding of her son's condition, if not his medical diagnosis, enables her to convey to him a highly complex political and cultural situation in words or rather, in sticks or strokes that he can understand; and yet, what the film proceeds to drive home is the fact that non-autistic humanity – hiding behind the sophisticated abstraction of historical, political and cultural theories, – fails to understand what Rizvan does. To paraphrase Oliver Sacks, then, it is not that we learn about Asperger's through Rizvan's narrative, but it is through Rizvan's narrative that we learn about ourselves. What *My Name Is Khan* opposes to diagnoses of the autism spectrum is the spectrum of humanity.

The film's expressly stated aim is thus to turn the concept of disability on its head: As Shah Rukh Khan himself has put it, "it's not about a disabled man's fight against disability. It's a disabled man's fight against the disability that exists in the world—terrorism, hatred, fighting" ("My Name is Khan." n. pag.). The politics of stick figures may hence be more than a way to teach a boy with Asperger's about the senselessness of religious violence; it may be a way of teaching the world about the disability of its cultural politics.

What *My Name Is Khan* plays out on American soil is the entire history of Hindu-Muslim relations in India. It is this history, then, which intersects with American distrust of Muslim communities after the attacks of 9/11. What's in a name, the film asks, when American lives have been disrupted by terrorist attacks unprecedented in their scope and their atrocity?

The tragedy which the film *My Name Is Khan* revolves around is that of mistaken identity: When Mandira agrees to marry Rizvan Khan, she also agrees to giving her son from her previous marriage to a Hindu man, a Muslim surname. In the wake of the 9/11 attacks, Sameer nicknamed Sam encounters rowdy American teenagers on a soccer field. When they tease him with racial, anti-Muslim slurs, he proceeds to retaliate in the most authentic American swear language, and they proceed to beat him to death. It is this tragedy of senseless violence and anti-Muslim sentiment fueled in the wake of 9/11 which is at the core of the film. In her despair over her son's death, Mandira proceeds to curse the day she married a Muslim:

> *On the soccer field where Sam was killed, MANDIRA kneels down on the spot.*
>
> MANDIRA: [*in tears*] Sam. My baby.
>
> KHAN: Mandira.
>
> MANDIRA: We killed him.
>
> KHAN: Mandira.
>
> MANDIRA: We killed him.
>
> KHAN: Let's go home.
>
> MANDIRA: Killed my baby.
>
> KHAN: It's time for dinner. [*informs her, in a monotonous voice*] Doctors say that post-traumatic stress disorder causes people to ignore their health.
>
> MANDIRA: Both of us killed him.

KHAN: You need to take care of your health.

MANDIRA: Just shut up! Just shut up! [*slapping him*] Are you listening to what I am saying? We killed him! It's all my fault. If I hadn't married you all this wouldn't have happened. I thought you loved me so much. Loved Sam so much. What difference would it make if his name is changed? What difference would it make if a "Khan" was added to his name? But I was wrong. It makes a difference. I should never have married a Muslim man! If Sam had been a Rathod, he would have been alive today. He was a Khan, so he died. He died because of your name.

KHAN: I don't understand what you are saying. You are not well.

MANDIRA: God. I want to die.

KHAN: [*worried*] Oh no, no, no. Please don't die. Please don't die.

MANDIRA: Just leave me alone, please? Leave me, please. I don't even want to see you. Whenever I see you I remember Sam's wounds. I can't do this. I can't do this anymore. I'm leaving you, Khan. I'm leaving you!

KHAN: Why should you leave? The house is yours. I will leave.

MANDIRA: Then go! Go right now! Go this instant! [*screaming*] Go right now! Go! Go! Go!

KHAN: Mandira. When should I come back, Mandira?

MANDIRA [*dismayed, shouting*]: When should you be back? You know Banville? It has a population of 30,000. And each of those 30,000 people hates you. They hate you. Tell all of them that you are not a terrorist. Why only them? Tell every person in America, "I'm not a terrorist." Can you do that? Can you? No, you can't. Why don't you tell the President of the United States, then? Mr. President, my name is Khan, and I'm not a terrorist. So he can tell all these people… that my Sam was not the terrorist son of a terrorist father. He was just a baby. My baby. When you do that… come back. [*pushes him*] Come back then! [*she leaves*]

KHAN [*speaking to the void*]: Mr. President, my name is Khan. I'm not a terrorist. Mr. President, my name is Khan, and I'm not a terrorist. (*My Name Is Khan)*

To the world, Mandira is well aware, she will be seen as the "wife of a fanatic", simply because her husband's last name is Khan. Her punishment for Khan, whom she holds responsible for her son's death, is quite simple: He is to tell the world, and the American president in particular, that his name may be Khan, but he is not a terrorist. In the single-minded manner typical of his condition, Rizvan proceeds to put Mandira's command into practice: He travels through the country in order to find the American president to tell him that his name may be Khan, but he is not a terrorist.

> KHAN [*voiceover*]: I'm in Santa Fe, New Mexico. I'm trying to meet the President. His motorcade has 12 cars, but no one tells me which car the President is in … [*standing on the parade grounds, now empty*]. Mandira, I don't know why, but I keep failing to meet the President. (*My Name Is Khan)*

It is the senselessness of anti-Muslim violence, then, which the film proceeds to cast through the prism of autism or rather, Asperger syndrome. Set on a mission to win back Mandira's love by telling the American president what Mandira wanted him to, Khan crosses the country trying to meet the American president. In a climate of fear and a universal distrust of brown faces, however, parts of his mission statement get lost: For a state in its war on terror, any sentence containing the word "terrorist" may be suspicious, even if the sentence in which the word occurs is a negation; there is no time for the intricacies of grammar.

> KHAN is trying to meet the president.
>
> VOICEOVER: I present to you the man, the legend, the President of the United States of America. [*George W. Bush is seen getting out of the car to greet the students*].
>
> KHAN [*in the crowd, trying to push in front*]: Excuse me, Mr. President! Mr. President! My name is Khan, and I'm not a terrorist.
>
> SECURITY GUARD: Did he just say Terrorist?
>
> KHAN: I'm not a terrorist.
>
> MAN [*standing next to Khan, screaming*]: Terrorist! He said he's a terrorist!
>
> SECURITY GUARD: We got code red! Can you get a visual on the suspect?

The President hurriedly gets back into the car. The security guard runs towards Khan and punches him in the face. Khan goes down. (*My Name Is Khan)*

It is on this mission to prove that he is not a terrorist that Khan becomes a suspect, an accusation which will eventually lead him to a Guantanamo fictionalized by Bollywood film.

It is at this point that the filmic narrative engages, and ultimately subverts, the limits of "common sense." If Khan had not been autistic, he would not have taken seriously Mandira's sarcastic suggestion that he tell the world and the American president in particular that he is not a terrorist in order to atone for the death of her son, Sameer. Because, as Temple Grandin has written in her autobiographical study *Thinking in Pictures*, it is hard for autistics to distinguish matter-of-fact statements from irony, Khan takes Mandira's words at face value; and because for him, social appropriateness is not a concept, he proceeds to tell the American president that his name is Khan. Yet, the feat which the filmic narrative accomplishes is that it is not Khan that we laugh at when it comes to inappropriateness; rather, what we shirk at is the paranoia of an entire nation which suddenly sees itself surrounded by brown faces which it is unable to tell apart. Within the logic of the film, Khan's Asperger syndrome makes for his inability to comprehend the nuances and maneuvers of a legal system engaged in a "war on terror"; and yet, it was only in 2014 that Diane Feinstein, head of the Senate Intelligence committee, has admitted that these maneuvers may in fact have been absurd. "The report concludes the agency [CIA] tortured suspects and gained little in valuable intelligence, leaving in Feinstein's words a "stain on our history that must never be allowed to happen again (Klapper n. pag.)." This is a verdict on the justice or rather, the injustice of American law which is also anticipated in Judith Butler's account. As Butler writes,

> The military tribunals that have, at this date, not been used, represent a breach of constitutional law that makes final judgments of life and death into the prerogative of the President. The decision to detain some, if not most, of the 680 inmates currently in Guantanamo is left to "officials" who will decide, on uncertain grounds, whether these individuals present a risk to U.S. security. Bound by no legal guidelines except those fabri-

> cated for the occasion, these officials garner sovereign power unto themselves. (*Precarious Life* xv)

The irony which *My Name Is Khan* drives home is that of a nation which, in its war on terror, has transgressed the limits of what can still make sense. A man with Asperger's who lacks common sense is put in prison because of this lack, of the inappropriateness of a Muslim man wanting to speak directly to the American President. And once in prison, he is at the mercy of a nation which has twisted its laws in ways in which torture can suddenly make sense. In highlighting the strangeness of the situation he finds himself in, Khan may in fact make more sense than an American legal system which has transgressed against itself:

> *Khan in his underwear, in a prison cell.*
>
> KHAN [*voiceover*]: This place is strange, Mandira. There are no windows to any room and the bathrooms don't have a door. And the toilet has a lock. My eyes burn and I feel sleepy, too. At times, it's very hot in here. At other times, it is very cold. I told them I would repair their air conditioner. ... but they won't let me. They don't even tell me the time so I can pray. That's why every time I feel scared I bow and pray. (*My Name Is Khan)*

It is in this sense that the film can also be said to engage Judith Butler's notion of "precarious lives," and her evoking Agamben's notion of "bare life." As the body of a Muslim man with Asperger's, Rizvan's body is doubly vulnerable, and doubly runs the risk of not being seen, by a dominant gaze in its war on terror, as fully human. As Butler writes, "Some lives are grievable, and others are not; the differential allocation of grievability that decides what kind of subject is and must be grieved, and which kind of subject must not, operates to produce certain exclusionary conceptions of who is normatively human; what counts as a livable life and a grievable death?" (*Precarious Life* xiv-xv). In Judith Butler's terms, Rizvan Khan's life is thus "precarious" in multiple ways. It is this precariousness, however, which the film proceeds to cast in the tragicomedy of Rizvan's own gaze. All his life, Rizvan has excelled at "fixing" things; it is with this talent that he offers to help the FBI fix its heating system, if only they would let him.

The twist which Bollywood film adds to its cynical persiflage of Guantanamo, then, is that because of the inhumane circumstances of this form of imprisonment of male Muslim bodies, Bollywood can actually catch two birds with one stone: It can condemn the U.S. for its inhuman practices of interrogation and it can showcase the body of Shah Rukh Khan the megastar. For when else would Bollywood film have had a pretext for showing Shah Rukh Khan in his briefs?

Uncannily, this is an instance where reality intersects with the politics of fiction in a way that could not have been scripted better by the ghostwriters of Bollywood film. As the previously mentioned scene has shown, the film thus both condemns the methods used in Abu Ghraib and capitalizes on the visual presence which such a depiction would allow for the film's main actor. Curiously enough, however, this is an instance in which reality turned out to surpass the fiction of film

> The 44-year-old pin-up, nicknamed 'SRK', said female security staff at the London airport had printed his naked image, as captured by the newly-installed body scanner. He even claimed he had autographed the pictures, although it is not clear if his comments were intended as a joke . . . . However, a BAA spokeswoman said the claims were "completely factually incorrect" because the body-scanning equipment had no capability to print images. She stressed that images captured by the equipment could not be stored or distributed in any form. (Jamieson n. pag.)

What the film engages, then, is precisely the scenario in which truth is stranger than fiction. When Khan the actor tried to promote his movie by the same name, he was held for questioning at LA airport. His name, the security guards eventually apologized, had triggered a security alert on their computer: "The star's claims have resonance because his latest film, *My Name Is Khan*, which is about racial profiling of Muslims at airports after the September 11 2001 terror attacks. A report last August that he was detained for questioning at Newark Liberty Airport near New York City sparked outrage in India. He said: "I'm always stopped by the security, because of the name" ("Airport Denies …" n. pag.).

As Khan wryly stated in retrospect, this was a promotion of the film's cultural accuracy that no advertising blog could have invented. Thus, the real life security guards came to star in a fuzzy form of post 9/11 reality where truth could no longer be distinguished from fiction. In another sequel to this incident which seems so uncanny it must have been invented, Arnold Schwarzenegger, the actor turned politician, proceeded to invite Shah Rukh Khan to dinner in order to apologize for what he termed the minor diplomatic crisis of a Bollywood star being mistaken for a terrorist at LA airport. Guess who's coming to dinner now?

> Shah Rukh Khan, the Bollywood actor who was detained for questioning at a US airport, has been invited for dinner by Californian Governor Arnold Schwarzenegger. The actor turned politician has offered to meet Shah Rukh Khan on September 20 in Washington in a bid to diffuse what has become a slight diplomatic row. Khan, 43, who is considered to be one of the icons of Indian cinema, was held up for almost two hours after falling foul of US border officials in a New York airport at the weekend. . . . It is not clear whether Khan will accept the California Governor's invitation. ("Arnold Schwarzenegger invites 'detained' Bollywood actor" n. pag.)

In this chapter, I am thus beset by all kinds of strange bedfellows both imagined and real. In this motley crew of strange bedfellows where reality meets fiction, Amitava Kumar has lunch with a bigot who used to work for the UN, and Arnold Schwarzenegger and Shah Rukh Khan go for dinner. Incidentally, Shah Rukh Khan the actor, of course, lives in Mumbai, not in the U.S.; for an Austrian governor who has opposed Proposition 187,[3] it is thus safe to invite him for dinner since he is by no means here to stay. And yet, we may do well to remember that the "ghosting" between reality and fiction has always been key to Shah Rukh Khan's life, the life of an actor who put into practice, in real life, the Hindu-Muslim romance which he had previously acted out on screen. Given the fact that *My Name Is Khan*, the film, is set in San Francisco, Shah Rukh Khan the person may thus do more than just stay for dinner, and Arnold Schwarzenegger the politician ghosted by the Hasta La Vista of his terminator stage persona, may want to think twice about whom he asks to stay for dinner.

[3] In 1994, California Proposition 187 was targeted at illegal immigrants, seeking to bar them from non-emergency health care, education and other public services. Approved through a referendum and translated into state legislation, the law was subsequently declared unconstitutional.

3.5 "Frontiers of Justice"

It is with the help of two student journalists, then, that Rizvan in the film is eventually cleared of the charge of terrorism. He returns to his mission of wanting to speak to the American president, this time with the entire Indian diaspora on his side, and with a diasporic media array hoping that yes, he can eventually speak to the American president.

It is at this point that I would once more relate the politics of Bollywood film to the prism of life writing. In her study, *Frontiers of Justice: Disability, Nationality and Species Membership* (2006), American philosopher Martha Nussbaum wonders about the question of access, and about who should and who should not have the right to speak to the American president. In this book, which is much more than an academic study, Martha Nussbaum the philosopher also writes about the life of her nephew, Arthur:

> My nephew Arthur is a big good-looking ten-year-old. He loves machines of all sorts, and by now he has impressive knowledge of their workings. I could talk with Arthur all day about the theory of relativity, if I understood it as well as he does. On the phone with Art, it's always, "Hi, Aunt Martha," and then right into the latest mechanical or scientific or historical issue that fascinates him. (*Frontiers of Justice* 97)

Like Bollywood's fictional Rizvan Khan, Martha Nussbaum's nephew has Asperger's. Like Rizvan, he knows, even at the age of ten, how to "fix" things given his astute understanding of the way in which technological mechanisms work. Like the fictional Rizvan Khan, Arthur would have been able to fix the air conditioning of the FBI, and may have been as astute in his diagnosing the senselessness of a legal system gone awry. Yet, Nussbaum asks, in what way would Arthur, like Rizvan, have been able to express his political will, and what are the channels which we supply to him for such expression?

Crucially, because Nussbaum's account of social justice is both necessarily abstract and deliberately specific in the examples she uses, her book itself can hence be seen as a form of life writing. It is thus much more than a philosophical, an academic study of the nature of justice in our contemporary world; it is also a book in which an aunt writes the life of her nephew. It is this shift from abstraction to the particular reality of a life lived by a disabled individual that seems to me one of the most memorable passages in Nussbaum's account. It is a deliberate shift in register that she herself addresses in the first sentences of her book:

> Theories of social justice should be abstract. They should, that is, have a generality and theoretical power that enables them to reach beyond the political conflicts of their time, even if they have their origins in such conflicts. . . . On the other hand, theories of social justice must also be responsive to the world and its most urgent problems. . . . Today there are three unsolved problems of social justice whose neglect in existing theories seems particularly problematic. . . . [One of them] is the problem of doing justice to people with physical and mental impairments. (Nussbaum, *Frontiers of Justice* 1)

What is at stake here is the very question of access and of participation in the social fabric. The "frontiers of [our] justice," Nussbaum points out, lie in just what access we provide to whom. She notes,

> Impairment and disability raise two distinct problems of social justice here, both of them urgent. First, there is the issue of the fair treatment of people with impairments, many of whom need atypical social arrangements, including varieties of care, if they are to live fully integrated and productive lives. (Nussbaum, *Frontiers of Justice* 99)

> Fifteen years ago, before Asperger's syndrome was recognized as a disease, Arthur would have been treated as a smart kid whose parents had messed him up emotionally. He would probably have been institutionalized, with no opportunity to learn, and they would have lived with crushing guilt. A just society, by contrast, would not stigmatize these children and stunt their development; it would support their health, education and full participation in social and even, when possible, political life. (Nussbaum, *Frontiers of Justice* 99-100)

The latter sentence is remarkable in a number of ways. First, it deliberately extends the question of justice to that of participation in social life; the problem, for Nussbaum, lies not only in "taking care" of disabled individuals like her nephew but in finding ways in which they can participate in the social fabric to the fullest extent of their possibilities. Secondly, the question, for Nussbaum, lies not only in social participation and, for instance, in the right to being educated (which, as she notes, can only be achieved at a specialized private school in Arthur's case), but it also includes the right of political participation. As Nussbaum goes on to say, Arthur has both Asperger's and Tourette's syndrome; at the same time, he has a distinct political opinion, even if he cannot always choose the "appropriate" ways of making this opinion known. What is at stake, Nussbaum emphasizes, is nothing less than the overall quality of the political and social citizenship which we accord to people like Arthur. For the notion of citizenship, she notes, has been predicated on the Kantian ideal and conception of personhood as such. Nussbaum writes,

> Arthur may or may not have the capacity for a sense of justice in Kant's sense. . . . Thus people with mental impairments and disabilities pose a double challenge to Rawls's theory. The contract doctrine seems unable to accommodate their needs for special social attention, for the reasons of social productivity and cost that pertain to all people with impairments. But they are disqualified from citizenship in a deeper way as well, because they do not conform to the rather idealized picture of moral rationality that is used to define the citizen in the Well-Ordered Society. (*Frontiers of Justice* 135)

As Nussbaum writes about Arthur, there is no question that he does have a political opinion; it is up to us, however, whether we enable him to make this opinion heard. If we privilege the *form* of political expression over its content, however, we will privilege appropriateness over the right to political access, and we will redraw the frontiers of our justice to exclude disability. As Nussbaum points out, people with Asperger's pose a special challenge to society's interaction with them because, like Bollywood's fictional Rizvan Khan, they "look normal." Nussbaum writes,

> One reason why integration is so difficult in Arthur's case is that he does not look different: thus, people expect "normal" behavior of him. And his social disabilities often take the form of rudeness and tantrums that seem inappropriate for a boy of his age who looks normal. Indeed, his cognitive gifts make it all the easier for people to think, when he says something that seems rude, that he must be a bad kid. (*Frontiers of Justice* 206)

In a striking if purely accidental convergence between Martha Nussbaum's nephew and Bollywood's fictional hero, Rizvan Khan, both

Arthur and Rizvan find fault not just with the American political system as such, but with one American president in particular: George W. Bush. As Nussbaum remembers,

> Take the example of Arthur's combination of cognitive advancement with behavioral rigidity. After the elections of 2000, Arthur decided that Bush had not been duly elected, and should therefore be called "the Resident" rather than "the President." After thinking up this quite subtle and impressive joke, he simply would not drop it, and every time the teacher referred to Bush as "President Bush," he insisted on correcting her. Such behavior obviously does not go down well in a public school classroom in a rather conservative state. (*Frontiers of Justice* 206-7)

I believe that in a sense *My Name Is Khan* continues where Nussbaum's account of Arthur's political will leaves off. First the film, like Arthur's brilliantly conceived joke, makes no secret of its criticism of George W. Bush. Not only was Bush "unduly elected" (Nussbaum, *Frontiers of Justice* 206), but the film proceeds to chronicle the neglect which Bush was guilty of once he had taken office, among them his dire disregard of African American communities hit by Katrina.

Hurricane Katrina, as Alondra Nelson has argued, emphasized the way in which social inequalities can be translated into forms of what has been called "medical apartheid" (xi). As Nelson points out, the government failure to help African Americans cope with the aftermath of Katrina reflected an entire system of inequality with regard to which lives should benefit from healthcare and which should not. According to Nelson, "Healthcare . . . discourse [has often been] couched in competing claims about what constituencies [matter], what lives [are] valued, and what bodies [are] deserving of medical care" (x). Existing inequalities can hence be translated into medical inequalities, or rather, into a lack of access to medical care. It is in this sense that, as Nelson points out, Katrina has been seen by many as a "man-made, state-exacerbated tragedy" (182). Nelson draws an explicit connection between the 1960s and the 1990s here, arguing that the reluctance of the government to take medical action to support the African American community in the wake of Katrina was only the most recent evidence of continued medical discrimination. She writes, "Just as the brutal facts of urban poverty, health inequality, and medical mistreatment showed the celebratory civil rights rhetoric of the late 1960s at its limits, the aftermath of Katrina confirmed that for vulnerable communities made up of lives deemed of little value, citizenship had indeed failed" (Nelson 183). What is significant for my purpose here is that the film *My Name Is Khan* is particularly astute in its laying bare precisely this disparateness in medical care when it comes to different ethnic communities in the U.S.. In its portrayal of the "state-exacerbated" horror of Katrina, the film astutely recognizes how social inequalities can be translated, as Nelson has described it, into medical inequality. In this sense, a Bollywood film can be seen both as a critique about the inequalities in medical care and a critique of the U.S. government which, particularly in the case of Katrina, exacerbates such inequalities. *My Name Is Khan* thus finds fault not just with the system, but with a particularly representative of the system: George W. Bush.

Given the contempt for George W. Bush which Rizvan Khan shares with Arthur, then, it may in fact have been for the better that Rizvan did not get to meet the President while George W. Bush was still in office. Like Arthur, he might just have told him that as President, Bush is a resident at best. In the end, then, the questions which Martha Nussbaum and the film *My Name Is Khan* ask are the same. Why should Arthur, Martha Nussbaum's nephew, and Bollywood's fictional Rizvan Khan *not* be allowed to speak to the American president? Why should people with Asperger's not be given the right to vote or make their political will known to the wider public? As Nussbaum writes, "Many other people with mental disabilities do aspire to hold a job, and vote, and tell their own story" (*Frontiers of Justice* 219). What, both Nussbaum and the film *My Name Is Khan* ask, are the ways in which we enable them to do so?

Remarkably, moreover, what is at stake in both cases, that of Nussbaum's nephew and that of Bollywood's fictional Rizvan Khan, is the question of disability versus the *universal* nature of our system of justice. The point which Nussbaum makes is that if we exclude her nephew from the political process, this says something not only about disability, but about the frontiers of *our* justice as well:

> All citizens should have the chance to develop the full range of human powers, at whatever level their condition allows, and to enjoy the sort of liberty and independence that their condition allows. (*Frontiers of Justice* 218)

> Then, having identified that (extreme) threshold, we seek a higher threshold, the level above which not just mere human life, but good life, becomes possible. (*Frontiers of Justice* 181)

By the same token, the master move which *My Name Is Khan* accomplishes is that it turns Khan's right to speak to the American president not into a question of Asperger syndrome, but into a discussion of the limits of American democracy as such. It is here that Khan's double exclusion as a man with Asperger's and as an Indian Muslim living in the U.S. are superimposed on one another by the filmic narrative. Just as Rizvan's "My name is Khan, and I'm not a terrorist" is echoed by anyone from a Hindu nationalist motel owner to an unkempt computer hacker, all of whom are proud to be what they are, so is the question of American democracy rephrased through a variety of voices and from a variety of perspectives: Why, the Indian Muslim community in the U.S. asks with one voice, should they not be allowed to speak to the American president?

> ZAKIR [*on a news report about his brother*]: The question over here is not why he's trying to meet the President. The question is what's wrong in an ordinary citizen wanting to meet the president of his country? Or is it just wrong for a Muslim man to even try?
>
> BOBBY AHUJA [*Sikh newscaster*]: And as Rizvan Khan continues to be treated as guilty until proven innocent, for PBS news, my name is Bobby Ahuja, and I am not a terrorist.
>
> *Dinner conversation at a Muslim home.*
>
> MAN: He is right. Zakir Bhai is right. We are told to report to the government any information we have on any terrorist activity. And when we do that, what happens is before you. Why is this being asked over and over again? "Why does Khan want to meet the President?" What's the harm if an ordinary citizen wants to meet the President? What's wrong? Or then tell us clearly that Muslims don't have the right to do so. (*My Name Is Khan*)

It is at this juncture that the film adds a particular twist to the question of who does and does not have the right to speak to the American president: Given the fact that he is a Muslim man, Khan's wanting to speak to the American president is deemed suspicious by an American nation coming out of the 9/11 attacks. At the same time, as a man with Asperger's, Khan, like Martha Nussbaum's nephew, lacks the appropriate social tools to make his political opinion known. In a shortcut which is logical but not socially appropriate, he simply proposes to speak to the president himself in order to tell him that his name is Khan, but he is by no means a terrorist.

Yet, the limits of Nussbaum's account, and of *My Name Is Khan*, is that the highest form of inclusion and social and political participation they can conceive of is the right to speak to the American president. U.S. democracy and the president as its representative thus becomes the epitome of democracy tout court – an idea which, of course, is highly fraught to begin with. The image and the imaginary scenario of speaking to or at least wanting to speak to the American president, of course, works precisely because of the American president's iconicity: It is in playing with the concept of inappropriateness that *My Name Is Khan* makes its point. As a person with Asperger's, Rizvan takes all things at face value; he has been told to tell the American president that he is not a terrorist, and so he will.

Yet, read through the prism of Arthur's political insight, the film goes one step further to critique the politics of the resident, George W. Bush. It proceeds to take issue not only with scapegoating of Muslim men in the wake of 9/11, but also with the universalizing of Christian religion as the only form of human justice. When Rizvan wants to meet the president at a charity event, he is turned away because charity, the receptionist informs him, is only for Christians.

It is in this context of mistaken Christianity that Bollywood film proceeds to retaliate: Against a racialized form of Christian charity from which Rizvan, the Indian Muslim, is clearly excluded, it proceeds to cast its own version of Christian hybridity: it proceeds to cast Shah Rukh Khan, the Indian actor who has founded his career on playing Hindu heroes on the Indian mainstream screen, not just as an Indian protagonist but as a Muslim Messiah as well. In creating a Muslim Messiah to fly in the face of white Christian fundamentalism, then, Bollywood film also demonstrates to an American mainstream audience that it is by no means culturally illiterate in terms of either Christian religion or Western cultural politics. No one can accuse Bollywood film of not knowing its Christian imagery, complete with Muslim messiahs.

In keeping with the Muslim messiah, then, Rizvan is also a savior figure: He is the man who perhaps the American president should have been. Bollywood would not be Bollywood and its narrative would not be Indian triumphalism on a global scale if the film denied itself this punchline. When the Resident George W. Bush deserted the African American community in the wake of Katrina, Rizvan Khan is there to take his place. When he hears on the news that Mama Jenny, the African American woman in Wilhelmina, Georgia, who once took him in when he was exhausted from his journey following the American president in order to finally speak to him, he takes the bus right into the eye of the storm. In an Afro-Asian encounter, to use Heike Raphael-Hernandez's term, the Indian community in Wilhelmina, Georgia, proceeds to do what the American president, George W. Bush, did not:

> *A woman is screaming because her child has died as a result of the flood. Her scream pierces the silence as some of the survivors have taken refuge in a church, trying to repair what they can.*
>
> WOMAN [*crying, in utter despair*]: Please don't take my baby away from me. Please don't take my baby away from me. Please!
>
> KHAN [*voiceover, reading out his diary entry*]: Mandira, people are suffering here and are very helpless. I wish I could take all of them from here. But I don't have the physical strength to do that. Mama Jenny is right. [*A hand is seen covering the face of the dead child*]. This one… This one I can't repair. Now we can only await the Lord's merciful eye. [*Night falls. When a new day is breaking, we hear Funny Hair Joel shouting*].
>
> FUNNY HAIR JOEL: Mama! Mama! Mama! Mama! [*Everyone runs to the church door to see what Joel is pointing to.*]
>
> *Led by Rizvan's brother and sister in law and the journalists who have helped bring about his release from jail, a group of helpers is wading through the flood towards them, carrying boxes of food and medical aid.*
>
> ZAKIR [*seeing his brother*]: Bhai.
>
> NEWSCASTER [*seen on television*]: While several hurricane-hit areas have suffered from government inaction, one small town in Georgia is slowly getting back on its feet. [*In Wilhelmina, we see streetlight being hoisted by up and pulled from the debris.*] This group has brought something more valuable than money. They've brought themselves.

> INDIAN NEWSCASTER [*in Hindi*]: The U.S. government may have forgotten the flood inflicted here in Wilhelmina, Georgia, but one man has refused to be indifferent to the plight of its inhabitants. This one man has spared no efforts in helping the rehabilitation of the population of Wilhelmina. Looking at him as an inspiration today many Americans have rushed to Wilhelmina and its neighboring towns to help in rebuilding the destroyed towns. [*The camera shows Muslim communities in India watching the news report about RIZVAN KHAN*]. And all this just because of one man whose name is Rizvan Khan and who, in his own words, is not a "terrorist." (*My Name Is Khan)*

3.6 Shaking Hands with the President

Bollywood, then, would not be Bollywood if Rizvan Khan did not eventually get to meet the American president, and to deliver his message. The telos of the filmic narrative is the very scenario which Martha Nussbaum envisions for her nephew. In the end, Rizvan Khan does get to speak to the American president. And yet, it is Bollywood's side blow on American politics that the president whom Rizvan eventually does get to meet is not George W. Bush, the resident who had continued to elude Rizvan on his travels across the country, but Barack Obama, the man whose campaign, we must remember, was also hampered by his Muslim name. If Rizvan Khan's mission is to tell the American president that despite his name, he is not a terrorist, it is with Barack Obama of all people that Rizvan can be imagined to preach to the choir. If Rizvan proceeds to complete his mission by telling Barack Obama that even though his name may be Khan, he is not a terrorist, Barack Obama could be said to have become president only by assuring an American public that his name may be Obama, but he is by no means un-American; and that his middle name may be Hussein, but he is not a Muslim.

In multiple ways, Barack Obama, the nation's first African American president, is the telos of *My Name Is Khan*. As President, Barack Obama did what the Resident George W. Bush did not: He helps the African American community in the wake of Katrina; by visiting Georgia, Obama, the African American president with the Muslim middle name, follows in the footsteps mapped out for him by Bollywood's Muslim Messiah whose name is Khan: What the film imagines as its telos is this moment of recognition, whose implications, for all of Bollywood's typical pathos, could not be more profound: In the end, the African

American president shakes the hand of an Indian Muslim, and of a man with Asperger's who refuses *not* to make his political will known to the President of the United States. In the end, Khan does get to shake hands with the president, and the president, it turns out, actually knows his name:

> AFRICAN-AMERICAN NEWSCASTER: After offering aid to the state of Georgia, the President will go to New York from here to participate in the United Nations' special summit.
>
> [*KHAN and MANDIRA arrive at the site only to see that the President has already left. They are dejected.*]
>
> SECURITY GUARD: Back up, please! Clear the area. Please, clear the area, folks, the president has left.
>
> INDIAN NEWSCASTER [*spotting Rizvan in the crowd; the camera swerves towards him*]: This is Rizvan Khan.
>
> SECURITY GUARD: Please. Back.
>
> RIZVAN: I want to meet the president.
>
> NEWSCASTER: Rizvan Khan who has been in the news for all his efforts in Wilhelmina, is now at the Governor's mansion. He has been trying to meet the President for a while now. It's sad he won't meet the President even today. Rizvan Khan's supporters are quite dejected at this prospect.
>
> AMERICAN NEWSCASTER: However, it looks like he will face disappointment all over again.
>
> MALE NEWSCASTER: A disappointed group of Khan's supporters are getting ready to turn back.
>
> SECURITY GUARD [*listening into his headset, surprised*]: Ten nine? Copy that. Regal is on foot. Repeat that please. [*Listening*]. Regal is on foot.
>
> SECURITY GUARD [*approaching RIZVAN and MANDIRA at the police barrier*]: Are you Rizvan Khan?
>
> KHAN: Yes, sir.
>
> MANDIRA: Yes.
>
> SECURITY GUARD: The President wants to meet you.

To the sounds of "We shall overcome" in Hindi, KHAN and MANDIRA ascend the stairs to where the President is standing, with his hand extended to welcome them.

KHAN [*to the PRESIDENT*]: Salaam aleikum! [*subtitled as: Greetings*].

PRESIDENT [*shaking Khan's hand*]: Rizvan Khan. Good to see you hale and hearty. You're on TV more than me now, huh?

KHAN [to MANDIRA]: Mandira. He knows my name. [to the PRESIDENT] You already know my name?

PRESIDENT: Yes, I do. Your name is Khan.

KHAN: Yes.

PRESIDENT: And you are not a terrorist.

KHAN: No, no. I'm not a terrorist. No. And [*reaching inside his jacket to produce a photo*] this is my son. He … he wasn't a terrorist either. My son.

PRESIDENT: I know.

KHAN: You know.

PRESIDENT [*laying his hand on MANDIRA's shoulder*]: I'm so sorry for your loss.

KHAN: Ok.

MANDIRA: Yes, thank you.

KHAN [*to MANDIRA*]: He's sorry.

PRESIDENT: [*to the public*]: All of us share this world but for a brief moment in time. And I am honored to share in the time of Rizvan Khan. Rizvan has reminded us…

MANDIRA [voiceover]: Sam. Our Khan has managed to achieve, with his love and humanity, what my hatred could never achieve. My anger threw us apart… but today his love has brought us together in a way where we remember you with renewed hope. Now I will never let him go anywhere again. I will keep this love with me. For me… For you.. forever.

PRESIDENT [*to the crowd*]: Yes, we can. [*To RIZVAN*]: Anything else, Rizvan?

KHAN: [*remembering the message which the racist security guard told him in order to make fun of his disability*]: Yes. John Marshall, Homeland Security, San Francisco, said today, "Howdy."

PRESIDENT [*raising an eyebrow*]: Howdy?

KHAN: Howdy.

PRESIDENT: I'll tell you what. If security has any other message, just call me.

KHAN: Good, good. Can I have your number, please?

MANDIRA [*gently pulling KHAN away*]: Thank you, Mr. President.

PRESIDENT: Thank *you*.

MANDIRA [*to KHAN*]: Shall we go home?

KHAN: Yes, let's go home.

PRESIDENT: Rizvan, pleasure. Thank you.

RIZVAN: Goodbye. (*My Name Is Khan*)

Would Barack Obama really have shaken the hand of Rizvan Khan if the latter had not been a fictional character? Be that as it may, what we do know is that in order to become the American president in the first place, the real Obama had to say precisely what Bollywood's fictional hero does: My name may be Obama, but I am not a terrorist. In this transnational, multi-ethnic, Afro-Asian credo, Bollywood imagines Rizvan Khan, an Indian Muslim man with Asperger's being welcomed by an African American president who was once attacked for his Muslim name. At the end of the film, Obama's campaign slogan – "Yes, we can" – evokes and transcends the frontiers of justice, frontiers which exclude persons with Asperger's by telling them that it is inappropriate to want to speak to the American president directly. In the end, Bollywood film joins the first African American president in American history in his credo of "Yes, we can" transcend the frontiers of our justice.

Moreover, the film ends with the recognition of both a man with Asperger's and a representative of the Indian-American community by the first African-American president in the history of the U.S., Barack Obama. It is in this sense, then, that the film also addresses the relationship between medical care and social inequality. As Alondra Nelson has argued, this relationship has historically been marked by a number of different parameters. First, even if biomedical progress was heralded as benefiting "humankind," thus abolishing all differences between different communities in terms of race, gender, or class, the benefits of such biomedical progress have not been extended to all Americans because of disparities in health care. It is in this sense, then, that it may be no coincidence that the first Bollywood film to address disabilities in the terms of medical humanities and with a disabled character as its protagonist should also revolve around President Barack Obama, the president who introduced a landmark reform in the American healthcare system, a reform named "Obamacare" (Nelson x). As Nelson observes,

> Health is also deemed to embody conceptions of the good society. In 2010, the administration of President Barack Obama ushered a historic healthcare reform with the Patient Protection and Affordable Care Act. At the time of its passage, this legislation marked the most sweeping changes in U.S. health policy since the establishment of Medicaid and Medicare in 1965. (ix)

Thus, through the seemingly trivial handshake between a (fictionalized) Barack Obama and a (fictional) Indian American man, Rizvan Khan, the Bollywood film *My Name Is Khan* can also be said to echo, if unconsciously so, the politics of Obamacare as a health care reform which counteracts practices in which social inequality is translated into a lack of access to medical care.

At the same time, it seems significant for my purposes here that Rizvan Khan should be both a non-white man and a person with Asperger's. For as Nelson has argued, the concept of biological citizenship – and, by extension, the citizenship rights called for by disabled communities in general – may run the risk of being counterproductive to the extent that it overlooks inequalities occasioned by race or class. In this context, Nelson draws attention to the work of Adriana Petryna, who had originally coined the term "biological citizenship" to refer to victims of the Chernobyl catastrophe. She emphasizes that there may be a need to

> return to the work of anthropologist Adriana Petryna and, in particular, to the milieu of catastrophe and deprivation that impelled her theorization of biological citizenship. . . . [It] is worth emphasizing that biologi-

> cal citizenship for Petryna is a vehicle of inclusion for "increasingly poor citizens" who, if not for their "damaged biology," might be otherwise lacking in social and economic rights. What happens when damaged biology or presumed biological pathology or disproportionate illness rates or disease identity come to stand in for citizenship? What are the transaction costs of biological citizenship? (Nelson 184-85)

What Nelson draws attention to here is the danger of pitting one concept of citizenship against another. Seen from this perspective, the concept of "biological citizenship" is meant as a way, through an alternative route or form of access, to counteract that fact that full citizenship rights are not extended towards poor communities. These communities, in turn, may often be communities of color. The point that the call for "biological citizenship" may obfuscate, in Nelson's terms, is the fact that these entire communities should have access to full citizenship rights, not only those who are eligible for these rights on the basis of a different "biology." Even as it may enfranchise some communities, Nelson implies, the concept of "biological citizenship" may end up perpetuating the inequalities of other communities.

Where the Bollywood film *My Name Is Khan* may be particularly evocative, then, is in its evoking of a kinship between various and variously disenfranchised social groups within the U.S.. Through imagining such kinship, I would argue, the film refuses to pit one form of citizenship another. It addresses the concept of biological citizenship and, by extension, of citizenship for disabled individuals by revolving around a protagonist with Asperger's; it calls for the inclusion of diasporic communities by recognizing an Indian American man and his right to speak to – and by implication, to be represented by – the American president; and it castigates the American medical system and the previous American president for failing to recognize the rights – in the sense of medical care as a fundamental human right – of African Americans in the wake of Katrina. In this sense, then, the film links medical humanities – as a representation of a man with Asperger's in a feature film – with a surprisingly nuanced discussion of social inequality and medical access in the U.S.. Even as the film does not directly address these issues, I nevertheless believe that it opens up a discussion about this very relationship between medicine, social equality, and forms of citizenship. This call for social and medical inclusion, I have tried to argue in this chapter, is also expressed through forms of life writing.

3.7 Conclusion

My point in this chapter, then, has been not only to re-read a fictional narrative – Bollywood's blockbusting feature film *My Name Is Khan* – through the prism of life writing, but also to re-read life writing through the prism, however inappropriate this may at first seem, of Bollywood film. In the end *My Name Is Khan* visualizes a life which Martha Nussbaum, the American philosopher, envisions for her nephew: a life which Indian philosopher Amartya Sen has called "the good life" and which in German we would term "gelingendes Leben," a life in which romance and disability are by no means mutually exclusive and a life in which Asperger's may be a form of deviance from the able-bodied norm, but not a difference so fundamental that it would become paramount to the telling of lives. In the end, *My Name Is Khan* is and is not a story about Asperger's, and it is by no means a story of *dis*ability. The frontiers of justice it calls on us to engage are the frontiers of our own thinking, the ways in which we separate some narratives from others, and some lives from the sum total of the lives which are said to be "good."

4 "An Anthropologist on Mars": Temple Grandin's *Thinking in Pictures*

4.1 Medicine and Its Others

What does it mean to be Other for and in medicine? This Otherness, first and foremost, seems to be that of the patient, whose Otherness would then be defined by or through medical categories. Yet, it is at this point already that we may run into a problem of definition, and of definitional categories. For there may be an error of categories if we were to assume that the Otherness of the patient is defined only by medicine; it is also brought about, we might argue, by his or her illness which causes him or her to seek medical assistance in the first place. The Otherness brought about by illness or disability is then translated into a diagnostic category, and whatever form of treatment is currently available ensues.

At the same time, biomedicine has long undergone a paradigmatic change from a diagnostic paradigm where the doctor, by virtue of his diagnosis, would observe and in a sense "Other" the patient and would then go on to prescribe a form of treatment. Today, we would assume what Norbert Paul has called a "co-construction of knowledge." In such a co-construction of knowledge, the physician would enter into a dialogue with his patient, and together they would determine the course of future treatment. This co-construction of knowledge may have been more common for some illnesses than others; it has, for instance, long been described for psychosomatic medicine, particularly in treating trauma and PTSD. As Waller and Scheidt observe, "In many respects, the object of psychosomatic medicine can be described as a narrative co-construction" (68; my trans.).

Yet, the question remains to what extent a certain degree of Otherness remains in the doctor-patient relationship. It is, after all, the physician who makes the diagnosis. What degree of alienness or Otherness would hence be part of the medical diagnostic framework? Following the work of Craig Irvine, I would like to begin this paper with a cartoon (Irvine, "Narrative Ethics" n. pag.). In this cartoon, the medical framework is itself portrayed as an encounter between humans and aliens. I want to argue that this cartoon invites two kinds of readings. In one reading, the patient is human and the doctor is the alien; it is the physician's face, after all, which bears a certain resemblance to E.T. In his recent work on narrative ethics, on the other hand, Craig Irvine has pointed to another reading of the cartoon. In his interpretation of the cartoon, the physician enters the hospital as he would enter a spaceship. In this reading of the cartoon, the physician, disguised by his space gear, is the human while the aliens are living in their natural habitat. The aliens, in this second reading of the cartoon, are the patients; and they are being observed by the physician-astronaut-ethnographer who sets out to study their alienness. This cartoon, in both its readings, is thus deliberately polemic. In distinguishing between doctors and aliens, it wants to call for a medical diagnostic framework which abolishes the human-alien dichotomy and allows for empathy and dialogue instead.

It is in this call for dialogue, in turn, that both readings of the cartoon converge. It is by no means coincidental, then, that Irvine has used this cartoon as a starting point for investigating the role of narrative in medicine: "the primacy of narrative is acknowledged across diverse disciplines: Historians, cognitive psychologists, social scientists, theologians, psychiatrists, and literary critics . . . have all 'come to recognize the central role narrative plays in the way we construct knowledge and interpret knowledge'" ("The Ethics of Self-Care" 47). There are a number of aspects in this passage here which are crucial for the ideas which I am trying to envision both in this chapter and in this study as a whole. First, Irvine points to the centrality of narrative not only for the humanities, but for other disciplines as well. In the above-cited passage, Irvine thus points to the importance of narrative knowledge – the idea that knowledge in various disciplines is not only, but also narratively constructed – in a variety of disciplines at the beginning of the twenty-first century. As Timothy Lenoir and Hans-Ulrich Gumbrecht have suggested in their concept of "writing science," moreover, we need to pay attention to the fact that scientific discourse is by no means devoid of narrative or metaphor; instead, we may focus on the ways in which science is *written*. As Lenoir and Gumbrecht state,

> Science is writing. The Writing Science series investigates the culture of science: its practice-and-instrument-laden character and its heterogene-

> ous, disunified nature. Studies in Writing Science treat scientific knowledge as always situated, local, and partial; they explore how the work of theorists, experimenters, and technicians is locally coordinated and the ways local contexts are multiplied in order to account for the striking capacity of science to capture supposedly universal features of the world. Writing Science volumes interrogate the ways in which different domains of practice mesh locally and translate globally to other sites, linking networks of heterogeneous actors and the literary technologies they employ to fashion arguments and enroll other social worlds into agreement. (n. pag.)

As an entry point into a discussion of Otherness in medicine, then, this cartoon – precisely because it points to the potential shortcomings of a medical-diagnostic framework – may thus be a useful starting point. It is this cartoon and its depiction of humans and aliens that I would like to apply to Temple Grandin's groundbreaking autobiography *Thinking in Pictures*. The book, I want to argue in this paper, is much more than a patient account. In fact, the fact that it resists being read only as a patient account is part of its very sabotaging of a traditional medical framework. It is in its sabotaging of various registers, I believe, that *Thinking in Pictures* is so fascinating. It can be read alternately as a patient account, an autobiography, an academic paper on brain research, and a piece of narrative advice for persons living with autism or their relatives. The book is also, however, the work of an animal scientist, who has compared the working of her own unusual mind to that of animals. As a biographical note which precedes Grandin's narrative puts it, "Temple Grandin has a Ph.D. in animal science from the University of Illinois and has designed one third of all the livestock-handling facilities in the United States, and many other countries. She is currently an associate professor of animal sciences at Colorado State University and a frequent lecturer at autism meetings throughout the country" (*Thinking in Pictures* n. pag.). It is these multiple positionalities through which, from the very outset, Grandin sabotages what might be construed as her own alienness – the alienness of a person with autism.

I would like to argue in this paper that this form of sabotage – the resistance, in a narrative that is only seemingly a patient narrative, to a diagnostic paradigm – has been instrumental in bringing about a change in medical diagnostics as such. *Thinking in Pictures* has been central to changing the ways in which we think about autism today. In what follows, I would like to focus on what I am reading as a signature moment in the study of Otherness in medicine: the conversation between Oliver Sacks, a neurologist renowned for the attention he paid to narrative detail in patient accounts, and Temple Grandin, whose emphasis on self-narration would turn the medical-diagnostic framework on its head. In this unusual dialogue, Sacks has commented on the ways in which Grandin proceeded to transform his diagnostic view of the Otherness of autism, a condition which, at the time in which Grandin's first autobiography, *Emergence: Labeled Autistic*, appeared in 1986, physicians were at a loss to explain. As Sacks writes,

> In 1986 a quite extraordinary, unprecedented and, in a way, unthinkable book was published, Temple Grandin's *Emergence: Labeled Autistic*. Unprecedented because there had never before been an "inside narrative" of autism; unthinkable because it had been medical dogma for forty years or more that there *was* no "inside," no inner life, in the autistic, and if there was it would be forever denied access or expression; extraordinary because of its extreme (and strange) directness and clarity. Temple Grandin's voice came from a place which had never had a voice, never been granted real existence, before – and she spoke not only for herself, but for thousands of other, often highly gifted, autistic adults in our midst. (Foreword xiii)

I believe that Sacks's reference to the "unthinkability" of Grandin's book is key here, and it is of key importance to an understanding of Otherness in medicine. As Sacks notes, prior to the publication of Grandin's narrative, it had been assumed by medical science that the interiority of an autistic mind, as well as its narrative creativeness, did not exist. Prior to Grandin's narrative, persons with autism would indeed have seemed alien to both medical practitioners and the general public. What this juncture in the history of medicine and in the history of narrative knowledge about autism reveals, then, is the extent to which our understanding of identity has relied on language and on narrative. Minus the ability to narrate herself, then, Grandin as a person with autism would have remained profoundly Other; she would have remained an alien because her mind would have been said to have no inside, simply because, outside of language, there would have been no way to make this inside *known*. What emerges at this critical juncture, I believe, are three aspects at once. First, there is the idea that identity can be conveyed through or perhaps only through narrative. Second, through this narrative conveying of her own identity, Grandin is able to dispel the presumed Otherness of her condition. Third, this disproving of the Otherness of Grandin's condition centers on proving, through narrative, that there is an *inside* to the autistic mind. Even more remarkable, however, is the fact that this redefinition of diagnostic categories should have been articulated not in an academic article, but in a narrative of life writing. Grandin succeeds in redefining medical definitions of autism, then, through writing an autobiography. Through the space created by Oliver Sacks, then, this autobiography indeed succeeds in entering into a dialogue with the life sciences.

It is in this sense, then, that Grandin's first autobiography, *Emergence: Labeled Autistic*, indeed gave a voice to a group of persons which had hitherto only been represented in medical discourse, never in life writing. The idea of giving a voice could not be more central here, and it could not be more complex in its manifold layers of meaning. For before the publication of *Emergence: Labeled Autistic* in 1986, it would have been unthinkable for medical practitioners that such a book could have been written by a person with autism. What Sacks's account is, then, is a profound moment of recognition. The signature moment which Sacks recalls is the recognition, by the human physician in space gear, that those whom he had deemed alien were in fact no less human than himself. As Sacks recalls, writing about the appearance of Grandin's first autobiography, *Emergence: Labeled Autistic*, "[Grandin] provided a glimpse, and indeed a revelation, that there might be *people no less human than ourselves*, who constructed their worlds, lived their lives, in unimaginably different ways" (Foreword xiii; emphasis added). I believe that this passage is remarkable for two reasons in particular. First, Sacks implicitly recognizes the human/alien dichotomy which had informed medical discourse about autism prior to the emergence of Grandin's voice. Second, this moment of recognition marks what I would read as a deliberate suspension, by Sacks the physician and neurologist, of his own medical authority. It is through this deliberate abandoning of his own authority, the humbling of the self as a medical practitioner, that Sacks creates a space for Temple Grandin to step into, and to step into as someone who is much more than a patient. It is from this suspension of medical power by Oliver Sacks the physician, who has turned himself simply into a listener and reader, that Temple Grandin's own powerful voice was able to emerge.

4.2 Taking off the Space-Gear

At this very juncture then, and in the unusual dialogue between Oliver Sacks and Temple Grandin about humans and aliens, the cartoon with which I began is turned on its head. How, then, might we read Sacks's divesting himself of his own medical authority in the visual terms of the cartoon? Sacks's groundbreaking gesture, first, is that on entering the spaceship, he refuses to don his space gear, the very gear protecting him from contact with the aliens. He meets the aliens, then, on their own terms. It is this simple divesting himself of the authority which comes with medical gear – here, with space-gear – that makes possible what Norbert Paul has called a co-construction of knowledge. It is a divestment of medical authority which enables the physician to meet on par with his patient, who in turn becomes more than a patient.

As Sacks himself goes on to recall in his foreword to Temple Grandin's *Thinking in Pictures,* it was only when he himself became, not a doctor but a *listener* that Grandin's own narrative and voice emerged; through this emergence, in turn, Sacks became aware of what, as a doctor, he had not known about autism, and what he had never believed a person with autism to be capable of. Sacks's emphasis on and attention to narrative in the practice of medicine, then, was instrumental in bringing about the paradigm shift in the encounter between humans and aliens. For Sacks in his emphasis on narrative in medicine, medical practice itself becomes an act of listening, of witnessing: As Sacks once put it in a lecture on the importance of narrative in medicine,

> I retain very little memory of medical lectures there, on the other hand, I remember all the patients I saw with vividness and affection. I'm not able to learn, except in a hands-on way or in the context of a relationship. One patient comes to mind, the professor of medicine has said to me: "Sacks, there is a delirium in room 6. Go see it." He felt that this would; this sort of talk is common in hospitals, one has 'the appendix in room 8', this was 'a delirium in room 6'; there was no mention of the person who had the delirium. ("Dr Oliver Sacks – Narrative and Medicine")

Central to Sacks's idea of what Sayantani DasGupta has called "narrative humility" (2006) is the idea of bearing witness. It is this idea, closely connected as it is to the idea of listening, which encapsulates the gist of Sacks's understanding of the interplay between narrative and medicine: "In a 1989 interview on *The MacNeil/Lehrer News Hour,* Joanna Simon asked Sacks 'how he would like to be remembered in 100 years,' the *Times* reports. He responded, 'I would like it to be thought that I had listened carefully to what patients and others have told me, that I've tried to imagine what it was like for them, and that I tried to convey this. And, to use a biblical term, bore witness'" (Ring n. pag.). It is in this sense that, if indeed we understand Sacks's gesture as the practice of narrative in medicine, there is a threefold development here. First, the physician divests himself of his medical diagnostic authority and becomes simply a listener; second, he listens to the patient-autobiographer's voice *with his diagnostic categories suspended.* Third, he proceeds to revise these diagnostic categories on the basis of Temple Grandin's narrative.

Where Sacks's work is so exemplary for the dialogue between life sciences and life writing which I am trying to envision in this book, then, is in the way he transforms the patient account or "case history" (Couser, *Vulnerable Subjects* 75) into a narrative akin to literature; he is hence acutely aware of the fact that patient accounts constitute autobiographies and forms of life writing in their own account. As Thomas Couser has noted, "As a neurologist, [Oliver Sacks] has created a distinctive ethos and even, one might say, a personal medical ethic. As a writer, Sacks is often credited with transforming a clinical genre, the case report (the written version of the case history), into a literary one, and in the process depathologizing his subjects" (*Vulnerable Subjects* 75). The dialogue between life sciences and life writing could not be more powerful here. In this framework, moreover, narrative in medicine is not only a form of medical practice, which Sacks intuitively employs, but it also has profound implications for the theory of illness and health, doctor-patient relationships, and the performance of medical authority. As a doctor turned listener, the physician has become the audience to his patient, who has now become the expert on her own condition – a condition which, in 1986 when Grandin first wrote her autobiography, *Emergence: Labeled Autistic*, was still little understood by biomedicine. Sacks, on the other hand, is quick to admit the deficiency of his own medical knowledge, and the extent of which deficiency was only made clear to him through Grandin's account. This account, in turn, had been able to emerge only when Sacks divested himself of his medical authority in the first place. The space which emerges here is that of a physician who is willing to enter the spaceship on the alien's terms: In fact, because the physician enters the room or the spaceship not as a diagnostician or an ethnographer, but simply as a listener, the human/alien dichotomy is suspended in the very act of listening. It is here that the logic of the cartoon has been fundamentally reversed. The doctor may have entered the spaceship, but he has done so without his protective gear.

4.3 An Anthropologist on Mars

How, then, does Grandin inhabit this space newly created by Oliver Sacks, the physician who has come to be her audience? The narrative stance which Grandin proceeds to assume, I would argue, could not be more powerful in its ironic reversal of the hierarchy embedded in the medical situation. In a powerful reversal of the doctor-patient-relationship, Grandin proceeds to turn the doctor into the alien who is now studied by the patient. Describing to Sacks and the general audience reading her book what it is like to live with autism, she describes herself as an "anthropologist on Mars" (Cohen n. pag.).

In order to make her way in the world of non-autistics, Grandin writes in *Thinking in Pictures,* she had to study non-autistics, alien as they might seem to her, as would an anthropologist on Mars. It is this image, the image of an anthropologist on Mars, through which she proceeds to turn the medical diagnostic framework captured in the cartoon upside down. Implicit in Grandin's image of herself as an anthropologist on Mars are two perspectives, one superimposed on the other. In this superimposition of perspectives, Grandin can be said to occupy both the position of the alien native and the human scientist at once.

First, in employing the idea of the anthropologist on Mars, Grandin can be said to embrace the human/alien dichotomy which she knows will accompany the encounter between autistics and non-autistics. Grandin could hence be said to employ what in the context of racial difference, American sociologist W.E.B. Du Bois has called the framework of double consciousness: In this double consciousness of autism, Grandin looks at herself the way she knows those without autism will look at her. She looks at herself, as it were, through a non-autistic gaze. It is this assuming of a "human" gaze which enables her to understand why others think of her as "alien." Growing up, Grandin recalls, she was well aware of how alien she appeared to her fellow students: "When I was a teenager I was called 'tape recorder' because I used scripted lines. As I gained experience, my conversation became less scripted because I could combine new information in new ways" (*Thinking in Pictures* 32). Similarly, Grandin describes the painful and painstaking ways in which she set out to teach herself "normalcy"; the ways she stored images and scripts in her head and then proceeded to copy them in her own actions: "The thing about being an autistic . . . I had to learn social skills like being in a play. We just have to learn it" ("The World needs all kinds of minds").

The reference to both irony and social skills is remarkable here, and it is remarkable for two reasons. First, it implies Grandin's knowledge of the fact that in a world of non-autistics, she might indeed seem alien; and second, because through an astonishing act of perseverance and self-discipline, she set out to learn the ways of those who had been deemed, by medical discourse and public opinion alike, more human than herself. What emerges here is a scenario in which the alien is aware of the response which her presence will trigger in the eyes of the humans, a response which she sets out to subvert by teaching herself the ways of "humanity."

Because, through the gift of medical double consciousness, Grandin knows how others will perceive her and what they find alien in her behavior, she can go on to disprove this alienness step by step. Again referring to the context of Africa American resistance to racism, then, Grandin can be said to use the master's tools to dismantle the master's house, to use Audre Lorde's memorable formulation. First, she knows that she will have to prove what Houston Baker has termed a "mastery of form": She knows, quite simply, that in order to no longer be called a tape recorder, she will have to use, not only inflection, but irony. She knows, in other words, that a supreme and a *human* mastery of language will be ascribed to her only once she can employ not only connotation, but *irony*. It is through the use of irony, then, that she disproves her alleged lack of humanity, her alienness in a world of non-autistics. As in other cases, it is Oliver Sacks, as Grandin's most devoted reader, who vouches for the success of this feat not only of narrative, but of the logic of ableism.

One of Grandin's most powerful gifts, not coincidentally, has been her irony, an irony that as she herself admits in *Thinking in Pictures,* persons with autism do not really possess. It is this sense of irony that is also apparent in an interview which Temple Grandin gave at a TED event in California:

> MODERATOR: You know you once wrote – I like this quote – "If by some magic autism had been eradicated from the face of the earth, then men would still be socializing in front of a woodfire at the entrance to a cave."
>
> GRANDIN [*turning to the audience*]: Who do you think made the first stone spear? It was an Asperger guy. And if you were to get rid of all the autism genetics, there would be no more Silicon Valley, and the energy crisis would not be solved. ("The World needs all kinds of minds")

Not only did Grandin's narrative thus prove that there was an inside to her mind, but the full humanity of this mind was constituted by the ability not only of conveying, but of *playing with* meaning. This was an ability, moreover, which, given her condition, had not come naturally to Grandin, but which she had painstakingly taught herself over the years. As Sacks is quick to note, in this irony as well, Grandin sets out to disprove medical characterizations of herself: "But many sorts of humanness have become available for Temple in the past ten years. Not least among these is a capacity for humor and even subterfuge which one would have thought impossible in someone who is autistic" (Foreword xvi-xvii). Yet, the notion of humanity is double-edged here: Even as there is solace in the idea that Grandin is able to prove her own humanity by demonstrating her ability to be ironic, and even as Sacks recognizes this achievement, both Sacks and Grandin leave the notion of normality embedded in this definition of the human intact. It is in this assumption, then, that notions of normality are subverted and confirmed at the same time. As Thomas Couser puts it, "Sacks seems reluctant to deconstruct received notions of normality – despite his own provision of cases that cry out for it – and he seems not much interested in the ways in which disabilities . . . may have cultural value" (*Vulnerable Subjects* 122).

Through mastering the use of irony, then, Grandin has succeeded in proving her own humanity. However, what is so remarkable about her narrative strategy is that she is not content with only proving her own humanity, but that she goes on to turn this humanity on its head by proving that those we deem human may in fact be the aliens. It is in this stance, the stance of an anthropologist on Mars, that she turns the power dynamics often embedded in the medical diagnostic framework on their head. As an *anthropologist on Mars*, she, as a person with autism, is indeed an alien who has come to study the humans. Crucially, however, Grandin does *not* say that as a person with autism, she feels that she is like a Martian among humans, but, rather, that she is an *anthropologist* on Mars. It is Grandin, then, who is the scientist here, a scientist who has come to study the natives – those living without autism – in their natural habitat. The reversal of the cartoon could not be more complete. It is the former patient who has become the scientist, with an authority of her own. It is she, then, who is a scientist in a twofold sense: first, as an expert on her own condition, which at the time that Grandin wrote her narrative, was little understood by medical science; and second, as an (autistic) anthropologist having set out to study the curious ways of the human natives.

Since it is Grandin who has now assumed the role of the scientist, moreover, Sacks the physician has been turned, if not quite into a patient, then at least into a native to be studied by the scientist/ethnographer. What I believe is so groundbreaking about Sacks's gesture of becoming a listener, a person who bears witness, is his willingness to be studied by Grandin, the anthropologist on Mars. In this unusual scenario, it is the physician himself who has become the object of scientific knowledge.

In this signature moment, Sacks, the physician, willingly turns himself into the alien who is now being studied by Temple Grandin, the autistic anthropologist. In this unusual situation which turns the medical scenario on its head, the native doctor looks at the patient ethnographer looking at him: The doctor, however, is quite at ease with having become the object of study. What Sacks emphasizes is his awareness that this change in hierarchy is necessary for an alternative knowledge to emerge. This alternative knowledge can be achieved, Sacks implies, only if the doctor recognizes, in the patient's gaze, his own alienness. Only if the doctor looks at himself through the patient's eyes and realizes how alien he must seem, will he be able to suspend his own categories of Otherness which he had previously employed looking at his patient. As Sacks writes, "And we get a glimpse – this perhaps the least imaginable of all – of her total bewilderment about other people's minds, her inability to decipher their expressions and intentions, along with her determination to study them, study *us*, our alien behaviors, scientifically and systematically, as if (in her own words) she were 'an anthropologist on Mars'" (Foreword xv; emphasis added). The physician's willingness to be studied, then, cannot be overemphasized here. The entire framework is now viewed and described from the perspective of those inhabiting and controlling the spaceship, it is the doctor who has become the alien; the humans, in other words, are those who had previously been considered alien by the medical authority of the doctors in spaceships.

Where the encounter between Temple Grandin and Oliver Sacks is so exemplary for a suspension of Otherness in medicine, I believe, is that each is able to occupy, if only temporarily, the place of the other. To speak only of a theory of mind would fall short of capturing the complexity of this encounter, and the role of narrative knowledge in it. In this encounter, both Grandin and Sacks occupy both the positions of human and alien at one and the same time. Sacks is aware that prior to the emergence of her voice and hence the proof of the inside of her mind, Grandin as a person with autism had indeed seemed alien to him. As he gains an insight into her mind, however, he is aware of how alien he will seem to her, with his strange, non-autistic ways of thinking. Grandin, on the other hand, had slowly taught herself to understand why she had always seemed alien to those around her. In order to understand her own alienness as seen from their perspective, however, she first needs to study and master their strange ways of being, thus becoming a scientific observer herself.

What is thus so striking about Grandin's narrative, however, is that she succeeds in turning the very concept of "weirdness" and the idea of normalcy on its head. It was Grandin herself, she recalls in her autobiography, who would go on to study the natives she was surrounded by; and it was she who became a scientific observer. As she recalls about her high school years, "When other students swooned over the Beatles, I called their reaction an ISP – interesting sociological phenomenon. I was a scientist trying to figure out the ways of the natives. I wanted to participate, but I did not know how" (Grandin, *Thinking in Pictures* 153). As Grandin illustrates both in her autobiographical prose and in lectures she gives touring around the country, she found herself surrounded by social clues she was unable to decipher. When the people she was working with were "rolling their eyes" when she spoke, she recalls, she was at a loss to know what this meant. It was these alien social cues, then, that she proceeded to study like an anthropologist on Mars. In this scenario which turns the concept of normalcy upside down, it is her colleagues who have suddenly become the aliens:

> When it comes to figuring out social interaction it's sort of being an anthropologist on Mars. Because when I was younger, we didn't have all the books that explained, you know, all the facial expressions. I didn't know what rolling the eyes meant. You know, these little eye signals. I didn't even know that people had these secret eye signals until I read about them when I was fifty years old in Simon Baron-Cohen's book *Mind-Blindness*. . . . Maybe not being able to recognize little things like eye-rolling actually helped. I think it did, because I think in most of the other feed guards I went to where I was not kicked out there was plenty of eye-rolling and stuff like that but they allowed me to stay, but I just didn't pay attention to the subtle social signals that they disapproved. ("Anthropologist on Mars")

Who, Grandin asks in this interview, is weird here? Grandin's narrative is hence the beginning of a new perspective on autism, a change in perspective that her autobiography *Thinking in Pictures* was instrumental in bringing about.

4.4 Autobiography as a Brain Scan of the Self

What is so central to Grandin's groundbreaking work, then, is that she writes about herself – a person with autism – from the perspectives of both the first and the third person. Not only does she study, as an autistic anthropologist on Mars, the curious ways, habits and ticks of the human native, but she is simultaneously aware of how odd she will seem to these natives. Assuming both a first and a third person perspective, then, Grandin is both the anthropologist and the native, continually taking turns with herself. It is in this sense that her autobiography, *Thinking in Pictures*, can be read both as a first-person account of what it was like to grow up with autism in the 1950s, and a medical history of the ways in which diagnoses of autism have changed over time. It is by pointing to the fallibility of diagnostic categories and their historical changeability that Grandin implicitly decenters medical knowledge, entering into a dialogue with the DSM and diagnosing herself as she knows medical practitioners would have done at various points in the history of medicine: "If I were two years old today, I would be diagnosed with classic Kanner's syndrome, because I had delayed abnormal speech development. However, as an adult I would probably be diagnosed as having Asperger's syndrome, because I can pass a simple theory-of-mind test and I have greater cognitive flexibility than a classic Kanner autistic" (*Thinking in Pictures* 49-50). Grandin knows that she possesses the ability to develop a "theory of mind," of imagining another person's perspective to an extent that a person with autism is often deemed incapable of. As a form of life writing, *Thinking in Pictures* is thus also a self-diagnosis. Time and again, Temple Grandin, who holds a degree in psychology, diagnoses herself in medical terms, but she then goes on to disprove this diagnosis by teaching herself skills that medical opinion deems beyond her reach. *Thinking in Pictures*, in this sense, is not only a stunning autobiography written by a person with autism, but also a highly ironical narrative.

Yet, Grandin takes the act of writing about herself in the third person one step further: At a recent lecture, she proceeds to show the audience a brain scan of herself:

> I got to have this brain scan done several years ago. And I used to joke about having a gigantic internet trunk like going into my visual cortex. [*pointing to the slide behind her*] This is Tenser imaging and my great big internet trunk line is twice as big as the controls. The red lines there are me and the blue lines are the sex and age matched control. [*switching to the next slide*] And there I got a gigantic one and the blue control as a really small one. And some of the research now is showing that people on the spectrum actually think with primary visual cortex. ("The World needs all kinds of minds")

It is here that Grandin can be said to assume three different perspectives at once. First, as a psychologist, she points to the fact that behavioral psychology has not been enough to understand or treat persons with autism and that recent research has stressed the necessity of bringing together classical psychology and brain science, as in the field of biological psychology. Second, referring to the use of imaging techniques such as Diffusion Tensor Imaging to provide an insight into the biological differences in the autistic brain, she uses imaging to describe the autistic brain from the third person perspective of the life sciences, particularly the neurosciences; and third, from a first person perspective, she proceeds to inform the audience that this autistic brain shown on the Power Point slide behind her is her own. In this superimposition of perspectives, then, Grandin can be said to be not only an anthropologist on Mars studying the alien ways of the humans, but she has simultaneously become an anthropologist or rather, a brain scientist of her own mind. Brain science has provided her, she stresses, with ways of understanding mechanisms of her own thinking (especially her thinking in visual terms) that she had previously been at a loss to explain. My point here is that Grandin's narrative stance here encapsulates four paradigm shifts at once. First, in the remarkable multiplying of perspectives, autobiography has become a brain scan of the self. Second, at this juncture in the history of medicine and the history of autism, Grandin's writing, as early as in *Thinking in Pictures*, published in 1995, anticipates the current emergence of fields such as biological psychology. It is hence noteworthy in this context that Eric Kandel, the founder of biological psychiatry, would be awarded the Nobel Prize for Physiology only in 2000. Third, in anticipating fields such as biological psychology, which set out to bridge the humanities and the life sciences, Grandin creates a dialogue between life sciences and life writing which could not be more memorable. And fourth, in creating this dialogue, she is able to bridge first person and third person perspectives. Prior to the possibility of brain imaging and the emergence of new brain imaging technologies, then, Grandin would only have been able to describe what Onur Güntürkün has called the "abstract level of thinking" ("Onur Güntürkün: Der Natur Fragen stellen"; my trans.), but she would have been unable to either understand the full complexity of her own thought processes or the ways in which, in the autistic brain, such thought processes are being generated. The knowledge gained through brain imaging and recent brain research, then, provides Grandin with an explanation for the thought processes in her own mind that she had previously only been able to describe through metaphors. It is the emergence of neuropsychology and neuropsychiatry, then, which enables her to link the metaphorical (her description of the workings of her mind) to the biological (an understanding on how her brain works). It is in this sense that *Thinking in Pictures* can be read both as an autobiography and a medical history charting the development of diagnoses of autism. In this medical history, Grandin anticipates, in 1995, the emergence of new fields such as biological psychology and neuropsychiatry.

Grandin invents or points to the necessity of fields such as biological psychology, however, not in an academic article but in a piece of life writing, an autobiography. Yet, the fact of anticipation remains: only if we refuse to separate life writing from life sciences, to separate autobiography from an academic paper on brain research, will we be able to grasp the full extent of Grandin's prophetic vision. It is this vision, I have tried to argue, which is recognized by Oliver Sacks's framing of Grandin's first and second autobiographies. What Sacks recognizes is that Grandin's work can be read both as life writing and as life science.

4.5 Beyond Space Odyssey

What remains for us to ask is whether this groundbreaking reversal of perspectives, the co-construction of knowledge, which depended on the mutual dialogue between an unusual physician, Oliver Sacks, M.D., and an autistic psychologist, Temple Grandin, can be true of and can be applied to other contexts within biomedicine as well. My aim in this paper has been to inquire into a framework in which such a reversal is possible. What, indeed, is Other in medicine and who is studied by whom?

What Sacks's foreword ends with, then, is not a dismissal of Otherness, but its redefinition: As Sacks is quick to acknowledge, Grandin's narrative, and her mind, will remain different; but as he immediately goes on to say, it is by no means "Other" is a sense as fundamental as medical science had believed it to be prior to the publication of *Emergence: Labeled Autistic*, in 1986. Where I would like to return to the initial discussion of Otherness in medicine, then, is in the recognition emphasized by Sacks. There is a sense in which, being autistic, Grandin's difference will remain; the Otherness, in other words, may be constituted not only by the physician's diagnosis, but by the condition itself. What is different, on the other hand, and what has to change, as Sacks emphasizes, is the relationship between doctor and patient which emerges from this difference. There can be no closure to this narrative about difference; the only closure available, Sacks emphasizes, lies in the need for a constant change in perspective: Time and again, sides have to be reversed in which the doctor and the patient takes turns in being the alien. Sacks writes,

> If Temple is profoundly different from most of us, she is no less human for being so, but rather, human in another way. *Thinking in Pictures* is finally a study of identity, the "who-ness" no less than the "what-ness" of a most gifted autistic person. It is a deeply moving and fascinating book because it provides a bridge between our world and hers, and allows us a glimpse into a quite other sort of mind. (Foreword xviii)

The "otherness" which Sacks refers to in this passage, then, is not capitalized; it is an otherness in degree, never in kind; it is an otherness which has nothing to do with the aliens, an otherness which can be found in a world where physicians and patients are living on the same planet and a spaceship is nowhere in sight.

The solace of this encounter, I have tried to argue in this chapter, lies in this utopian turn-taking, in which both the doctor and the patient get to be the anthropologist on Mars: Each of these participants knows how alien he or she will appear to the other; but they also know that this otherness is not to be feared. It is never an Otherness with a capital "O." There are no aliens here, and the only otherness which exists is that of a difference whose knowledge the physician and his patient set out to co-construct. In this instance, unlike in the carton, the medical encounter is by no means, to quote David Bowie, a space odyssey. Even if the medical condition at stake – autism – is to some extent, alien to both the physician and the patient, they each take turns in being the expert. Each of these two – the medical practitioner and the person with autism – in turn gets to be the anthropologist studying the native. The autistic observer studies the alien ways of humans rolling their eyes; and the non-autistic physician marvels at a brain whose mechanisms are so different from, and in some ways far superior to, his own. In this turn-taking which is certainly unique in the history of autism, both the physician and the patient at times get to be the "anthropologist on Mars." The spaceship, on the other hand, is only the location of the humanity which we all share.

4.6 Against the Biomedicalization of Culture?

So far, this chapter seems to have been rather welcoming of what may be termed a "biomedicalization of culture." In the subchapters above, I have been intrigued by and welcoming of the roles played by both Oliver Sacks and Temple Grandin in what I have read as a dialogue between life sciences and life writing. In this last part of the chapter, however, I would like to take up what I see not only as loose ends to my initial arguments, but rather, counter-narratives which would seem to eclipse the very argument from within. At the intersection between life writing and forms of agency in a biomedical context, both Sacks's and Grandin's roles have elicited not only praise and recognition, but also controversy. Thus, some critics have claimed that Sacks exploits patient narratives as mere freak shows, parading examples of "abnormality" in front of a mainstream audience whose normalcy is hence confirmed (Couser, *Vulnerable Subjects* 75). As Couser goes on to observe, then, the danger of Sacks's appropriation of patient narratives is most acute where these patients cannot represent themselves (*Vulnerable Subjects* 75). It is this absence of representation, then, which is emphatically different from what I have read as a dialogue between Oliver Sacks and Temple Grandin: In this context, Sacks's personal stance as a neurologist turned listener creates a space and critical framework for Grandin's own voice to emerge. This shift, I have suggested, is key for the third person narrative of the life sciences and the first person narrative of patient account/autobiography to enter into a dialogue with each other. It is this necessary fusion of perspective, then, which Couser refers to as the telos in the work of Oliver Sacks. He writes,

> It may be, however, that the full undoing of the metonymic imperialism of the encasement of people with neurological conditions can be accomplished only by those subjects themselves – through first-person testimony – or by those who know them more intimately than Sacks's house calls permit. Perhaps, as a physician first and foremost, Sacks cannot be expected to produce genuine biography without a trace of pathography – that is, narrative entirely free of medical perspective. (Couser, *Vulnerable Subjects* 121-22)

As I have tried to argue in this chapter, then, there is in Sacks's writing about Temple Grandin's work precisely that essential gesture to what lies beyond the medical gaze. Sacks is a neurologist, in other words, who in his narratives constantly gestures to what is beyond neurology. It is in this sense that it is so significant that Sacks himself, explicitly taking up Grandin's image of an "anthropologist on Mars," has termed himself a "neuroanthropologist" (qtd. in Couser, *Vulnerable Subjects* 122): This reinvention of the neurologist as a neuroanthropologist, I believe, is significant for a variety of reasons. First, it can be read as a complete reversal of what Couser terms the "metonymic imperialism" of the clinic, in which identity is constructed solely on the basis of a biomedical framework (*Vulnerable Subjects* 122): In this reversal of perspectives, the neurologist reinvents himself in the terms prescribed by his patient; it is Grandin, in other words, who supplies to Sacks a terminology in which to reinvent himself. This act of renaming, then, could not be more crucial for an analysis of a potential dialogue between life sciences and life writing. Moreover, there is at the core of Sacks's version of neuroanthropology the same idea of "taking off the space gear" which I have explored above: What is at stake is the explicit and material act of the neurologist's leaving the clinic and venturing into the unknown terrain of the patient's everyday life. It is this immersion into the patient's everyday routine and his or her surroundings which has also been key to the work of Deepu Gowda in the context of narrative medicine ("Bearing Witness to Yourself"). According to Couser,

> Oliver Sacks should be credited with seeing and showing that the representation of neurological anomaly can take the form of ethnography rather than pathography. He has gone a considerable distance toward demonstrating what neuroanthropology might look like in practice. For example, immersion in a community of people with a neurological condition should erase or at least erode the power differential that obtains between neurologist and patient in the clinic. (*Vulnerable Subjects* 122)

In Couser's reading of him, then, Sacks has transformed the clinic from within; and he has done so by reading patient accounts and case histories as autobiographies in the full sense of the term. It is this vision of life writing beyond the medical gaze which makes his work so exemplary for any discussion of a dialogue between life sciences and life writing.

If Sacks's work has generated considerable controversy, this is even truer of Temple Grandin. I believe that Temple Grandin's work can be located at a critical and highly controversial juncture at the intersection between life writing and life science. Her work has been highly controversial for a number of reasons. First, through her writing on autism, she has herself become a celebrity: Not coincidentally, her life has recently been turned into a motion picture in 2010.[1] This celebrity status, of course, comes at a price for the representation of autism in the public sphere. This dilemma has been true of all forms of minority representation: If a certain author is taken by public discourse to be a spokesperson for the community she comes from, this may lead to a disenfranchisement of other parts of the community; the problem, in short, is what Linda Alcoff, in another context, has called "the problem of speaking for others." Precisely because what is at stake is the autism *spectrum*, then, Grandin as a "high-functioning" person on this spectrum, may have come to be understood as the yard stick against which all others on the spectrum come to be measured. Even more problematically, as a narrative about cognitive difference,[2] Grandin's autobiographical accounts may in fact correspond to what many critics, above all Leonard Davis, have termed heroic narratives: by informing her audience in minute detail of the ways in which she has succeeded in overcoming the obstacles arising from her condition, Grandin seems to have signaled to the public that cognitive difference is really only an obstacle to be overcome through hard work and self-discipline. There is hence a certain closure to both Grandin's autobiographies and her representation of her own biography, a closure which may be far beyond the reach of most individuals on the spectrum. In this context, it is also significant that Asperger's syndrome has itself dropped out of the most recent DSM, thus depriving Grandin, according to some critics, of the very legitimation for representing persons with autism.

Moreover, Grandin's references to and embracing of biomedicine, about which, in the passages above, I have been highly positive, have also been very controversial. This is a debate, however, which has also been at the heart of disability studies. As I have suggested in the preface,

[1] The "biopic" *Temple Grandin* was directed by Mick Jackson and produced by HBO.

[2] Throughout this study, my distinction between illness, disability, impairment and difference, has been informed by my discussions with Danielle Spencer, who argues that "difference" may be understood as an umbrella terms under which other concepts, such as disability or impairment, may be subsumed and investigated in relation to one another. See also Spencer, "The Art of Medicine."

some proponents of disability studies argue that disability is, first and foremost, a social impairment: In this view, disability arises from society's reluctance to accommodate and become accessible to different bodies. These bodies' differences or the physical or biological causes for their differences are hence seen as secondary to the changes which societies have to make. Yet, other critics such as Hille Haker have suggested that a progressive vision of disability can only lie in linking an awareness of both social and physical constraints which persons with disability have to face (77).

What, then, has been Temple Grandin's role in this discussion of difference? What has been especially controversial in this context has been Grandin's conviction that there is a genetic cause to autism; her view has been criticized by the autism community as a reduction of autism to biological and above all, to genetic causes. Moreover, critics have cautioned that Grandin's emphasis on the dichotomy between "high functioning" and "low functioning" persons on the spectrum itself plays into an ableist logic. As Lydia X. Z. Brown observes,

> Temple Grandin believes that "high-functioning" autistics are talented, intelligent, and necessary to human survival, while "low-functioning" autistics cannot function or live independently, and thus should be cured in the present and prevented from existing in the future. Both I and others have thoroughly deconstructed the false dichotomy of high and low functioning, but suffice it to say that such claims not only reinforce ableist hegemony, but also reinforce a capitalist notion of success and value in that only people who can produce are worthy of inclusion in society; all others are burdens. (n. pag.)

It is in light of a critique of social usefulness, also, that we may need to revisit the passage quoted above in which Grandin, demonstrating her ability to be ironic, suggests that if autism were to be eliminated from the face of the earth, "there would be no Silicon Valley and the energy crisis would not be solved" ("The World needs all kinds of minds"). Here, too, there is an emphasis on the social and economic usefulness of the autistic subject; a logic which, as Brown suggest, implicitly marginalizes those persons with autism who are not on the high-functioning end of the spectrum. Crucially, the logic of "social usefulness" can also be seen to inform some of Tito Mukhopadhyay's work, and the ways in which his success has been framed by his mother in interviews. What emerges at this juncture is the dilemma between social or economic inclusion and the cost at which such inclusion is achieved. This dilemma is also at the heart of what I am reading as a cognitive citizenship test in Kingsley and Levitz's co-authored autobiography *Count Us In* in Chapter 7. At this juncture, the dialogue between life sciences and life writing may in fact be detrimental: For in order to enter this dialogue, the person engaging in life writing (here, a person on the autism spectrum) has to espouse the language in which such inclusion seems possible. Thus, as I have argued above, Grandin sets out to prove her humanity, but she sets out to prove her humanity in Oliver Sacks's terms. It is owing to this matching terminology, then, that this dialogue (of which the initial part of this chapter has been much more positive) becomes possible. The match in dialogue and in the normative parameters it assumed, however, may at the same time be a severe limiting of agency for the disenfranchised person thus included. It is here, I believe, that the discussion is doomed to be trapped in a dead end. The only way to overcome this impasse, I believe, is to continue to point to its shortcomings: to the problems of assuming a primacy of language and of autobiographical self-representation; to the pitfalls in embracing the terminology which make a conversation with the life sciences possible. Yet, I believe that to be stuck at the opposite end of the dilemma may be equally fruitless: In this sense, the emergence of Temple Grandin's voice can only be a beginning. What historical, social, economic and discursive conditions are necessary, then, for other voices to be heard? As Lydia Brown goes on to suggest, moreover, the focus on Grandin's position as a person on the spectrum may have obfuscated her privilege in terms of social location. As Brown goes on to say, "her experiences are inextricably linked to her race, her class, and the time period during which she came of age . . . " (n. pag.). Brown's critique of Temple Grandin's use of her own biography as exemplary for the autism community is crucial. It is important to note that in order to achieve this entry into "normality," a normality proved through both irony and eloquence, Grandin has certainly benefitted from her social and economic privilege. As a member of a white middle-class community, Grandin had access to speech therapy, and later on, to college education; what is left out of the discussion, then, is to what extent access to forms of therapy, social and medical support make such progress possible in the first place. Grandin's autobiographical narratives run the risk of suggesting that her remarkable progress was based solely on her intellectual abilities; while she does refer to mentors and role models such as her aunt and her high-school teacher, the social and economic underpinnings of her success largely remain unexamined. It is in this sense that Brown rightly suggests that Grandin's narrative be read not only as a narrative about living with autism, but also as a narrative about whiteness and social and economic privilege.

I believe that "the problem of speaking for others" may be at the heart of a dilemma which is ultimately insoluble: For Grandin's own opinion about the causes for autism would not be half as detrimental for the public perception of the entire community of persons on the spectrum were it not for the ways in which her self-representation has circulated in the public domain. As Brown puts it in the above-cited blog, "Because Temple Grandin is functionally the world's only famous autistic person (and certainly the most famous), what she says about autism is taken as gospel, regarded as absolute truth, and frequently generalized as if representative of the experiences and views of every other autistic person on the planet" (n. pag.). If, in other words, other voices of persons on the spectrum were made visible, Grandin's account of causes for autism would be recognized to be what they are: one author's personal opinion. They would not be taken as a pars pro toto for the entire community of people living with autism. It is in this sense, then, that I have included in this discussion of medical humanities in American Studies not only an autobiography by Temple Grandin, but also a collection of poems and prose by Tito Mukhopadhyay, whose location, in many different ways, is vastly different from Grandin's. To return to Grandin's celebrity status, it would, of course, be too simple to argue that a book cannot be blamed for the politics of its circulation; agency ensues from both textual politics and the politics of public reception. At the same time, I think that it is significant that Grandin, throughout her text *Thinking in Pictures*, continues to draw attention to the fact that she cannot claim to represent all persons on the spectrum. For instance, she writes, "More severely impaired people, who can speak but are unable to explain how they think, have highly associational thought patterns" (Grandin, *Thinking in Pictures* 9). While this passage upholds the distinction between "high-functioning" and "low-functioning" autism, it can nevertheless be read as an indication of Grandin's awareness that she cannot assume to speak for the entire autism community. At the same time, I think that it is essential that we take into account the historical moment from which Grandin's work arises. If indeed, following Oliver Sacks's comment, Grandin's writing was able to change medical opinion on autism, then it can be seen as a crucial intervention, by a work of life writing, into the paradigms known at the time to the life sciences. It is the significance of this intervention that I have tried to chart in the first subsections of this chapter. As both Sacks's response to Grandin's writing and Grandin's own autobiographical narrative in *Thinking in Pictures* emphasize, then, the history of autism in the U.S. was also marked by a politics of institutionalization. Arguably, if the politics of institutionalizing persons with cognitive differences is justified by the assumption that the minds of such persons have no "inside," to paraphrase Oliver Sacks, interventions such as Grandin's are indeed indispensable. To argue that Grandin's narratives must by no means be seen as the ultimate telos of the self-representation of the autism community, then, is decidedly different from saying that Grandin's books should never have been written, or should not continue to be read. What is necessary, rather, is the urgency of reading them with both their merits and limitations in mind. If we follow Linda Alcoff's model of the stages involved in "speaking for others," however, this initial phase of making spaces for persons on the spectrum must then be proceeded by the spokesperson's stepping aside.[3] It is this next step of stepping down, it could be argued, which has been prevented by Grandin's assuming a celebrity status. As Thomas Couser notes, then, the double bind between giving a face or voice to a community which would otherwise remain invisible and the spokesperson's assuming celebrity status in the process is ultimately insoluble: "To some, the use of such venerated – and exceptional – figures will seem rhetorically unfair; but the essential division in this dialogue is between those who think of disability in terms of generic conditions "suffered" by nameless, faceless people, on the one

[3] While Alcoff is concerned with the politics of Native American (self-) representation ("The Problem of Speaking For Others"), I believe that the paradigm she outlines can also be applied to other minority contexts. This is by no means to argue, of course, that these different instances of minority representation (the representation, that is, of ethnicity, disability, and cognitive difference) can be collapsed into one another; yet what connects them, I would argue, are the power dynamics and the relationship between minority community and dominant culture.

hand, and those who think of it in terms of actual individuals living with these conditions, on the other" (*Vulnerable Subjects* 195).

At the same time, I am interested throughout this study in the preconditions – historical, cultural, and epistemological – which make a dialogue between life writing and life sciences possible. Such a dialogue is facilitated, I believe, precisely through Grandin's own expertise in the fields of psychology and the neurosciences. It is only through her knowledgeability in the terminology of these fields, it could be argued, that she was able to initiate, in her life writing, a dialogue which depended on medical discourse engaging *with* her self-representation. Here, too, my argument is admittedly circular: A dialogue between life writing and life sciences, and, by implications, between the humanities and the life sciences, seems to be possible only if the former adopt the terminology of the latter. And yet, Oliver Sacks's genuine admiration for Grandin's narrative subjectivity and the personhood which emerges from her narrative, suggests at least a degree of reciprocity. Even if I acknowledge the severe limitations of both Sacks's and Grandin's position, then, it is this reciprocity between life sciences and life writing which remains the utopian telos I would like to envision here.

What is key in this context, I believe, is a dialogue between mind and brain: As Grandin herself has argued, brain imaging techniques may provide, for her own understanding of how her mind works, some way of comprehending what she sees as a "different" mind. Yet, the dilemma of rendering the body or brain of a person on the spectrum translucent (a term I have used with regard to Mikhail Baryshnikov's connecting his own heart to an on-stage monitor), may be a "biomedicalization" of the self. What if, in other words, individuals come to be understood only through brain scans? What if the brain scan comes to replace the autobiography, if the brain comes to replace (an account of) the mind? Yet, in this as in many other instances, I believe that it would be counter-productive, on the part of the humanities, if, for fear of the ways in which a certain (biomedical) paradigm might be used or abused, they refuse to engage with this paradigm in the first place. To argue that brain research must not become the be-all and end-all of the ways in which we define what it means to be human at the beginning of the twenty-first century, is by no means to say that we should simply refuse to say what brain research has to say about the different cognitive mechanisms of the human brain. To continue to argue for the importance of the human mind, in other words, is not to say that there is no brain.

My own reading of Grandin's autobiography *Thinking in Pictures* has been that her vision accommodates both mind and brain, both first and third person perspectives. Such a balance may not be true, however, of the ways in which her argument has come to circulate in the public domain. As some critics have warned, then, it may actually play into a biomedicalization of culture. Yet, following the work of Nikolas Rose and Joelle M. Abi-Rached in *Neuro: The New Brain Sciences and the Management of the Mind* (2013), which I will take up again in my conclusion, I would argue that it would be short-sighted for the humanities not to take recent developments in brain research into account. Precisely by entering into a dialogue with the life sciences, the humanities would not, as some critics argue, jettison their moral function as a commentator on new scientific developments, but they may, on the contrary, be even more mindful of that function. What may be necessary, in other words, is a balanced account of how living with autism may be affected by both social obstacles and physical difference. To speak of such difference, a difference in neurobiology, is decidedly different from neurobiologism, from reducing human behavior to brain functions and brain scans. As I will elaborate in the conclusion to this book, neuroscientists themselves have drawn attention to the fact that they are, as of yet, at a loss to explain the interrelationship between mind and brain, between different brain functions and the unique mind of an individual, which emerges only out of the intersection of biological factors and social environment. Thus, Grandin's autobiographies as well as her public appearances may serve less as a role model for understanding autism – an idea which the first part of this chapter may perhaps run the risk of embracing – than as an exemplary case of representing cognitive difference at a specific historical moment: a historical moment in which the relationship between the life sciences and the humanities may be undergoing a change which seems unprecedented since the initial specialization of both fields in the nineteenth century. It is in this sense, then, that the inquiry into the relationship and potential dialogue between the life sciences and the humanities may be fruitful not only for the field of life writing research, but also for the history of science. Throughout these chapters, one of my aims is to locate narratives of life writing in the history of science by looking at the ways in which they have been read, or not read, by, practitioners in the life sciences. The telos, which any discussion of the intersection between life sciences and life writing has to envision, then, is the striking of a balance between the medical and the social model of disability. What is at stake, as Hille Haker has outlined, is the idea that individuals with disability need to be able to avail themselves of whatever biomedicine has to offer ("Medizinische Hilfe"), while at the same time not subscribing to the biomedical model of "'cure, correct, or eliminate'" (Couser, *Vulnerable Subjects* 164). It is this latter emphasis on what Couser calls a "robust disability narrative [of a] life without cure" (*Vulnerable Subjects* 164) which Grandin's emphasis on the benefits of biomedicine runs the risk of obscuring. Yet, as I have tried to propose in this chapter, there is a difference between referring to the discourse of the life sciences in order to explain the way a different brain works, and of assuming biomedicine to be the sole framework of reference. What is at stake, in other words, is the difference between using biomedicine as an explanatory framework, on the one hand, and the be-all and end-all of describing a life lived with difference on the other hand. What remains central, however, is the ways in which, at the beginning of the twenty-first century, biomedicine cannot be separated from the ways in which we conceive of what it means to be human.

As I will argue in the next chapter on the work of Russian-American dancer Mikhail Baryshnikov, the terminology and the logic of the life sciences has been indelibly inscribed on the ways in which we conceive of our own humanity, and the materiality of our own bodies. Both art and life writing, however, also respond to the nature of such inscription; as I will try to illustrate in the following discussion of Baryshnikov's experiment in modern dance, they can appropriate, resist and reshape biomedical technology in their own turn.

5 "Living Autobiographically" in Modern Dance: Concepts of Aging in Mikhail Baryshnikov's "HeartBeat: mb" Performance

5.1 Biomedicalizing the Artist's Body

In 1998, Russian dancer Mikhail Baryshnikov took a decision which not only seemed far-reaching for the history of dance, but which can also shed light on the question of how "aging" – as the loss, to some extent, of physical capabilities – is incorporated into art. What Baryshnikov did was to connect his body to an on-stage cardiac monitor so the audience could witness, via medical technology, the *limits* of Baryshnikov's physical ability.[1] The graphic image of his heart beat would draw the audience's attention to, rather than conceal, the limits that, at this age, Baryshnikov's body could no longer go beyond. According to Margo Jefferson, in his "HeartBeat: mb" performance, Baryshnikov "is scrupulous about what kinds of movement his body can and cannot – well, what's the right word? Accommodate, endure, master, submit to, express" (Jefferson n. pag.). In "HeartBeat: mb," the physical process of aging, and the limits beyond which the aging body is no longer able to go, is directly inscribed into the performance, rather than being concealed by it.

In a number of ways and for any study concerned with the interface between life sciences and life writing, this performance could not have been more evocative. First, Baryshnikov makes explicit what is in fact one of the biggest obstacles in the realm of sports and physical perfor-

[1] The ideas discussed in this chapter appear, in a different version, in the paper "'Living Autobiographically': Concepts of Aging and Artistic Expression in Painting and Modern Dance," co-authored with Ralf Dahm and Anita Wohlmann.

mance: the loss of capabilities brought about through aging or illness. For any professional athlete, aging seems to be the ultimate sign of physical decay, the gradual decrease (or, in the case of an illness, the sudden loss) of physical faculties which, in the arena of sports competition, can only be comprehended as a decrease in performance and competitiveness. Dance, to be sure, is not only a sport but an aesthetic performance; it links the physical performance, in the utmost disciplining of the human body, to aesthetic performance. Nonetheless, the fact that Baryshnikov should have made explicit the limits of his own physical capability draws attention to the fact that classical ballet, too, is based on physical ability.

What, then, does this chapter have to do with American Studies? Mikhail Baryshnikov's move into modern dance was paralleled, and to some extent informed by, his move from Russia to the West; the North American dance scene, the framework in which he developed a concept which Stanley Keleman has called "aging authentically," was Berkeley, not St. Petersburg. While I would by no means like to imply a teleology here, I am nevertheless concerned with the frameworks in which a given artistic performance – and, in this case, the history of dance – unfolds. As a biography housed on the Kennedy Center website puts it, "Baryshnikov defected from the Soviet Union in 1974 in search for artistic and personal freedom in the West." Moving to Canada and then to the U.S., and becoming a naturalized U.S. citizen in 1986, Baryshnikov has defined himself as a citizen of the world: "I'm Mikhail Baryshnikov and I'm a citizen of humanity, or I hope I'm one" ("Mikhail Baryshnikov: Charity and art video for Citizens of Humanity").

Thus, I am concerned with the role of American Studies with regard to conceptions of interdisciplinarity between life sciences and life writing. Arguably, the field of medical humanities itself has received many of its impetus from research based in the U.S.. Conversely, if American Studies are conceived as a framework which not only investigates U.S. cultural production, but also the scientific and theoretical framework developed by American scholars, then concepts such as Eakins' "living autobiographically," as well as Stanley Keleman's "aging authentically" could also be explored through the framework of American Studies. At the same time, beyond the framework of American Studies, I believe that looking at Baryshnikov dance also has profound implications for studies both of autobiography and of the recording or coping with aging in autobiography.

Not only is this paper thus concerned with concepts of aging in American Studies, but also with the role of dance for autobiography. Crucially, recent studies in the field of life writing have drawn attention to the fact that investigations of the autobiographical mode need to go far beyond the written text; not only can they comprise oral testimonies, but they can also explore performances of the body, and the role of "dance in self-performances" (Hornung xii). One of the aims of this paper is thus to link a consideration of the history of dance – conceived, as Baryshnikov's own vita indicates, transnationally and involving the concept of a transnational American Studies – to a study of autobiography, and the genre of what has been called "age narratives" within this tradition.

Crucially, even before his body started aging, Baryshnikov's physical appearance was cast by classical ballet dance critics in terms of deficiency. He was described as a "short, stocky and quick 'hockey puck'" (Aria, "Nonfiction Book Review: Misha" n. pag.). Clearly enough, it does not bode well for the career of a classical ballet dancer to be compared to a hockey puck. What was worse, these critics held, than a principal dancer who could not tenderly look down on the prima ballerina standing beside him? According to critics, "He was shorter than most dancers, he couln't tower over a ballerina en pointe and was therefore relegated to secondary parts" ("Michael Baryshnikov" n. pag.). From the very beginning, then, Baryshnikov's physical body, the raw material he was to turn into the basis of his art – classical ballet –, seemed to be ill-suited for the endeavor. But it was this very material that Baryshnikov proceeded to work with. As he once put it in an interview, "It's undescribable, you can't ask why a cello player plays his instrument; I'm playing my instrument, my body" ("Mikhail Baryshnikov: Charity and art video for Citizens of Humanity"). If classical ballet is concerned with the perfection, the perfect disciplining, of the human body, then it is significant for the purposes of this paper that Baryshnikov should conceive of "perfection" not as an end result, but a process in and of itself: "Perfection, it's a theory; I think in any failure there are a lot of positive aspects. You cannot be a perfect human being, a perfect artist, a perfect husband, you cannot be a perfect father probably. And probably I'm not, but go through your day with the hope that you will be a little better, in all respects, and do something meaningful" ("Mikhail Baryshnikov: Charity and art video for Citizens of Humanity").

It is this processual understanding of the perfection of the human body that has profound implications, I would like to argue, for the notion of aging. Aging, as it has been traditionally defined, is the very antithesis to perfection; a potential deterioration of human faculties (Kampf and Botelho 2009). Crucially, age studies have long shifted from speaking of "periods in life" (such as childhood, adulthood, old age) to aging as a perpetual process. Baryshnikov's on-stage monitor thus makes explicit the processual quality of aging; it records the process, not the result. Similarly, to conceive, as Baryshnikov does, of the human body as an instrument that is re-tuned every day, at once implies a departure from this conception of aging. What is at stake, rather, is the musician's being attuned to his instrument, to the state that it happens to be in at a given moment in time. It hence comes as no surprise that in the attempt to define Baryshnikov's oeuvre, critics have come up with no bottom line: "He has been, and continues to be, a surprise. He embodies so many different and impossibly beautiful things to so many people that it is next to impossible to define him save to say this: Mikhail Baryshnikov is a dancer" ("Mikhail Baryshnikov" n. pag.). If dance is an art form and Baryshnikov's instrument is his own body, his artistic genius consists in making the form comply to the (limits of the) instrument, and not vice versa.

Baryshnikov's "HeartBeat: mb" performance can hence be seen as the breaking of a taboo: through an on-stage monitor, he makes explicit what is supposed to be hidden from the audience. In making explicit the limits of physical performance brought about by processes of aging, moreover, Baryshnikov deliberately adulterates the genre in which he performs: A cardio-monitor, of course, has no place in a ballet performance. Baryshnikov's "medicalizing" of his own body, whose unruliness the monitor both records and exhibits to the audience, is thus also a deliberate shift in register. The performance of classical ballet has been hybridized through the monitor which is jarringly out of place in a classical ballet performance. Baryshnikov's performance hence plays with, and flaunts, the concept of the inappropriate: a heart-rate monitor is inappropriate on a ballet stage. Yet, this biotechnological inappropriateness – the inappropriateness of technological devices on a stage which is supposed to feature only human bodies – broaches a subject even more tabooed: the assumption that an aging body is inappropriate on a ballet stage. Baryshnikov's involvement with the White Oak Dance Project, then, incorporated "aging" bodies into its very design: "Nevertheless, his fascination with the new has stood him in good stead. As he observed, 'It doesn't matter how high you lift your leg. The technique is about transparency, simplicity and making an earnest attempt.' The White Oak Project was formed to create original work for older dancers" ("Mikhail Baryshnikov" n. pag.). Baryshnikov's making the form of his dance conform to the changed nature of his own body, making the tune fit the instrument so the instrument can excel at playing the tune, has helped shape the history of modern dance. As his biographers have noted, "In 1990, he teamed up with Mark Morris and founded the White Oak Project, a unique dance company that reflects Baryshnikov's passion for modern dance and embodies the extraordinary transformation of a paragon of Russian ballet into the very model of perfection in American modern dance" ("Mikhail Baryshnikov" n. pag.). The inappropriateness of the monitor thus mirrors that of the body it is connected to. Up to this point, then, the inappropriateness of a body that no longer lived up to its prior performance was cloaked only by the fact that this was not just an aging body, but the body of one of the most celebrated dance performers in the world. Baryshnikov's celebrity status as principal dancer thus served to both conceal and excuse his loss of physical capability. His bringing on stage of a heart-rate monitor can thus be seen, at first, as scandalizing the audience's expectations: He makes explicit, visible, what the audience tacitly agreed not to notice.

Baryshnikov's "HeartBeat: mb" performance thus centers on the notion of vulnerability. By biomedicalizing his own body, by showing to the audience what is supposed to be hidden – the limits that the dancer's body, in middle-age, cannot go beyond – Baryshnikov, the celebrity dancer, makes explicit – indeed, he makes both visible and audible – the vulnerability of his body which is due to his human form. As Anna Kisselgoff has written in a New York Times Review of "HeartBeat: mb":

> At the end of the fourth and last solo on the program he is performing this week with a chamber music group, Mikhail Baryshnikov stands alone on the darkening stage at City Center. It isn't a case of me and my shadow but of me and my heartbeat. Suddenly, a conceptual work about a dancer generating sound in front of a sensor that amplifies electrical

> impulses from the brain to the heart becomes a touching study in vulnerability. (n. pag.)

Quite crucially and on a number of different levels, then, "HeartBeat: mb" can be seen as a form of life writing, of the dancer engaging, on stage, in a reflection of his own mortality. Not only does he "medicalize" his own body, then, but he engages in a dialogue with himself – and the audience – of what such medical surveillance – as well as medical self-surveillance – may mean for the conceptions of human lives at the turn of the twenty-first century. As Kisselgoff goes on to say,

> Nonetheless, a solo like "HeartBeat: mb" suggests that mortality is on his mind. Only his cardiologist knows for sure if the crackles, rumbles and beats that accelerate or change in volume, depending on his movement, accurately measure the rhythm of his heart. But for a visibly nervous audience, the solo becomes more than a metaphor for human existence. What if the dancer felt faint or ill? Many another dancer has crumpled onstage, having pulled an Achilles tendon or worse. (n. pag.)

One of the goals of the performance, then, is to unsettle the audience, which is made "nervous" in its inability to decode the signals of the cardiac monitor. What emerges from this connection of the dancer's body to an on-stage monitor, then, is a visual and acoustic depiction of the ways in which the life sciences have come to permeate the ways in which we come to conceive of our lives, but also an addressing of the ways in which we make sense of these inscriptions. The metaphor used by Kisselgoff in her review of "HeartBeat: mb" is a crucial one here: the audience, she implies, is holding their breath, waiting for or at least fearing that the dancer may "crumple onstage." What Baryshnikov does in his performance, then, is to expose this very vulnerability of the dancer's body as one of the most significant taboos in the performance of classical ballet. For the discipline which classical ballet requires, arguably, is that the dancer conceal the vulnerability that his human body makes him prone to, a vulnerability and human fallibility which he must try to transcend at all cost.

It is thus significant that "HeartBeat: mb" should be a solo performance; it is the physical enactment, in the form of modern dance, of a dancer who is contemplating his own mortality. In "HeartBeat: mb", Baryshnikov is looking at his own body, and the ways in which this body has been aging, as if from the outside; an externalizing of the gaze which is also effected through the cardiac monitor. As Eleanor Randolph writes in another review,

> As of this rainy afternoon, Baryshnikov has twice danced a new all-solo program--his first ever--in New York. The notices, just published, are raves, echoes of reviews that accompanied much the same show in Europe last fall. . . . What all the reviews have focused on is the finale of "An Evening of Music and Dance," a work called "HeartBeat: mb" In it, a bare-chested Baryshnikov dances to the amplified sound of his own heartbeat. The audience can not only see his 50-year-old physique (his birthday was last Monday), it can experience his every pulse. (n. pag.)

Many of the narratives which I discuss in this study return, time and again, to the notion of vulnerability. Thus, Michael J. Fox addresses, in both his first autobiography *Lucky Man* (2002) and its sequel *Always Looking Up* (2009), the fears and doubts he was facing when trying to decide whether or not to go public about his Parkinson's diagnosis. It is this vulnerability, then, which Baryshnikov exposes when literally baring his chest. It is this gesture of baring, of laying open and visually exposing the dancer's body, which Baryshnikov's memorable performance can be said to engage in on two levels. On one level, he addresses the fact that at the age of fifty, he is still a sex symbol to a worldwide audience; he is still, in other words, Mikhail Baryshnikov. At the same time, however, – and this is an idea to which I will return in more detail below – the exposing of his bare chest is not only a gesture of masculine self-assurance, but quite the opposite: by medicalizing the audience's gaze onto his bare chest, he addresses the possible "waning" of desirability and the physical prowess of his dancer's body due to age. The audience's gaze, then, becomes that of the cardiologist; and yet, the audience, unlike the cardiologist, cannot decode the signals which the monitor records. Moreover, there is an immediate link which the performance creates between the performer and his audience: both his own body and the body of the spectator, the performance makes explicit, are linked through the vulnerability of their human form. As Randolph states in an interview with Baryshnikov, the audience was worried that the dancer's heart beat was too accelerated, and was reminded of its own vulnerability in the process. Randolph writes, "Yes, on opening night, I thought it couldn't be your heart, it was too fast. People in the audience kept touching their necks to check by comparison" (n. pag.). Thus, by biomedicalizing his own body through an onstage monitor, Baryshnikov has succeeded in making his audience biomedicalize themselves. Not incidentally, as Christopher Janney, the sound engineer who co-created "HeartBeat: mb" and to whom I will return in more detail below, has noted, the device taped to Baryshnikov's chest is originally a biomedical device. According to Janney, "This is actually a device that was developed for biomedical purposes, for post-operative heart patients to be able to get up out of bed and walk down the hall or do various kinds of exercises and not be connected via wires to a normal EKG machine" ("Janney and Baryshnikov" n. pag.). Faced with such biomedical surveillance of the dancer's body, particularly the pace of his heart, the audience is called upon to reflect on what is "normal" and what is not. In fact, the suspense the performance creates stems from the blurring of lines between the normal and the pathological; the audience, mesmerized by the body onstage which it, uncannily, can inspect from within, is not quite sure what this body can endure: "The instrument that is his heart plays more quickly as he moves, which sets an even faster pace for his dancing, which raises his heart beat even more" "Baryshnikov Dancing from the Heart"). In this sense, "HeartBeat: mb" is a dialogue by a dancer with his own heart, a heart which literally enables him to dance in the first place.

In this performance, to use Margo Jefferson's term, Baryshnikov has made his own body "translucent" (n. pag.); he has enabled the audience not only to look at his bare chest, but to see inside it. At the beginning of the performance, the dancer is nervous; it is this nervousness, in turn, which makes the audience hold its breath, unsure, given the medical framework which the performance deliberately creates, whether this accelerated heart beat is due to nervousness or a failure in health:

> BARYSHNIKOV: The heart is attached to your emotions and your mental state, and obviously at this performance, I was a bit nervous. No matter that I was not, you know, breathing deeply. Just [to have] one thought at the beginning of the piece is to push your heartbeat up, and it [was] probably about 150 before I did one step, before one single move.
>
> RANDOLPH: The audience gets inside you in a way. (Randolph n. pag.)

In this sense, "HeartBeat: mb" is clearly the complete antidote to the ideal of classical ballet; not only is it modern dance, with a completely different repertoire and content, but it refuses to uphold the tenet of classical ballet, the axiom that the dancer, in the perfection of his art, transcends the fact that he is merely human. What could be further from this ideal than a dancer who lets the audience see inside his chest, and to witness the beating of his own heart? What is significant here, then, is that Baryshnikov, in his own interpretation of "HeartBeat: mb" goes on to compare this dance performance to a cardiologist's inspection: in both instances, it is vulnerability that is at stake. At the same time, he addresses a question which is crucial in many of the narratives discussed in this study: the fact that the cardiac monitor "objectifies" the patient-dancer's condition. What is so memorable, and so courageous, about Baryshnikov's performance is that he creates a concept which is in fact unthinkable in classical dance: that of the patient-performer. The performer, in the sense of classical dance, is the exact opposite of the patient; he embodies the ideal of human form in the ideal of individual health. Not so in the case of Baryshnikov's performance:

> BARYSHNIKOV: It's an unusual "instrument." When you lie down for a simple cardiology test, you know, you look at those little blue arrows going up and down and this is already a weird feeling--that one thing that actually your heart is producing. Can you imagine a lie detector test? But listening [to] yourself, it is probably even more disturbing than listening to the sound of your voice [on a tape recorder]. It's scary in a way: It's me--no, it couldn't be me. It's the technology which has really transformed my beautiful voice into this ugly, squeaky, illiterate sound.
>
> It becomes a kind of pingpong game, your partial ability to control your heartbeat. You can slow it down with breathing, you know, and exercising, but [onstage] it's more a state of mind than some kind of gimmick . . . and that adds a certain mystery to this piece. (Randolph n. pag.)

What Baryshnikov does in his performance, then, is to point not only to the dancer's mental state in connection to his body's performance – a connection which is made explicit and visible to the audience, through the cardiac monitor, but also the imperfection of his health. What the audience sees on the monitor, holding its breath and comparing the dancer's heat beat to their own, is the arrhythmia of the dancer's heart.

As Baryshnikov goes on to say, "Dancing is very much a reflection of your state of mind in the present--in a split second. [In this piece] you hear the heartbeat [as well as some electrical impulses], and you hear the changes and skips, because I have arrhythmia—it's normal, a lot of other dancers have this, too--and it will say, uh, oops, blip, plop" (Randolph n. pag.). Thus, Baryshnikov deliberately superimposes his medical history – the medical description of the beating and the rhythm of his heart – onto his dance performance, which in turn becomes palpable as a form of life writing. Baryshnikov writes into the performance of "HeartBeat: mb" the medical history of his own heart, as well as the memory of the loss of close friends to heart disease. As he states in an interview,

> It is, however, deeply personal for Baryshnikov, who in recent years has lost several close friends to heart disease – among them the writer Joseph Brodsky and paper company owner Howard Gilman; Baryshnikov named his company after Gilman's Florida plantation. "I have been in hospital after open heart surgeries, and I know people who have lived with heart conditions for many years. And you can't avoid that mortality aspect of it – let's face it, we are all afraid of death." (Kaufman n. pag.)

In his performance, Baryshnikov takes up the materiality of the "open heart" in a way that is much more than metaphorical: Instead, he inscribes the memory of the actual experience of having had to undergo open heart surgery into his art. There is a direct line from his bare chest, the "translucency" of his body, the cardiac monitor, to the recording – through modern dance as a form of life writing – of the experience of open-heart surgery. What "HeartBeat: mb" as a performance dramatizes is the vulnerability of the human dancer to conditions brought about by aging, a vulnerability from which the dancer's body is by no means exempt. As Kaufman goes on to write, "It isn't lost on the dancer that many men his age may also be wearing electrodes – hooked up to a nurse's station, not a stage" (n. pag.).

5.2 Biotechnology as Life Writing

What is remarkable about this passage is that concepts of life writing can be inscribed not only into narratives or dance performance, as in Baryshnikov's case, but also into biotechnology. Thus, an article in MIT News about "HeartBeat: mb" stresses the fact that Baryshnikov's onstage performance may have been a solo performance, but it was also a collaborative endeavor:

> When Mikhail Baryshnikov performs "HeartBeat: mb" this week as part of the White Oak Dance Project, he won't be dancing to classical ballet music by Tchaikovsky or Copland. Instead, he'll be accompanied by sounds generated by his own body through a device created by interactive architecture artist and composer Chris Janney, who received his SM in visual studies from MIT's Center for Advanced Visual Studies (CAVS) in 1978. The bioengineering device, developed by Transkinetics, Inc. captures the electrical impulses to the heart and surrounding muscles via wireless telemetry. Placed on the performer's chest and amplified through filters and a sound system designed by Mr. Janney, the machine provides a percussive track layered over music based on jazz scat and Indian tabla rhythms and Mr. Janney's recitation of medical texts. ("Janney and Baryshnikov" n. pag.)

To be sure, Janney's creation exceeds mere biotechnology, combining technological devices with artistic ones; not incidentally, as the MIT news article points out, Janney had majored at MIT in a very specific and highly interdisciplinary program. If "HeartBeat: mb" is a co-authored performance, then, it is also the writing of Baryshnikov's and Janney's lives, respectively. The tragedy which Janney, the MIT graduate, writes into his part of the performance is the fact that the artificial heart was only developed in 1983; his father, however, died of a heart attack four years earlier. As Janney states in the MIT news interview,

> When I developed the piece, my father had recently died of a heart attack (in 1979) and the Jarvik-7 artificial heart had been invented (in 1983). These coincidental events made me ponder the juxtaposition of the heart as both a sophisticated pump and as the seat of the soul, as we've read in literature and poetry. The medical-text section of the score is about the heart's function as an almost totally sold, anesthetic machine. The other end of the spectrum is the score's inclusion of the music

> of Barber and the whispered track singing jazz scat phrases. The heart is really a machine that gives life, just as rhythm is the foundation of life. ("Janney and Baryshnikov" n. pag.)

The beating of a human heart thus plays a specific role in both Baryshnikov's and Janney's life; both these meanings converge in "HeartBeat: mb" as a dance performance in which life sciences meet life writing in a very specific way. What Janney's contextualization of the history of his part of the performance piece reveals, however, is that the very dichotomy implied in the opposition between life sciences and life writing may be a misleading one. As his account of the relevance of "HeartBeat: mb" for the writing of his own life and that of his father implies, lives can also be written through biotechnological innovations; these innovations, can also write or rewrite their creators' lives. What Janney's account of the invention of the artificial heart stresses is the interrelatedness of material science, biomedical technology, and life writing. Material science invents new materials which can then be incorporated into biomedical technology; indeed, some of these new materials make new technologies possible.[2] At the same time, the invention of these materials and their incorporation into medical technology can in turn be seen as a form of life writing. For Janney, the impetus for trying to create new technology was profoundly interconnected with his own life and his relationship to his father. In the interface between life sciences and life writing, then, lives can be written and re-written not only through biographical accounts, but also through the invention of new materials and new biomedical technologies. This idea is intriguing in that it complicates the very opposition between life sciences and life writing, as it proliferates the meaning of each of these fields. First, the notion of the life sciences is extended towards the investigation of new materials; second, the definition of life writing is extended from the textual or narrative (life writing as autobiography) to the inclusion of biotechnological invention as a form of life writing. Such an inclusion, I would like to argue here, has profound consequences not only for the forms and genres which may be investigated under the rubric of "life

[2] See, for instance, Christof Niemeyer et al., "Nanopartikel, Proteine und Nucleinsäuren."

writing," but also for the relationship of life writing research to science and technology studies.

It is in this context that the concept of life writing may prove especially fruitful to an investigation of the nexus between life sciences and life writing. Life writing research opens up new avenues for the humanities precisely in its openness to a variety of different genres. Thus, dance can also be seen as a form of life writing. This idea can be seen to take very specific shape in Baryshnikov's "HeartBeat: mb" performance, which explicitly addresses the interface between life sciences and life writing in a variety of ways: by calling attention to the aging process from which the dancer's body is by no means immune, and by exploring a particular sense of haunting: the haunting, to use Carlson's term, of the male virtuoso[3] of modern dance by the classical ballet dancer. It is this layering of ghosts and of ghostings that Baryshnikov deliberately inscribes into his performance. Yet, like Michael J. Fox, in a way which I will discuss in the following chapter, Baryshnikov refuses to conceal or deny this haunting: Unlike Nureyev, he does not deny that his present-day self, at the age of fifty-one, cannot quite live up to the "ghost" of his previous self. What Baryshnikov's "HeartBeat: mb" performance can be said to do, then, is not only that he engages, quite literally, what Marvin Carlson has called the concept of the "haunted stage" (here, the haunted stage of classical ballet), but that he includes the concept of aging in this performance of haunting. What Baryshnikov's "HeartBeat: mb" performance may add to Carlson's understanding of ghosting may be the "authorship" of ghosting by the dancer or actor himself. Carlson, exploring the idea of the audience's reception of a given performance by a stage actor, argues that the audience will superimpose their memory of this actor's previous performances onto his current appearance on stage. What Baryshnikov adds to this notion of audience reception, I would argue, is that he deliberately engages this superimposition for the purposes of his "HeartBeat: mb" performance. He is aware that the audience will superimpose on "HeartBeat: mb" the

[3] At the beginning of the twentieth century, the male virtuoso emerged as the male counterpart to the ballerina in classical ballet. The Russian dancer Rudolf Nijinsky is often credited with creating the role and image of the male virtuoso in classical ballet. See Thomas, "Male Virtuosos."

"ghosts" of his previous performances in classical ballet, as the star of the Kirov Ballet. The effect of "HeartBeat: mb," then, also rests on a certain jarring between the original image (or ghost) of classical ballet and the current "HeartBeat: mb" performance. In this performance, "ghosting" occurs on a number of levels: First, the audience recognizes the actor/dancer (Mikhail Baryshnikov) whose current appearance on stage is ghosted by the audience's memory of innumerable previous performances; indeed, it is this ghosting which accounts for Baryshnikov's "star" persona. The White Oak Project largely revolves around his celebrity status as a key protagonist in the history of classical ballet, as a world famous dancer. Second, however, there is a form of ghosting at work in the notion of genres that "HeartBeat: mb" engages. In "HeartBeat: mb," modern dance is "ghosted" by classical ballet. In each of Baryshnikov's moves, the modern dance form is haunted by movements from classical ballet which modern dance cites but alters for its own purposes. Thirdly and finally, "HeartBeat: mb" plays with the "material" or instrument which makes this performance possible: the dancer's own body. It is the dancer's present, middle-aged body which is being ghosted by the body of his younger self; a body whose physical versatility it cannot quite live up to.

While the other chapters in this book may be situated more squarely in the domain of medical humanities, a discussion of Mikhail Baryhshnikov's "HeartBeat: mb" performance at first glance seems to be ill-suited in this context, because the performance has nothing whatsoever to do with illness in the first place. However, I have included this chapter on Baryshnikov's shift from classical ballet to modern dance since the performance, too, talks about the "biomedicalizing" of the artist's body, and the forms in which the body may "write back" at such a biomedicalizing. What is at issue, then, is the ways in which our writing and understanding of our bodies, as the twenty-first century opens, may have been "biomedicalized" to an unprecedented extent.

Yet, Baryshnikov's "HeartBeat: mb" performance can be seen not only as a performance about aging and our conceptions of "aging well," but also as a performance which playfully takes up the entire discourse and practice of medical surveillance and self-surveillance that marks the beginning of the twenty-first century. If our contemporary life-world as well as the market of consumer choices has been swamped with self-tracking devices, it is this "self-tracking" which Baryshnikov playfully incorporates into his performance. Even more ironically, he does so at a time when, in 1998, these self-tracking devices had not yet come into existence. What Baryshnikov's "HeartBeat: mb" performance does, then, is that it anticipates the logic of self-tracking which has come to be the basis of a contemporary debate of the "optimization" of personal health. As Thomas Lemke has argued, part of the discussion around "biological citizenship" involves the fact that we are urged to be responsible guardians of our own bodies, thus preventing potential costs this body – if not carefully monitored – may impose on the social system. According to Lemke and Wehling,

> Yet, it is not only the prioritizing of biomedical knowledge over everyday rationality and cultural values as well as the focus on imperatives of prevention, which may give rise to some misgivings here. Above all, the emphasis on the individual's responsibility for his or her health, especially in the context of the dismantling of systems of social security, triggers existential uncertainties, since the causes of an illness, its treatment, and the costs of treatment are being individualized. (86-87; my trans.)

Baryshnikov's biomedicalizing of his own body, it could be argued, takes up and anticipates this very logic of self-control. The self-control of the artist's body as a dancer and performer of classical ballet mirrors that of the dancer as biological citizen of a world steeped in the personal responsibility of individual health.

What may be at stake when the humanities meet the medical humanities, then, may be a sliding scale of such biomedicalization. As Michael Bérubé writes in his memorable description of his son, Jamie was a "medical narrative" long before he came home from the hospital (x). What reading Mikhail Baryshnikov's performance and Michael Bérubé's written account, not in discontinuity but in continuity with one another may yield, then, is the idea that, in the era of biomedicine, all bodies have become biomedicalized to a certain extent. Indeed, as Bérubé puts it, the biomedicalizing of "disabled" bodies may only make us aware of the degrees to which "normal" bodies, too, have come to be inscribed through biomedical discourse. What taking a look at Baryshnikov's performance reveals, then, is a glimpse into the practices (practices both performative and narrative in scope) through which such a biomedicalization may be resisted, refracted, or reformed. As importantly, Baryshnikov's collaboration with Chris Janney and the technology through which "HeartBeat: mb" is made possible, reveals another layer of life writing. I argue throughout these chapters that life sciences and life writing should not be seen as separate from one another but as mutually constitutive. To look at Chris Janney's coping with his father's death by inscribing the technological monitoring of a human heart into a dance performance, then, may reveal some of the artificiality of separating (medical) technology from life writing, and the productive ways in which each of these spheres may inform the other.

5.3 "On Beauty": The Dancer's Body and the "Human" Form

"HeartBeat: mb," by the bringing on stage of inappropriate objects – above all, a cardiac monitor – signals a shift in register: a shift, indeed, from classical ballet to modern dance. It is this shift in register, in fact, that may have proved to be the saving of Baryshnikov's career: the next logical conclusion following from the inclusion of the heart-beat monitor was not only to make the limits of one's own body explicit, but to respect them: to respect the limits to physical performance brought about by aging processes and to step into a medium in which such processes would be permissible: modern dance. Arguably, in comparison to classical ballet, modern dance privileges the aesthetic over the physical performance.

What "HeartBeat: mb" as a performance of modern dance illustrates is the very dialogue between the art form of dance and the "instrument" which makes this art form possible: the human body. Crucially, this is a dialogue which Mikhail Baryshnikov has engaged in long before he changed the style of his art to classical ballet; precisely because, as I have suggested above, his body did not seem to fit the requirements of classical ballet. He had been faced, since the beginning of his career, with the challenge of how to bend the principles of classical ballet to fit the shape of his own body, not vice versa. He thus had to come to terms with the "material" and the materiality of his body at the very onset of his career. From the very beginning, then, Baryshnikov engaged in a debate over the form of classical ballet and the ideal of the human body that this form seems to imply and perpetuate. Crucially, it is this nexus between dance and the materiality of the dancer's body which Baryshnikov addressed long before he embarked on his second career, shifting from classical ballet to modern dance. While "HeartBeat: mb" makes this debate explicit, it is crucial to note that the antecedents of this debate were present in Baryshnikov's art from the very beginning.

It is this debate, incidentally, which may link "HeartBeat: mb" to other forms of dance which similarly make explicit the link between physical materiality and the form of dance. Crucially, what these performances, diverse as they may be at first glance, have in common is that they can be said to denaturalize the link between the dancer's body as the material of his art and the art form of modern dance or classical ballet itself. It is significant here that the history of Western dance has rendered this very nexus invisible, looking at the dancer's body as a mere vehicle of his art and thus making invisible the requirements which this body has to fulfill. This, arguably, is the ultimate implication of the notion of "discipline" in classical ballet: The dancer must discipline his body to make it fit the ideal of the human body which is inscribed into and required by classical ballet. According to Sabine Kim, "Ballet, as *the* cultural form associated with a strict code of prescribed movements and tableaux, aligns itself with the gaze of the spectator as a disciplinary power, as Christiane Berger has argued. . . . In classical ballet, the purity of the line of the dancer's body is privileged" (144). What is crucial, then, is that Baryshnikov, both in early interviews in which he addresses the "deficiencies" of his own body (his short, "stocky" build), and in the way in which he makes such deficiencies – exacerbated by age – explicit in his "HeartBeat: mb" performance, resists this scripting of the ideal human body by classical ballet. His intervention is crucial in that he reads the human materiality required by classical dance against the grain by making the art fit the instrument and not vice versa.

It is in this context that "HeartBeat: mb" as an alternative performance of human physicality, perhaps counterintuitively at first, can be seen as being in dialogue with other alternative dance forms such as, for instance, Down Syndrome ballet. What is at stake here is *not* the disciplining of one's body as a form of physical and aesthetic performance, but an art form that is more attuned, arguably, to the multiple shapes which human bodies can come in. Otherwise, the very genre of Down Syndrome ballet would be unthinkable. Crucially, the art form of Down Syndrome ballet, developed in the Adaptive Dance Program through a collaboration between the Children's Hospital Boston and the Boston ballet, defies the assumption that the human bodies that classical ballet can be performed by have to conform to expectations of beauty and perfection. Crucially, the incorporation of children with Down Syndrome into the art form of classical ballet can be conceived within the larger framework of what Renato Rosaldo has called "cultural citizenship" (402). The artistic participation mirrors social participation here; if Baryshnikov, the dancer who became, alongside Nijinski and Nureyev, one of the most celebrated dancers of our time, succeeded in his art form despite his seeming physical deficiencies – his "shortness" and his "stockiness" of build –, children with Down Syndrome too claim access to classical ballet as an art form ("Boy With Down Syndrome") for which their bodies have long been seen as "inappropriate."

By the same token, Baryshnikov's deliberate hybridizing of art forms and his shifts in register (from the genre of classical ballet to that of modern dance) is key to any reading seeking to link the life sciences and the humanities, medicine and the arts. If Baryshnikov, the Russian dancer who moved from Russia to the U.S. and from classical ballet into modern dance, conceives of himself as a "citizen of humanity," these children, too, by appropriating an art form that has never included the conception of their own bodies, have become "honest-to-God citizens of our culture." Moreover, as Hans-Ulrich Gumbrecht has argued in a different yet related context, to conceive of Down Syndrome ballet as somehow "inappropriate" or incongruous, is at once to enshrine a particular idea of human beauty and perfection. By contrast, to take Down Syndrome ballet seriously not only as a form of empowerment but an art form in itself, is to profoundly recast concepts of human perfection: According to Gumbrecht, "In order to be able to answer this question, we have to abandon the Appollonian ideal of the human body" ("Körper und Technik" n. pag.; my trans.). What is at stake, then, is the question of the congruence between a given art form and the *bodies* which engage in it. From the view of the art critic, the question is one of appropriateness and of artistic perfection; from the perspective of the dancer – *with or without* disabilities – it is a matter of authenticity.

As I would like to argue here, Baryshnikov's "HeartBeat: mb" performance opens up and participates in recent debates about the bodies suitable for classical ballet. By incorporating into his "HeartBeat: mb" performance the forms in which our bodies have become "biomedicalized," and the ways in which biomedicine has come to hold interpretive power over the meaning of certain lives, Baryshnikov defies such biomedical definitions by opposing them to a different conception of aging and of ability. As dissimilar as Baryshnikov's "HeartBeat: mb" performance may at first seem from the Adaptive Dance Program referred to above, there can nevertheless be said to be a continuum between the two. Both intervene with what they see as the dominant definition of the bodies suitable for classical ballet, a "suitability" which has been defined as the opposite of both age and disability. It is this definition which both Baryshnikov's White Oak Project and the Adaptive Dance Program can be seen to contest.

Moreover, Down Syndrome ballet, too, can be said to deliberately engage – and defy – the notion of "ghosting." Seen through the master narrative of classical ballet, Down Syndrome ballet would be said to be inappropriate, because the bodies which execute the script differ from the ideal human body that a given script in classical ballet has been intended for. It is by insisting on the specificity of their own bodies, then, that the bodies of the dancers of Down Syndrome ballet resist that very scripting, arguing instead for the legitimacy, necessity and urgency of their own bodies to be included in that script. Like Baryshnikov, who, despite the alleged initial "inappropriateness" or lack of suitability of his body for a career in classical ballet, went on to become a world famous dancer, the performers of Down Syndrome ballet go on to master an art form which has implicitly excluded them from the very beginning. What is at stake here, I would argue, is more than the appropriation of an art form by subjects who have been excluded by this art form. Rather, the intervention that Down Syndrome ballet can be said to perform is a much more profound interrogation of the concept of human materiality that can be said to underlie classical dance, and hence also some of the ideal of Western ("high") art.

At the same time, both Baryshnikov's "HeartBeat: mb" performance and Down Syndrome ballet address a question which has been tabooed: the question of the desirability of bodies which have been conceived of as "deviant." One of the questions which Baryshnikov addresses and which he plays with in his "HeartBeat: mb" performance is the relationship between aging and desirability. Precisely by daring to engage the concept of ghosting, by deliberately superimposing the image of his younger self on his present-day performance by his middle-aged body, Baryshnikov dares the audience by asking whether or not his body is still desirable. If age has been conceived as a waning of physical faculties, even a decline of masculinity, then Baryshnikov calls the audience's bluff, knowing full well that his body will still be, to the members of the audience, desirable. As Margo Jefferson has put it, "He was a beauty, in his quicksilver way. And he is still wonderful to look at, but he is fully mortal now. The body seems smaller; the hair has thinned, and the ears are a little big. The intangibles are there in the face: pains, pleasures, responsibilities, things done and not done. Everything leaves its trace" (n. pag.). As Jefferson goes on to note, then, what may be at stake is the concept of what she calls "aging gracefully": embodying the process of aging in such a way that the self is constantly in touch with the material changes of the body in which this self is "housed." She writes,

> 'Aging gracefully' that modest little phrase doesn't begin to capture the shock and struggle involved. ... Performers radically dramatize questions and strategies we all have to maneuver through. What is revealing itself? How does sexual desire play out against the marks of decline and decay? What do you do with the kinds of power that can only be gained once you admit to certain losses? (qtd. in Keleman 1)

By literally baring his chest, Baryshnikov thus urges his audience to define just what they understand by the "beauty" of the male physical form. The desirability of this form, he implies in his "HeartBeat: mb" performance, has to be negotiated against processes of aging, and – as the onstage monitor suggests – possible also by a waning of health. What, Baryshnikov asks by literally pointing at his middle-aged body, does it mean to be physically attractive?

It is in this context, once again, that Gumbrecht has intervened in discussions about the ideals of Western beauty, using the form of photography as a case in point. One of the photographs contained in an article entitled "Bodies and Technique" is an image of the legs of a beautiful woman in a white dress and black high heels; a close-up which evokes what Laura Mulvey has once termed the "visual pleasure" of an image which caters to a male gaze (Mulvey 1975). This image, then, would be a "classical" example of such a male gaze were it not for the fact that on her left leg, the woman is wearing a prosthesis. As the caption reads, this is a photograph of the legs of Viktoria Modesta, who sang at the 2012 London Paralympics dressed as the snow queen. This image, Gumbrecht is well aware, will be seen as the image of a beautiful woman in conventional terms – if it were not, he adds, for the leg prosthesis that the woman is wearing. Thus, Gumbrecht urges us to own up to the physical ideals – the ideal, in this context, of femininity ("Körper und Technik" n. pag.)[4] – which have been enshrined in, and perpetuated by, concepts of beauty. In what way, Gumbrecht dares us to admit, has disability compromised these understandings of ideal female beauty? Is the woman in the photograph, Gumbrecht asks quite simply, beautiful? With regard to media representations of the Paralympics, Gumbrecht writes, "For the erotic appeal of such partial substitution or of such a marking of absent limbs, there are numerous historical examples. . . . At the beginning of a different discussion, what emerges is the question whether there is an affinity of the Paralympic body to the horizon of the Dionysian (and perhaps also, beyond beauty, to the overwhelming effect of the sublime)" ("Körper und Technik" n. pag.; my trans.). This subject, the relationship between disability and beauty, captured in the image of a prosthetic leg in high heels, has long been tabooed. As I will elaborate in Chapter 6 with regard to the self-representation of Michael J. Fox, what is at stake here is the relationship between illness or disability on the one hand and sexual attractiveness on the other. To the extent that, as in the image discussed by Hans-Ulrich Gumbrecht, a prosthetic leg and the image of female beauty are no longer seen as incompatible, we may indeed be witnessing a historical period where, as Leonard Davis has claimed, we have reached the "end of normal" (1).

It is in the sense of these repercussions, I believe, that Baryshnikov's "HeartBeat: mb" performance is central to a contemporary debate which links concepts of age, disability, and beauty; which links Western art – one of whose central concerns, arguably, has been to investigate the concept of the beautiful – to the physical ideal of a (universalized) human body. Baryshnikov's modern dance, Down Syndrome ballet, and the photography cited by Gumbrecht all set out to challenge this ideal.

[4] A further layer could be added to Gumbrecht's discussion here given the fact that the woman in the photograph is a white woman. Whiteness, of course, has also been key to Western concepts of feminine beauty, a fact which has been contested not only by postcolonial writers from the very beginning. See, for instance, Jamaica Kincaid's early postcolonial novel *Lucy* (1990), as well as Zadie Smith's more recent novel, *On Beauty* (2005).

They all intervene into a debate which links the life sciences to a discussion of art, as an expression of human "beauty."

It is thus no coincidence that Baryshnikov, whose exposure of the vulnerability of his own body to processes of aging was considered by critics to have been singularly courageous, addresses the question of disability head-on. His future career, Baryshnikov states in an interview, will depend on the ways he can devise on inventing new art forms for the changing materiality of his own body. As Kaufman writes about her interview with Mikhail Baryshnikov, "He pauses, eyes distant; you wonder if he's having a flash of regret. But he suddenly breaks into a grin. 'Okay, wheelchair! Good idea. I'd like to do one piece just sitting in a chair, just moving arms. Right in front of audience.' It is conceivable that people would fill a theater to see him do this. It is also conceivable that he would make it worth their while" (n. pag.). What Baryshnikov addresses in "HeartBeat: mb" and beyond is no less than an ethics of dance, an ethics, I would argue, which can be situated at the very nexus of life science and life writing. Both, in fact, are inseparable in his "Heart Beat" performance. As Kaufman goes on to quote Baryshnikov, "'Dance is not the peak of physical form – jump, turn, balance and all those elements. Dance is something else,'" he says (n. pag.). Working with the veteran choreographers "'gave me true inside knowledge about what dance, and the ethics of dance, is about'" (Kaufman n. pag.). What Baryshnikov is implying here, then, is that we may come to rethink the very genre or medium of dance precisely through deviant bodies, such as the bodies of veterans; "the ethics of danced" may be captured not by the bodies that ideally fulfill the requirements of dance as an art form – evoking, as Berger has written, the "purity of the line of the dancer's body" (qtd. in Kim 144) –, but by the bodies which are unable to fulfill these requirements. In making us reconsider the link between the genre of dance and the ideal of the human body that this genre can be said to have been premised on, these artists – the members of the Down Syndrome ballet project "Boston Ballet Adaptive Dance Program" ("Boston Ballet – Education" n. pag.) at Boston Children's Hospital and the virtuoso dancer Mikhail Baryshnikov – address a concept which has been problematic in many different contexts, but which may have resurged in the nexus between life writing and life sciences in a new light: the concept of authenticity. While this concept, arguably, has been suspect due to the ways in which it has historically been misused – especially, for instance, in representatives of ethnic groups being urged to convey an "authentic" picture of "their" culture, leading them towards essentializing their cultures and towards a practice of autoethnography[5] –, it has been taken up in a more productive way in discussions of an appropriation, by patient groups, of the medical discourse about their "condition." What Baryshnikov's use of "authenticity" in "HeartBeat: mb" seems to imply, I would like to argue, is the idea of developing an artistic expression which is attuned to the specificity of his own body, and his experience of the way in which this body is aging.

5.4 "HeartBeat: mb" and Notions of Aging

Thus, it seems remarkable that Baryshnikov's scandalous performance should have been taken up by psychosomatic medicine as a key example of the concept of "authenticity," of "aging authentically" or, in Margo Jefferson's terms, of "aging gracefully." Stanley Keleman, founder of the Berkeley Center of Somatic Medicine, has conceived of aging as a perpetual process of the changing of the human body into an evolving continuity of shapes. Keleman writes,

> [throughout] our lives we form bodies appropriate to the age we are. A somatic-emotional approach offers a way to work with the feelings and challenges of each emerging shape. Somatic work begins with discovering our individual patterns of self-use and the emotional body states that give us a primary reality. With this self- knowledge, we learn to grow an interior presence, to be bounded in ourselves and to sustain our process in relationship to others. (2)

Keleman sees in Baryshnikov's "HeartBeat: mb" performance a direct link to his own work in the field of psychosomatic medicine. According to Keleman, there is much more to Baryshnikov's performance than the

[5] See, for instance, Ty and Verduyn's *Asian Canadian Writing Beyond Autoethnography* (2008) for a detailed discussion of the politics of autoethnography. For a strident critique of the notion of cultural "authenticity," see Gerald Vizenor's *Manifest Manners: Postindian Warriors and Survivance* (1999).

mere idea of "coping" with processes of aging; in Keleman's view, what is at stake is the act of embodying these changes related to aging, and of translating such embodied experience into art. He writes, "Artists like Baryshnikov show us how they live the inevitable transitions of life" (1). Keleman has contrasted Mikhail Baryshnikov's biography with that of a second Russian celebrity dancer, Rudolf Nureyev. Unlike Baryshnikov, Keleman argues, Nureyev strove to conceal the fact that his body, too, was aging. The result of such concealment, Keleman suggests, was the failure of embodiment: Eventually, as the loss of the dancer's abilities could no longer be concealed, the dance performance became a farce. This farce, moreover, can also be seen in photograph taken of Nureyev at the time. The face in the photograph, it could be suggested, is a mask; it is mask-like in its attempt to exhibit a universal, an ageless face of an iconic dancer. This, it could be suggested, is a form of ghosting gone awry. As Keleman writes about what he sees as a key contrast between two of the world's most famous dancers, Mikhail Baryshnikov and Rudolph Nureyev,

> Baryshnikov embraces and embodies his aging and deepening self. In contrast, Jefferson points out, Rudolf Nureyev became feverish and hysterical as he aged and fought against changes in his body. Baryshnikov gets better and better at what he does without trying to look or act like his younger self. He shows no sexual posturing or arrogance, but as Jefferson concludes, "he is using time and himself in ways that seem transcendent and possible. (2)

Authenticity, in this context, is defined as a form of being attuned to one's physical body, to the ways in which this body changes and evolves. As Baryshnikov himself puts it, "'Be yourself and dance with your mind and your body, the way it is right now,' he says. 'Don't try to fight the image of yourself from 20 years ago'" (Kaufman n. pag.). Baryshnikov's "HeartBeat: mb" performance, then, can be seen as a way of integrating the concept of "ghosting" on both levels: on the level of the actor's being haunted by his previous performance, and on the level of the body of the older dancer being haunted by that of his younger self. Nureyev, as Keleman puts it, sought to conceal the implications of such ghosting, denying the fact of superimposition and trying to make the ghost fit its original: While Baryshnikov deliberately draws attention, both through the shift from classical ballet to modern dance and through the device of the onstage monitor, to the limits of what his body, at 51, cannot quite "endure" (Jefferson n. pag.), Nureyev sought to erase these very limits. The result, both Keleman and Jefferson write, was grotesque. What the audience witnessed, in Nureyev's case, was a dancer denying the aging process of his body, rather than inscribing, as Baryshnikov dares to do, this process into his art.

Crucially, the notion of aging and the aging process which the body of the actor is by no means exempt from has also been addressed by Marvin Carlson in *The Haunted Stage* (2001). If we were to look at Nureyev's refusal to acknowledge the aging process of his own body through Marvin Carlson's idea of the "haunted body" (52) of the actor, then, the fact of ghosting might account for Nureyev's continuing to perform the parts that his own body had once so effortlessly been able to meet. If we follow Carlson's argument, then the audience would at first not have resisted such a performance of make-believe agelessness, counterintuitive as this may at first seem. According to Carlson, "we tend to dismiss as grotesque or foolish an actor who similarly maintains youthful roles into advanced age" (57). Precisely because Nureyev could count on the way in which his performance would be "ghosted" for the audience which had made him a star, however, this grotesqueness would initially be kept at bay. Carlson writes,

> Before we too hastily condemn the apparent folly and vanity of an aging actor still playing youthful roles, we must recall that every new performance of these roles will be ghosted by a theatrical recollection of the previous performances, so that audience reception of each new performance is conditioned by inevitable memories of this actor playing similar roles in the past. The voice that might seem to an outsider grown thin with age may still to a faithful public echo with the resonances of decades of theatergoing, that slightly bent body still be ghosted by years of memories of it in its full vigor. (58)

What is crucial to note here is that Carlson directly addresses not only the way in which any actor is haunted by his previous on-stage appearances, but that he argues that this haunting is of particular significance once the actor's body changes to the extent that he may simply no longer "look" the part. In the case of Nureyev, however, it is important to note the difference between the dancer and the actor: for the professional dancer, there may be a limit that his (aging) body refuses to go beyond. The incorporation of the process of aging into the art of dance, then, may necessitate a change not in the performance (let alone the performer himself), but a change in the script that he sets out to perform. If, in an adaptation of Carlson's concept, the script is the "haunted text," which the actor/performer used to be able to deliver with ease, the incorporation of and the owning up to the process of the aging of the dancer's body necessitates a modification, or complete exchange of, this script. It is this change in script, in register, then, that Baryshnikov performs, while Nureyev chooses to ignore the ways in which both his body and the script are haunted by previous on-stage performances of his younger self.

Arguably, it is this incorporation of aging, of the dancer owning up to the changes of his body, that increases rather than diminishes the attractiveness of this body to an audience to whom the dancer has created, by virtue of an onstage cardiac monitor, the most intimate of relationships. As Jefferson concludes, Baryshnikov toys with the very notion of sexual attractiveness, knowing fully well that it is himself that the audience has come to see. Jefferson writes, "Enough. Back to Baryshnikov, onstage with five lovely dancers, all young women. He gives off nary a hint of professional arrogance (I'm the master here) or of sexual grandstanding. He is using time and himself in ways that seem transcendent and yet, if the rest of us are willing to take risks on our own scale, possible" (n. pag). What resurfaces here is the notion of "taking risks": Exposing his body to the gaze of the audience and laying bare this body's vulnerability, Baryshnikov is well aware, is a courageous endeavor. This is a juncture which, as I will elaborate in Chapter 6, recurs in the autobiography of Michael J. Fox. He, too, is faced with a difficult decision: whether or not to "go public" with the fact that his body has been, and will be, changing in ways that neither he nor the audience could have anticipated. What both Baryshnikov and Fox reveal, however, is that the result of such courageousness, the addressing, head-on, of physical changes in the performer's body which may interfere with traditional notions of "attractiveness," may at first seem surprising. If anything, in both cases, the audience's esteem for the performer seems to have been increased by the courageousness he has displayed by taking risks: The bond between performer and audience, in both cases, has been strengthened, and it has been strengthened by the performer's stressing, and laying open in his art, the bond of human mortality that he shares with the audience. He has reached out to the audience on a somatic level, a level which exceeds the layer of art or performance and is yet inseparable from it.

What is crucial here is that this approach taken from the field of psychosomatic medicine implies that an individual can sense or learn to be attuned to the changes in his or her own body. This sense of being in touch with one's own materiality, then, mirrors or parallels the function of the heart-rate monitor. To an extent, it resists the biomedicalizing of the human body in the age of biomedical technologies and opposes to them that the body has a sense of its own materiality, or that the owner of the body, too, can monitor its functions.

Keleman's is hence a notion of the *embodiment* of aging, of making the narrative of identity – or in, Baryshnikov's case, of an identity expressed through art – conform to the age of the body that this person inhabits. There are some overlaps here between Keleman's notion of somatic identity and John Paul Eakin's notion of "living autobiographically." Crucially, Eakin takes as his point of departure not a state of embodiment when the "storying" of one's own life is physically possible, but when this "storying" is being disrupted by an age-related process of impairment. According to Janis Breckenridge,

> Underlying this recognition that a sense of personhood is derived from the creation of identity in narrative oral and written) is the haunting question regarding those who are unable to provide the coherent, stable life story society has come to expect. Eakin remains especially concerned with the increasing occurrence of Alzheimer's in an aging population and asks if a de-storied person (one who has suffered memory loss) thus loses his or her identity and becomes *de-selved*. Uncomfortable with this notion, the author ultimately concludes that there is a self beyond language -- for we are embodied selves. (135)

At the core of Eakin's concern is thus also the relationship between the (autobiographical) story that is being told and the material body from which this telling emanates, or by which it is being obstructed. Telling one's story is hence a narrative as much as a material act, just as human identity is at once an "embodied" entity. It is in the notion of embodiment that Eakin's and Keleman's argument, if from profoundly different disciplinary directions, can be seen to converge. Not incidentally and crucially for our investigation of the convergences between life sciences and life writing, Eakin draws, among others, on the disciplines of both psychology and neurobiology. As Breckenridge goes on to state, "*Living Autobiographically* draws upon a vast array of texts and research findings across a variety of disciplines: art and literature, literary theory, developmental psychology, cultural anthropology, and neurobiology" (134; emphasis in original).

Telling one's story is hence a narrative as much as a material act, just as human identity is at once an "embodied" entity. Eakin is concerned with age-related illnesses such as Alzheimer's in which the telling of one's own story in verbal terms may no longer be possible, a condition which leads Eakin to look for alternative forms of expressions. Thus, life writing research has recently drawn attention to the ways in which a life can also be expressed through gestures, gestures which an Alzheimer patient may remember from the time he or she was still working in a particular profession or trade. For life writing research as much as for studies of age-related illness, it is essential to recognize such forms of expression as alternative forms of life writing and autobiography. Eakin's research can thus be seen to challenge, as many scholars in the field of medical humanities have done, the primacy of the verbal. As Angela Woods has noted, the field of medical humanities may have been centered on narrative to an extent that it may have tended to exclude other, non-narrative forms. She writes, "[It can be argued that studies such as Galen Strawson's] 'Against Narrativity' can and should stimulate robust debate within the medical humanities regarding the limits of narrative, [and the need for] discussing a range of possibilities for venturing 'beyond narrative'" (Woods 73). It is this challenge, from a profoundly different direction, which Mikhail Baryshnikov's "HeartBeat: mb" performance may also take up. If dance can be conceived as a form of "storying" in its own right, a medium in which Baryshnikov expresses the story of his own aging, "HeartBeat: mb" is intriguing because the dancer inscribes into it an implicit dialogue between his present-day self and his younger self. He creates a hybrid space in which classical ballet meets modern dance, in which the self he once was (the male virtuoso of classical ballet) is in dialogue with the older self he has come to embody. What is at stake is hence not a state in which the individual has been "de-selved" by aging, to use Eakin's terms, but in which one's self has been transformed into another. The risk of being "de-selved", what is more, is only at issue if the dancer refuses to change the medium in which such de-selving will be impending. Recognizing this risk, Baryshnikov chooses instead to change the medium. He shifts from classical ballet to modern dance. As we have suggested above, this shift is itself related to a particular conception of the aging process: the ability, as Stanley Keleman has put it, to "age authentically" or, in John Paul Eakin's words, to "live autobiographically" and to incorporate this process of living into artistic expression. What is implicit in Baryshnikov's artistic development is that such modern dance lends itself to the expression of the aging experience to an extent that classical ballet may not. An individual artist's attempt to translate an embodied experience into his art hence poses a challenge to the individual in which he may come to re-assess the restrictions imposed on him by the medium in which he has chosen to work. What this means in more abstract terms is that it is through deviance – the difference by which certain bodies come to be defined through processes of aging or age-related illness – that the parameters of the "normal" can be assessed or made visible in the first place.

5.5 Conclusion

In this chapter, I have drawn on disciplines as diverse as sociology of sports, sociology of dance, psychosomatic medicine, molecular biology and cultural studies. All these fields, I have argued, create their own readings of aging processes of the human body. Yet, these interpretations are often read independently of one another, each within its own specific discipline and disciplinary epistemologies. Resisting what Snow once called the "two cultures" split between the natural sciences and the humanities, this chapter has explored convergences between different disciplinary narratives of aging. Such an interdisciplinary approach, I have suggested, can shed light on the way in which a specific phenomenon in the history of dance or of modern painting, can be read on multiple levels which, ultimately, reveal much more than mono-disciplinary frameworks could have done. Moreover, I have argued that such a genuinely interdisciplinary approach may add another layer of meaning to the concept of "living autobiographically" proposed by John Paul Eakin. Mikhail Baryshnikov's performance in which he hooks the dancing body – his own body – up to a medical monitor may prove to be a fitting illustration of how to live autobiographically. Dance, in this context, can also be seen as a form of life writing. In Baryshnikov's performances, neither is the body reduced to its "identity" as a famous ballet dancer nor is its physical aging allowed to eclipse this identity. Rather, the "ideational" and the material body, the dancer's identity and his material body permeate each other in a way in which one can no longer be separated from the other. Thus, Baryshnikov's performance becomes a manual of how to "live autobiographically": how to incorporate and listen to changes in the *material biography* of one's body, not just the biography of one's life made up of profession, identity, and performance.

6 "Like a Hole in the Head": Comedy and Parkinson's Disease in Michael J. Fox's Autobiographies *Always Looking Up* and *Lucky Man*

6.1 "Playing in the Dark": Disability, Autobiography and the Suspension of the Senses

Especially in my discussion of Tito Mukhopadhyay's book *Beyond the Silence* in Chapter 2, I have wondered not only what is to be gained, but also what may be lost by a "medicalizing" of literary analysis. In this chapter, I will be concerned with the ways in which life writing, as in Tito Mukhopadhyay's "case," may offer us a way out of this dilemma. What, life writing as a genre may implicitly come to ask, are the ways in which we can suspend our medical gaze, a gaze – as a lay person's gaze – which has long been informed by discourses of the life sciences as they have filtered, in a perhaps unexamined ubiquity into our life worlds? In the chapter on Tito Mukhopadhyay's writing, I have thus explored the question of how particular senses – visuality above all – may trigger a medicalizing of particular bodies conceived as "deviant," as different. What does it mean for us, I have asked, to read Mukhopadhyay's story without witnessing the difference in his body, by being sidetracked, as it were, by the visual and the acoustic "deviance" of the body telling the story of a life? I have argued that, precisely as in the arena of race studies, the power of (life) writing may lie in suspending our visual perception of difference. By enabling us to imagine a body *without* witnessing its physical materiality – a materiality that may trigger a preconceived set of associations and assumptions –, writing may open up a powerful sense of perception, and of *alternative* perception. Writing – both in the sense of writing fiction and of writing lives – may hence open up new spaces through the curious alternation between embodiment and disembodiment. It is Tito Mukhopadhyay's body that we imagine through his writing on the page. Our imagination of his body –

a body which is disabled, to an extent, by autism – is unhampered by visual and acoustic cues. One of the most significant interventions of literary portrayal into conceptions of disability, I suggest in this book, is the literal *disabling* of what I would call a medico-ethnographic gaze. By translating embodiment into written text, our perception of this physical form of disability is altered significantly. What, then, would be the disability studies equivalent of Toni Morrison's memorable phrase, coined for the arena of race studies, of "playing in the dark" (1992)?

It is in this suspension of some of our senses that the power of life writing may lie. Taking my cue from Thomas Couser's groundbreaking work on disability, then, I am interested in the ways in which American Studies, in exploring concepts and practices of disability, may draw from other areas in which the deviance of certain bodies from an implicitly or explicitly defined norm has already been explored. Thus, Toni Morrison writes at the beginning of *Playing in the Dark* (1992), that she had experimented, in earlier phases of her career, with a narrative which is not coded by color (xi).

What, then, might the notion of color-blindness mean when applied to discourses of disability? It may mean, above all, the suspension of ability (let alone "ableism") as a category of knowledge and of meaning-making. It is such an attempt at constructing "ability-blindness," I would argue, which we may achieve by suspending some of the senses through which disability is perceived. This, moreover, would also be the difference between literary studies and narrative medicine in the sense that an autobiography is different from a patient narrative because, first and foremost, the former is meant to be read instead of listened to. A patient narrative, on the other hand, is mostly heard by a medical practitioner, who sees the patient before him or her; here, the corporeality of the patient and her narrative converge. There is no sense, in this respect, of disembodiment. This, as I have also argued in Chapter 2 with regard to Tito Mukhopadhyay's life writing, is the power of autobiography, which can conceal or reveal the narrative subject's vulnerability, as it can be brought about by illness, age, or disability. What is at stake, then, is the relationship of a given difference – a difference which, at first glance, seems to be physically manifest – and its presence in what Morrison calls the "literary imagination" (*Playing in the Dark* x). Moreover, it may seem significant here that the beginning of Morrison's award-winning collection of essays, *Playing in the Dark: Whiteness and the*

Literary Imagination, should start with reference to a life writing narrative concerned not with race but with mental illness: "Some years ago, in 1983 I believe, I read Marie Cardinal's *The Words to Say It*. . . . Cardinal's project was not fictional, however; it was to document her madness, her therapy, and the complicated process of healing in language as exact and as evocative as possible in order to make both her experience and her understanding of it accessible to a stranger" (v). At the same time, Morrison goes on to discuss how in Cardinal's narrative and her recollection of her illness, race figures prominently: "In Cardinal's narrative, black or colored people and symbolic figurations of blackness are markers for the benevolent and the wicked . . ." (*Playing in the Dark* ix). Cardinal's narrative is thus highly complex in that it addresses the conveying of two differences – race and mental illness – in and through narrative, a narrative which Morrison calls an "autobiographical novel" (*Playing in the Dark* v). In this process, however, one difference seems to become subservient to the telling of the other: Mental illness is conveyed through tropes of blackness. Blackness, in turn, becomes metaphorized in the process; it is at the service of what is, after all, a white imagination of illness.

At the same time, it is significant for my purposes here that Morrison engages the ways in which differences can be imagined through language, and in which a given narrative can play with the embodiment or disembodiment of a given difference. The notion of what I would call "*literary disembodiment*" is hence crucial for the narratives I am discussing in this study. Crucially, then, Morrison herself experiments, in her short story "Recitatif" (1983) with the notion of the literary concealment – literally, the refusal to embody a specific difference in the narrative – of both race and disability. Morrison notes,

> The kind of work I have always wanted to do requires me to learn how to maneuver ways to free up the language from its sometimes sinister, frequently lazy, almost always predictable employment of racially informed and determined chains. (The only short story I have ever written, "Recitatif," was an experiment in the removal of all racial codes from a narrative about two characters of different races for whom racial identity is crucial.) (*Playing in the Dark* xi)

The power of "autobiographical novels" (Morrison, *Playing in the Dark* v) in conveying age, illness or disability, I believe, lies precisely in the deliberate undoing of what Morrison calls the social codes embedded in language. In this respect, of course, approaches such as Critical Race Theory converge with disability in emphasizing that the difference (of race, of disability) is not biological, but social. It is, first and foremost, a constructed difference. Applying Morrison's idea of race to literary imaginations of disability, then, I am interested in the extent to which these literary autobiographies can undo or strive to deconstruct the ways in which they know illness or disability will be coded by the reader. At the same time, it must be noted that Morrison is concerned with the role of blackness in white literary imagination. By the same token, such an approach clearly intersects with approaches from disability studies, which, as Leonard Davis has done, look at the ways in which metaphors of disability, to paraphrase Morrison, are made "serviceable" for the ableist imagination. Conversely and drawing on these deconstructive practices of race and disability, then, I am interested in the ways in which these autobiographical accounts, which are much more than stories about illness or disability, deconstruct both ideas of normalcy and the "service" to which their difference may be put to.

By the same token, a literary narrative, like a camera, can choose what parts of a human body it zooms in on. What parts of this body – and, by extension, what aspects of a person's life – does the literary narrative zoom in on? To use Hans-Ulrich Gumbrecht's discussion of beauty and disability as a case in point, a discussion which I have already explored in Chapter 5 with regard to Mikhail Baryshnikov's "HeartBeat: mb" performance, what would it have meant for us to have two photographs, one of this beautiful woman's torso and one full portrait of her body, a body which now comes to be defined through its disability and no longer through its beauty? To the extent that "beauty" presupposes the universality of the non-disabled subject, what are the ways in which we may suspend such universality? The device of the lens or zoom employed by the camera may be an important one here. As I suggest throughout these chapters, I am concerned with the way in which these narratives, precisely by being autobiographies, play with a variety of different "zooms," refusing to "zoom in" only in questions of aging, illness or disability. Rather, their articulation of a given condition – a condition which, all of the narratives are quick to ask, has been completely medicalized – emerges only in the conjunction they deliberately create with other pictures, other aspects of their bodies and their lives which have nothing whatsoever to do with this "medical" condition. They confound the reader, I would argue, with this variety of zooms, of objectives, thus paradoxically, refusing to have their bodies reduced precisely be first fragmenting and then reassembling this body in different ways. One of the key strategies employed by these texts, I am trying to argue in this book, is the project of medical sabotage; the insistence on including, in an autobiography which the author knows will be read as a "patient" account, chapters which will seem inappropriate to such a medical gaze. The aim of these autobiographies, I argue, is to sabotage the very ways in which they know they will be read. In this sense, they can be seen to undo, to deconstruct, what Leonard Davis has called "normalcy." They deconstruct notions of normalcy, which in turn seek to medicalize the reading of these narratives. What I am calling for, then, is the paradox of resisting to read a narrative about illness as an illness narrative. What does it mean, as I have also asked in Chapter 2 with regard to Tito Mukhopadhyay's narrative, to resist medicalizing the autobiography of a person with autism, or, in the case of Michael J. Fox, of an actor affected by Parkinson's Disease? Paradoxically, then, I am aware that the circulation of these narratives is itself fueled by the increasing institutionalization of, for instance, medical humanities programs and the acceptance of the genre of illness narratives. Yet, I believe that these narratives, while benefiting from these new frameworks in which they know they will be read, also set out to sabotage these frameworks, insisting on the surplus, the excess in their narrative content which cannot be subsumed under notions of illness or disability. It is here, I argue throughout this study, that the concept of "autobiography" can be a useful antidote to what I understand as a restrictive use of these narratives. It is in this sense, then, that the title of my study *Medical Humanities in American Studies*, is deliberately ambivalent, especially since this title, to some extent, is at odds with the subtitle, *Narrative Medicine, Life Writing and the Power of Autobiography*. I am thus interested in the ways in which current frameworks, especially medical humanities and the notion of illness narratives, may at one and the same time be useful and counterproductive. This paradox, I argue, is written into the narratives who embrace but are also wary of their own canonization.

It is at this point, moreover, that I would like to return to another aspect of applying Rita Charon's concept of "narrative medicine" to literary analysis, a practice that I would see as a form of methodological re-import. Charon is concerned with the ways in which doctors "read" their patients' stories, and with the ways in which, minus narrative knowledge and the knowledge of narrative, they may not be sufficiently equipped to read these stories:

> Health professionals and patients are at a crossroads. Together, we have to discover means of sustaining the tremendous capabilities of our biomedical sciences while trying to ease the suffering and loss occasioned by serious illness. The price for a technologically sophisticated medicine seems to be impersonal, calculating treatment from revolving sets of specialists who, because they are consumed with the scientific elements in health care, seem divided from the ordinary human experiences that surround pain, suffering, and dying. (*Narrative Medicine* 6)

Charon is thus trying to change the face of medicine, and of a contemporary medical practice geared towards cost-efficiency and increasing technologization. "Re-importing" her methodology of narrative medicine to literary analysis, especially the literary analysis of life writing narratives, I am interested in the ways in which narratives themselves can invite, trigger or sabotage certain readings of themselves. Like Charon, if in a very different context, I am concerned with the "unruliness" of narratives. The very nature of narratives is that they exceed the factual and the utilitarian; this is what makes narratives, we may argue, narratives. What Charon draws attention to, then, is the difference between listening – or, in the context that I am discussing here, reading – to a given narrative about illness: The doctor's way of listening to the narrative is different from the practice of the literary critic; whereas the former must translate metaphor into diagnosis, the latter may be able to listen in a less goal-oriented way. As Charon recalls her early practice as a doctor, "I had to do what all doctors – ideally – do, whether they realize it or not. I had to follow the patient's narrative threat, identify the metaphors or images used in the telling, tolerate ambiguity and uncertainty as the story unfolded. . . . I was the interpreter of these accounts of events of illness that are, by definition, unruly and elusive" (*Narrative Medicine* 4). The ideal that Charon envisions for medical practice, then, is a practice in which the reading or listening skills of the physician and the literary critic are not at odds with one another, but can actually be akin to one another. This ideal, in turn, may be exemplary of the future of humanities research. Charon's concept of narrative medicine *applies* literary methodologies to medical practice without, however, reducing the humanities to their application value. While Charon is concerned with the practice of listening and of reading narratives of illness, she is quick to include the practice of telling: "I saw that, while I had very demanding 'listening' tasks, the patient's 'telling' tasks were even more demanding, because pain, suffering, worry, anguish, and the sense of something not being right are conditions very difficult, if not impossible, to put into words" (*Narrative Medicine* 4). Adding to the question of "telling tasks," I would like to explore not only what it means to be telling an (autobiographical) story of illness, but also with the ways in which such autobiographical narratives can write into themselves knowledge of the ways in which they will be read. In how far, in other words, do these narratives play with the role of the implied medical reader here, and with the reading routes they know his or her reading will be liable to follow? In how far can they sabotage the directions of such reading? Throughout this study, then, I am concerned with the ways in which we read and in which we may come to canonize stories of illness. Alternative forms of canonization, I argue, may provide room precisely for what Charon calls "honoring the stories of illness" (*Narrative Medicine*): The minute we canonize, anthologize or simply file a given narrative under the rubric of autobiography rather than illness narrative or medical humanities, we may be able to honor the narrative for the life narrative it is, and for the unruliness it contains. In this sense, moreover, the autobiographies inscribe, in their specific aesthetic and narrative construction, what Rita Charon has called "honoring the story of illness" (*Narrative Medicine*). To construct an autobiography as being much more than a patient account, to construct it as an autobiography in the sense "proper" of the term, is precisely to honor such stories of illness; to inscribe into the aesthetics of writing and of autobiography what Rita Charon has also called for in medical practice.

6.2 The Translucency of the Self: Onstage Monitors and Stage Directions

The way in which Michael J. Fox describes, in his first autobiography, *Lucky Man* (2002), the beginning of his disease, is in fact highly similar to the way in which Baryshnikov dramatizes, in his "HeartBeat: mb" performance, the ways in which his body sabotages the script of classical ballet which his younger self could so effortlessly perform. In Fox's life writing, the notion of "scripting" is twofold: Long before his body refuses to "act in" the scripts of the films that Fox had agreed to act in, his body "acts up" in a different, quite material sense. It is this "acting up," this moment in which the materiality of his body takes on a life of its own, that Fox describes, in his autobiography, as a "wake-up call" (*Lucky Man* 1): "*I woke up to find the message in my left hand. It had me trembling. It wasn't a fax, telegram, memo, or the usual sort of missive bringing disturbing news. In fact, my hand held nothing at all. The trembling was the message*" (*Lucky Man* 1; emphasis in original). In the irony characteristic of both his autobiographies, Fox plays on the idea of the "message" in his left hand: As he soon realizes, the message is "in" his left hand in quite a literal sense; in fact, the message is his left hand which has started to tremble. What Fox addresses in his memoir is the ways in which we have learned to conceive of our bodies only as vehicles for something much more important, as a passive entity to be controlled by our minds. It is this subjugation, the severing of body from mind in which the body is subordinate to the mind, which may be revealed only in the process of malfunctioning. Yet, as Fox's autobiography makes clear, there may in fact be a continuity between "health" and "illness" here: the subordination of the body to the mind is as common to those affected by illness as it is to those who are not: the illness only makes explicit what we may otherwise refuse to acknowledge. As Fox goes on to note, "Ten years later, knowing what I do now, this mind-body divorce strikes me as a serviceable metaphor – though at the time it was a concept well beyond my grasp" (*Lucky Man* 4). As Fox describe in the account of his own condition, Parkinson's Disease, this malfunctioning revealed to him, with a vengeance, the manifold ways in which he had refused to take his body into account in his life as a Hollywood megastar. Fox describes the moment in which his hand, or more specifically, his pinkie, had taken on a life of its own, acting quite independently of its owner: "That's when I noticed my pinkie. It was trembling, twitching, auto-animated. How long this had been going on I wasn't exactly sure. But now that I noticed it, I was surprised to discover that I couldn't stop it. . . . I didn't have to see the underlying skeletal structure; the information I was looking for was right there in the flesh: a thumb, three stock-still fingers, and out there on a lunatic fringe, a spastic pinkie" (*Lucky Man* 2-3). What Fox's narrative draws attention to is the moment of prognosis, and the temporality which may arise from such prognosis. The realization that he would have to live with chronic illness, and a disease which would involve the increasing deterioration of his mind's control over his body, changed Fox's attitude towards his life, and to the body that he had so far taken for granted. It is for this reason that, quite counterintuitively, he entitles his first autobiography *Lucky Man*:

> Unbeknownst to me, things had been deteriorating long before the morning of the pinkie rebellion. But by declaring its dysfunction in such an arresting fashion, my brain now had my mind's full attention. It would be a year of questions and false answers that would satisfy me for a time. . . . The answer came from a doctor who would inform me that I had a progressive, degenerative, and incurable neurological disorder; one that I may have been living with for as long as a decade before suspecting there might be anything wrong. This doctor would also tell me that I could probably continue acting for "another ten good years," and he would be right about that, almost to the day. What he did not tell me – what no one could – is that these last ten years of coming to terms with my disease would turn out to be the best ten years of my life – not in spite of my illness, but because of it. (Fox, *Lucky Man* 4-5)

Autobiographies, from the very beginning, have been explorations of human life on two levels. First, they have addressed, as in the case of Benjamin Franklin, the representativeness of an individual's life for that of his nation, and have explored the question whether the life described in the autobiography might be seen as a model life to be emulated by those who read the autobiography. Yet, beyond such a national context which would take on a particular significance in the era of nation-building, autobiographies, particularly in a Western context, have been concerned with what it means to be human. This notion of humanity has, of course, taken on particular significance at the beginning of the twenty-first century, where human life can increasingly be reshaped by the technologies made available by the life sciences. What does autobiography mean, then, in the era of the "technological reproducibility of human life" (Weiß 2009; my trans.)? Where Fox's autobiography *Lucky Man* is exemplary of this nexus, I believe, is in its insistence that the narrative cannot be reduced to pathography, to being an account only of

Parkinson's Disease or an actor's "coping" with this disease. Quite on the contrary: *Lucky Man* is an engagement with the temporality and the materiality of human life; even as this engagement was born, Fox readily admits, of a medical diagnosis, it is at the same time independent of this diagnosis. As Fox writes, "It is one of the great ironies of my life that only when it became virtually impossible for me to keep my body from moving would I find the peace, security, and spiritual strength to stand in one place. I couldn't be still until I could – literally – no longer keep still" (*Lucky Man* 17).

6.3 Acting as Life Writing: *Spin City*

It is this suspension of a medicalizing gaze through life writing and its power of disembodiment that I would now like to turn to a reading of Michael J. Fox's award-winning TV show, *Spin City* (1996-2002). What, exactly, do we see when we look at Michael J. Fox in *Spin City* after the disclosure of his PD diagnosis? It is through his autobiographies, *Lucky Man* (2002) and *Always Looking Up* (2009), that Fox himself has given us stage directions for reading or rather, for re-reading *Spin City*. What is at stake in these stage directions? I would argue, it is something much more profound than an author seeking to determine and to define, the ways in which his writing is or should be read. Rather, Fox's reminder of his subjectivity outside his diagnosis cuts to the heart of what I would call a "medicalizing" of cultural production. The worst thing for us to do, Fox asserts, is to re-watch *Spin City* in its last season starring Michael J. Fox, and look for clues and symptoms of the actor's PD: As Fox puts it in *Always Looking Up*, "When people first found out I had PD, I remember feeling uncomfortable that they might be inspired to rent old movies in an effort to trade the accumulating effects of the disease. I'm sure many did" (67). Much of the same reductionist reading, I propose, would be at stake if we read Tito Mukhopadhyay's autobiography only through the "category" or diagnosis of autism, thereby reducing its author to his disability.

Rather, what Fox suggests is a dialogue between life sciences and life writing; a dialogue between the way in which his body has begun to change through Young Onset Parkinson's Disease *and* his power as an actor, a power which can by no means be reduced to the symptoms of his disease. There is a sense, to be sure, in which Fox's performance in

Spin City may be "ghosted," in Carlson's terms, by performances that he gave before being affected by PD. Yet, the power of Fox's life writing – and of his *acting as a form of life writing* – , lies precisely in incorporating the changes in his body into his art. It is here that I would locate a parallel between Mikhail Baryshnikov's memorable dance performance in "HeartBeat: mb" – in which he incorporates the aging process of his body into his art – and Fox's performance in *Spin City*. What is key to Baryshnikov's performance – as different as it may at first sight be from the context of Michael J. Fox's acting in *Spin City* – is that aging is conceived not as a deterioration from a young, able-bodied norm, but as a gradual process in which the human body changes. Crucially, Baryshnikov's performance makes clear that aging is not to be conceived as a process, let alone a clearly definable moment, of *loss*. Rather, it is a *normal* change of the human body which it would hence, in fact, be absurd to judge. By the same token, Fox describes the way in which PD involves a gradual diminishing of physical control. The telos which Fox's life writing describes, then, is the actor's ability to incorporate his illness into his art, and in so doing, much as in Baryshnikov's memorable performance, change the nature of his craft. Yet, while Baryshnikov went from classical ballet to modern dance and was hence able to change the format in which he performed, this was not quite true for Michael J. Fox. As Fox puts it, "Although everyone – cast, crew, and audience – knew by this point that I had Parkinson's, I was still attempting to play a character who did not" (*Always Looking Up* 10).

I am hence interested in the dialogue between the actor and his role; in the ways in which aspects not just of the actor's identity informs his interpretation of his role but the ways in which the materiality of his body may impose constraints on his performance. To be sure, Fox, in his life writing, is quick to stress the point that it was a privilege that, given his previous career and celebrity status, he was able to define the parameters of production in which such a transformation of the *context* of his acting and in fact, of the entire show, was possible. He was, after all, the show's protagonist:

> I never logged out of the online PD forums without realizing how fortunate I was. My family, my relative youth, my financial situation, as well as my public position gave me a tremendous advantage in dealing with my illness. While Parkinson's did have a direct impact on my ability to do my job, I was, to all intents and purposes, my own boss. So for me,

> decisions on whether or not to disclose my illness were not as fraught with risk. (Fox, *Always Looking Up* 26)

What Fox gives us in his life writing, in a remarkably candid fashion, is a glimpse back stage of *Spin City*. It is here, through the curious palimpsestic layering of on-stage and back-stage performance, that Fox describes the ways in which – much like Baryshnikov – he was able to tailor his performance to what his body was physically able to perform. As Fox recalls,

> I discovered that, for short periods of time, I could direct all the energy coursing through my body to one particular extremity – a hand, leg, or foot. So when blocking a scene, I would position myself (and the rest of the cast as well) in such a way as to best conceal the appendix in which the surge of Parkinsonian energy was manifest. Like I said, it's the same sort of thing I'd been doing for years, and my thinking was once I could explain to people why I was doing it, it would make the whole process that much smoother. (*Always Looking Up* 10)

In this inscribing of the performer's biological materiality into his art – an art, predicated, in Baryshnikov's case, on the ageless/youthful, able-bodied universality of the dancer – Fox's acting in fact mirrors Baryshnikov's memorable "cardiac" performance. Yet at the same time, Fox's performance in *Spin City* can be located half-way between the inscription and the concealment of Parkinson's Disease: While in Baryshnikov's case, there is no dichotomy between the script in which he is performing and the body which is doing the performance, Fox, in *Spin City*, is still not playing a character who also has PD.

However, what can be gained from juxtaposing Baryshnikov's performance with a reading of *Spin City*, I believe, is also a decentering of disability: The fact that our bodies change as we age is due to our own physicality as human beings; the question asked by both Fox and Baryshnikov, is how we incorporate these changes into our practices of living. What is more, a comparison between Baryshnikov's dance performance and Fox's *Spin City* would enable us to conceive of these performances as differences in degree, not in kind; in a sense which would resist or center on disability studies readings of *Spin City*. What may be at stake, then, is a context for cultural studies analysis in which, for instance, medical humanities and film studies would no longer be a variance with each other. As in Baryshnikov's case, if in profoundly different ways, Fox's inability to perform certain roles has changed the nature of his acting. By inscribing the change of his aging body into his dance performance, Baryshnikov changed the history of modern dance. Similarly, on the level of the history of popular culture, Fox (literally) reworked *Spin City* to tailor it in such a way that he would still be able to perform; he was, after all, the show's producer. What matters here, I believe, is more than a simple distinction between "high" art (classical ballet, modern dance) and popular culture, or the legitimacy of comparing Mikhail Baryshnikov to Michael J. Fox, their matching first names notwithstanding. What is at stake, as I have argued with regard to "HeartBeat: mb" is the dialogue of an artist with an instrument, his body.

There is a curious parallel here to Baryshnikov's on-stage cardiac monitor: By not only changing the nature of the dance (script) but by having a cardiac monitor on stage, Baryshnikov exposes the vulnerability of his own body, making the audience see the limits beyond which his body is now unable to go. Yet, since Spin City is, after all, a comedy about a character who does not have Parkinson's, this is impossible for Michael J. Fox. Yet, it could be argue that his second autobiography, *Always Looking Up*, is in fact the equivalent of Baryshnikov's cardiac monitor. In this autobiography, Fox himself provides the stage commentary on his acting style in this season of *Spin City*: As in Baryshnikov's cardiac monitor, his own commentary on his acting style expose to the audience the vulnerability, brought about by dyskinesias, that determined his acting in *Spin City*. While in Baryshnikov's "HeartBeat: mb" performance, both the monitor and the dancer are simultaneously present on stage, Fox provides the "monitoring" of his own body in an autobiography in which he looks back on his performance in *Spin City*. Nonetheless, I would argue, the "translucency" of a body changed by age or illness is strikingly similar in both performances.

Fox's supplying the back-stage commentary to the making of *Spin City*, then, fulfills the same function as the monitor in "HeartBeat: mb": in a way, Fox's autobiography is Baryshnikov's cardiac monitor. Both attest to the actor's physical vulnerability, the vulnerability of his material body which is, however, not hidden from the audience's view but inscribed in the very nature of the performance. By including a cardiac monitor in his performance, Baryshnikov makes his body "translucent"

(Jefferson n. pag.) to his audience. By the same token, by making visible those movements of his body, within his performance on *Spin City*, which were due less to his acting style than to his physical condition, Fox engages in precisely such an act of the translucency of the self. Paradoxically, then, it is by medicalizing their own bodies – through an onstage cardiac monitor, through stage directions – that both Baryshnikov and Fox succeed in *resisting* the audience's medicalization of their own bodies.

What is equally significant is that his comments in his autobiography, which provide the audience with a back-stage glimpse of the acting, also include the predicament which he is aware he put his fellow actors through:

> Those around me had a difficult time reconciling the energetic, expressive Mike Flaherty that they would see in front of the camera with the shuffling, mask-faced Mike Fox that they would encounter as he went about his business behind the scenes. My producing partner, Nelle Fortenberry, remembers more than a few occasions when department heads and other members of the cast would step into her office, close the door, and beg her to tell them why I was mad at them. . . . Nelle would repeatedly explain that one of the symptoms of PD is a dearth of facial animation – the Parkinson's mask. (Fox, *Always Looking Up* 12)

Yet, Fox is also quick to note his appreciation of his actor colleagues' sense of solidarity, which enabled him to go on with *Spin City* in the first place.

What Fox calls for in his autobiography *Lucky Man*, then, may in fact be a blueprint for "reading" all of the texts discussed in this book, a strategy of reading which I have attempted, to some extent, in my previous chapter on Tito Mukhopadhyay's *The Mind Tree*: We should, first, read *Spin City* without the knowledge of the main actor's PD diagnosis, or recall our perception of *Spin City* prior to this knowledge. Second, we should re-watch the show and be attuned to what the diagnosis – Parkinson's Disease – does to our reading of Fox's acting performance. The third, comprehensive reading which Fox calls for in *Lucky Man* is a reading which would take his PD as one characteristic among many. It is this sense of downgrading illness, of refusing to give it precedence over other characteristics of the acting style of Michael J. Fox that has, in fact, informed the public reaction to Fox's PD disclosure. What Fox describes in *Lucky Man*, is that the disclosure of his own vulnerability made people aware not of his difference or diagnosis, but of the vulnerability and the proneness to physical change which we share as human beings. The point that Fox makes is hence not only that in his performance in the third season of *Spin City*, he is being ghosted by his younger self, by a self before the PD diagnosis, but that there is a sense in which as human beings, we are being "ghosted" by one another: Fox's particular form of ghosting, brought about by Parkinson's Disease, may foreshadow the way in which we will also come to be ghosted by our younger, able-bodied selves, the way in which aging and illness are specific to our human condition.

What is at stake in this reading, then, is to allow for the text to choose its own melody, to determine the background music which it wants to go with its theme: As Michael J. Fox has written in *Always Looking Up*, his second autobiography, published eight years after his first autobiography *Lucky Man*, what matters is not only the inclusion of illness or disability, but the *terms* on which this inclusion takes place. As he writes,

> In a recently published *New York Times* article, "Clearly, Frankly, Unabashedly Disabled," Mireya Navarro asserts that "the public image of people with disabilities," which "often hinged on the heroic or the tragic," is changing. . . . At once the same and the opposite of the shrieking violins in the shower scene of *Psycho*, [representations of disability often] root our reaction to what we are seeing away from thinking and directly towards emotion. . . . It's dehumanizing and marginalizing. . . . If society is encouraged to view you in a certain way, you come with theme music not of your choosing and perhaps not suited to your point of view. (Fox, *Always Looking Up* 143)

An autobiography, then, is implied by Fox to be the possibility to orchestrate one's own theme music; to set the tone, in one's own account of illness or disability, to the story of one's life. For Fox, his worst fear is that the audience will not be susceptible to the potential of ghosting; that it will conceive of the difference between his healthier self and his present condition as an absolute split. What Fox fears worst, then, is for the audience to compose his eulogy: "A lot of it [the news coverage of Fox's 'outing' himself as a person with PD] was in slow motion, giving the piece a somber tone: *This is the Michael J. Fox that was*. Any public figure will tell you, you know you're in trouble – dead, sick, or under indictment – whenever they start running footage of you in slow motion. It was as close to watching my own obituary as I ever want to get" (*Lucky Man* 229). Conversely, the way out of the impasse which his illness could have been, Fox implies, is to engage actively a form of ghosting in which the potential for his future acting career – and his future relationship to his fan community – may lie in constantly negotiating the nature of the ghosts; in creating a dialogue between his younger and his present-day self. It is in this sense too, I would argue, that the politics of ghosting may by no means only be directed towards the past; they may come to include the future as well. What emerges here, I believe, is much more than the intersection between celebrity autobiography and illness narrative. Rather, what may be at stake here is another instance of what Charon calls "honoring the stories of illness" (*Narrative Medicine* x). Precisely because Michael J. Fox is a celebrity, the audience – as his fan base – has known and connected to the story of his life, a life that cannot be reduced to illness. Because of his celebrity status, then, the narrative of his illness which he has now made public continues to be ghosted, in Carlson's terms, by his celebrity persona. It is because of this celebrity status, Fox himself implies in his first autobiography, *Lucky Man*, that the public will honor the story of his life beyond the narrative of his illness. Conversely, this latter narrative enables PD patients to speak up about their illness; their stories, too, may now be honored in a different way given the public's sudden interest in a disease that Michael J. Fox is also affected by. Fox notes, "I distinctly remember one person writing, 'I went to the market this morning and the cashier asked me why my hand was shaking. I told her it was Parkinson's, and she was really interested. "Oh, just like Michael J. Fox." For the first time in years, I didn't feel embarrassed'" (*Lucky Man* 229). The problem with this form of ghosting, of course, is that there is a certain amount of unfairness: the experience of a fellow blogger outlined by Fox is that the story of one's illness is not "honored" to the same extent unless one is a celebrity in the first place. This is a paradox, then, that Fox's narrative seems to be well aware of. Yet, what emerges is a form of narrative midwifery: By telling his own story, Fox creates a new space for other narratives – narratives by the entire "patient community" (*Lucky Man* 229), as he puts it – will also be heard. Moreover, what Fox's account also points to is the relevance of blogs for coming to terms especially with the experience of illness. Two forms of life writing converge here: In his written autobiography, Fox emphasizes the power of the blogs shared by other persons affected by PD; for him, the blogs create a space of solidarity in which narratives can be shared: "It was an online chat room for P.D. patients. I lurked there for a while, eavesdropping on their conversations. To a person, these patients were heralding my announcement and enthusing over the welcome turn in coverage, away from the celebrity angle and toward the patient community" (*Lucky Man* 229). For Fox, the practice of eavesdropping soon gives way to a more open dialogue with P.D. patients who, unlike him, cannot rely on the current narratives of their lives being ghosted, for the observer, by who they once were. Moreover, by creating the Michael J. Fox foundation, the actor has gone on to translate his celebrity status into seeking funding for Parkinson's research. What emerges here is a form of communal life writing, a life writing which encompasses, even as it transcends, the PD community. Fox observes,

> My greatest teachers now came from within the P.D. community itself. My coming out had an impact on their lives, as it turned out, but even before that, their stories – gleaned from what I read on P.D. websites suddenly lit up by conversation – had at least as profound an impact on mine. It was as if I was looking in a window, and to my comfort and relief, there were lights on and people inside – people just like me. (*Lucky Man* 230)

It is thus the most memorable part of the memoir that in exposing his vulnerability, Fox uses his own body as a pars pro toto for the entire Parkinson community. At the same time, he is keenly aware that this ability to go public with his diagnosis at a time of his own choosing was itself owed to his celebrity status.

It is in this sense that being the lead star of Spin City enables Fox to inscribe his subjectivity – and physical subjectivity – as an actor into his role in *Spin City*. Quite self-ironically, one of the episodes plays with the idea that for Fox, one of the key features of his identity, physical as well as emotional, has been his height. It is his height as well as his youthful looks which made Fox a media celebrity in the first place through his award-winning performance in *Back to the Future* (1985). It is this height, however, which caused him to conceive of his body as "deviant" well before the onset of PD. Yet, as he indicates in *Lucky Man*, Fox has long been able to inscribe this deviance into his acting in a manner that is both self-ironic and supremely self-confident. As he himself makes clear, dealing with his deviance in statue may have prepared him for incorporating the unruliness of his body into his art, if under much more serious circumstances. Ghosting, in this context, takes on a very specific quality: the ghost of his shortness of statue, in fact, paves the way for Fox's coming to terms with Parkinson's Disease. He has had time, he writes in both *Lucky Man* and *Always Looking Up*, to get used to the deviance, the unruliness of his own body. Why else should the title of his second autobiography, *Always Looking Up*, be a "short joke"? As Fox notes about the titles of both his first and second autobiographies, "As the title for this new book, *Always Looking Up* works on a couple of levels. First off – let's just get this one out of the way – it's a short joke. At a fraction of an inch under five-foot-five, much of my interaction with the world and the people in it has required that I tilt my head backward and direct my gaze upward" (*Always Looking Up* 4). For Fox, coming to terms with his PD diagnosis was made possible, then, by his previously having come to terms with his shortness. He had already had time to become used to, he writes in characteristic self-irony, the experience of having a body which did not quite match the requirements of physical "normalcy." It is this shortness of statue, incidentally, which links Fox's experience to that of Mikhail Baryshnikov, as I have argued in the previous chapter. Fox may not have quite looked like a "hockey puck," then, but his height seemed to bode ill for a future career in acting; and yet, it was his shortness which, as he points out in *Always Looking Up*, would be the reason for his breakthrough when, at the age of twenty-four, he was cast for the role of teenaged Alex Keaton in *Back to the Future.*

As Fox is quick to point out in a curious mixture of modesty and ironic self-assurance, however, his lack of height did not interfere with the audience's attitude towards his physical attractiveness. As he is well aware, he was simply seen by the audience as "pretty damn cute" (*Lucky Man* 237). What permeates Fox's discussion of his illness, and the way in which it has informed and changed his acting, is a sense in which he reflects on the different "ghostings" of his performance on this last season of *Spin City*: His performance, he makes clear, was ghosted as much by his previous break-through role on *Back to the Future* or *Family Ties* as it was affected by his previous, healthier self. It is this other "ghosting," quite independently from his diagnosis, which Fox mobilizes to retain and renew his bond with his audience. As Fox writes about his relationship to his studio audience after disclosing that he was affected by Parkinson's Disease,

> I feel I need to give them permission to laugh. So I say hello, tell a few jokes, and ask if there are any questions. One young woman puts it very simply: "How are you feeling?" "Better than I look," I answer her quickly and with a smile. "And I don't know about you, but I find me pretty damn cute." There is a brief delay and then, mercifully, a wave of warm laughter. Maybe this is going to be all right. (*Lucky Man* 237)

This reference to his own "cuteness", then, is both self-mockery and the knowledge that, to his audience, Fox has always been attractive. This phrase is remarkable for a number of reasons. First, it addresses, as Baryshnikov has done, the relationship between disability and sexual attractiveness. Baryshnikov, at fifty-one and despite baring his chest to the audience in a "medicalizing" gesture, is confident in the knowledge that it is him that the audience has come to see; it is this same confidence that, pace his PD diagnosis, Michael J. Fox may also be said to share.

What links Mikhail Baryshnikov's performance to Michael J. Fox's appearance on *Spin City*, for all the differences between these two men, is the knowledge of their own physical attractiveness impaired by the ways in which this body has changed through age or, in Fox's case, through illness. At the end of Baryshnikov's performance, and in deliberate contrast to the cardiac monitor which records the aging process – and hence, by social implication, the waning of physical attractiveness –, there may be, as Margo Jefferson notes, no "sexual grandstanding" (n. pag.), but there is the awareness and confidence by the master of dance that he may be aging, but he is still attractive. Similarly, Fox inscribes into his autobiography *Always Looking Up*, as well as into his acting performance, the fact that he may have dyskinesias (122), but he is still, as he puts it, "pretty damn cute" (*Lucky Man* 237). It is this "grandstanding" of a different kind on the part of both celebrity personae, which forces us to reconsider the interface, or the disconnect, between sexual attractiveness on the one hand and physical impairment on the other. This impairment, of course, may be gender specific; as Kathleen

Woodward and a host of other critics have argued, the aging of the human body is seen as different in men than in women (*Figuring Age*).

In the previous chapter on Mikhail Baryshnikov's modern dance, of the dancer's incorporating the aging process of his own body into his art through a cardiac monitor, I have tried to explore, first, the extent to which artistic production can be a form of life writing, and a form of life writing which is not only about a person's identity, but about the physical materiality of a life. Secondly, I have explored the ways in which life writing can also be a way of coming to terms with an illness, perhaps in the most literal sense of writing a life. What Michael J. Fox's memoirs do, then, is that they deliberately expose the actor's vulnerability, a vulnerability that, Fox is quick to point out, emerges quite simply from the actor's humanity. It is the universality of human vulnerability, which Fox's account of his own PD diagnosis drives home. In this sense, any life – the life of an able-boded, healthy individual, is always-already haunted by a sense of this person's vulnerability. It is in this sense, Fox points out, that he, the person afflicted by PD, ended up reassuring those who had come up to him originally to voice their sympathy with him, the patient.

Subsequently to his going public as a person suffering from Parkinson's Disease, Fox proceeded to work on a show in which both these personae – Fox the actor and Fox the person who had been diagnose with PD, would merge. Like Baryshnikov, then, Fox incorporates the change in his body's ability into his art – dissimilar as the process of aging and that of Parkinson's Disease are, there is at the heart of both performances – Baryshnikov's modern dance and Michael J. Fox's television comedy – the possibility, indeed, the quest to incorporate the materiality of the artist-actor's life into his artistic performance. With keen irony, Fox stresses the fact that it has been quite a feat to incorporate his PD diagnosis – and the body visibly affected by PD not just into any art form, but into *comedy* of all genres. In his reference to a *New York Times* article by Mireya Navarro, Fox himself draws a comparison between illness and disability; and muses about ways to convey experiences of difference in and through art. In this same article, Navarro writes about the stand-up comedian Josh Blue:

> "My right arm does a lot of crazy stuff. Like the other day, I thought someone had stolen my wallet."

> It's funny only if you know that Mr. Blue has cerebral palsy.
>
> The public image of people with disabilities has often hinged on the heroic or the tragic. But Mr. Blue, 28, represents the broader portrait of disability now infusing television and film. This new, sometimes confrontational stance reflects the higher expectations among many members of the disabled population that they be treated as people who happen to have a disability, rather than as people defined by disability. (Navarro, "Clearly, Frankly" n. pag.)

I am interested, then, in the ways in which a linguistic convention can be translated into narrative: The shift outlined by Navarro, the re-thinking of disability in significantly new ways, first works by transforming social criticism into linguistic conventions: What, Navarro asks, is the difference between "people defined by disability" and "people who happen to have a disability"? This, then, is the difference between the terminology of "disabled persons" and "persons with disability." Josh Blue, we may argue – as he himself does – is first and foremost a comedian; a comedian who happens to have cerebral palsy. It is this condition, then, which Blue inscribes – as one aspect among many – into his art. This, in essence, is what I am trying to argue with regard to our reading of autobiographical narratives of persons with illness or disability: The minute we regard these narratives not so much as illness narratives but as narratives by persons who are also affected by illness or disability, aspects of these narratives emerge which would otherwise have gone unnoticed. (This is an idea to which I will return below with regard to Michael J. Fox's embrace of Jewishness.) It is only in this way that these narratives *become* autobiographies in the full sense of the term.

What I am concerned with, then, is a shift both in representation and in reception. As Navarro notes, recent casting practices have opened up spaces for actors of disability in the sense that these actors have no longer been confined to acting out roles about disability. As Navarro notes,

> In Hollywood, disabled members of the Screen Actors Guild and other entertainment groups are agitating for plots that include more disabled characters and for the hiring of more disabled actors to play both disabled and nondisabled roles. . . . "It used to be that if you were disabled and on television, they'd play soft piano music behind you," said Robert

> David Hall, a double amputee who plays a coroner on "CSI." "The thing I love about 'CSI' is that I'm just Dr. Robbins." ("Clearly, Frankly" n. pag.)

What does it mean, then, for an actor with disability to play a non-disabled character? I believe that the shift indicated here could not be more profound. Precisely by making this form of casting possible, perception changes: the actor cast in a certain role is seen as an actor, first and foremost, and not an actor defined by his or her disability. What would happen, then, if we were to translate this politics of (media) representation into narrative? It would mean, quite simply, that aspects in the narrative would emerge which are not "about" illness or disability at all. In this way, I will argue below, Michael J. Fox's autobiographies can be read about growing up Irish Canadian, marrying into a Jewish community, or being short.

6.4 Michael J. Fox and "Biopolitics from Below"

Fox's autobiographies, and the politics of intervention that they are predicated on, correspond to one parameter in particular which has been raised in the debate around biological citizenship. In his book and with explicit reference to this debate, Fox establishes himself as a patient, who is implicitly part of a patient group whose intention it may be – and historically has been – to lobby for the funding of more research (in Fox's case, stem cell research) which might eventually lead to the discovery of a cure for Parkinson's Disease. Yet if in this context, Lemke has argued that patient groups have been chronically underfunded, this is emphatically not the case for Michael J. Fox. In fact, as his narrative makes clear, he uses his own considerable wealth and his prestige as a world-famous actor to generate research funds which, on the level of patient initiatives, have been unparalleled.

Crucially, Fox's role with regard to both the representation of the PD community and with regard to basic research about PD can be read as what Lemke has called "biopolitics from below" (129; my trans.). As in the concept of "genetic citizenship" espoused by Rapp and others (Lemke 126; my trans.), what is central to the idea of "biopolitics from below" is that the focus is not on the negative consequences of biomedical knowledge and the power of definition it may hold over our identities and life worlds, but, by contrast, the ways in which such biomedical knowledge can be appropriated by patient communities themselves. Explicitly referring to the link between concepts of "genetic citizenship" (Lemke 127; my trans.) and "biopolitics from below" (Lemke 129; my trans.), Lemke notes:

> What is common to these concepts is the idea of a systematic correlation between a biomedical production of knowledge, self-relations and political forms of articulation. For this reason, patients' associations, self-help groups and groups formed by relatives are said to attain growing political importance. Through these developments, it is assumed, new collective subjects emerge which shift the boundary between laymen and experts . . . . (127-28; my trans.)

There is an interesting dialogue here between the role of Temple Grandin as a (controversial) spokesperson for the autism community, on the one hand, and Michael J. Fox's advocacy and financial support for PD research on the other. While Grandin has been ascribed celebrity status on account of her representation of autism to a mainstream audience, Fox has used his celebrity status – a status he held prior to being diagnosed with PD – in order to lobby for more funding to be given to PD research. It is this celebrity status, then, which he has deliberately used in order to gain more visibility for the PD community and explicitly to influence funding policies. I would like to argue that Fox's description of his own role in this context can be read as an empirical case study for the role of "biopolitics from below" with regard to Parkinson's Disease. Lemke writes,

> So far, only few studies exist which have investigated this "biopolitics from below," which have empirically studied the relationship between collective forms of action, group identities and political activism by patient groups and relatives associations. Only to some extent do we know which rules for membership and which criteria for belonging inform the actions of those involved, what channels of influence and agencies of mediation they use and what alliances they form. (129; my trans.)

It is in the sense envisioned by Lemke, then, that Michael J. Fox's autobiography *Lucky Man* can be read as an in-depth description of how such a "biopolitics from below" can be put into practice.

How, then, does Fox set out to lobby for stem cell research? First, he deliberately uses his own body in his call for a change in policy; he uses himself as his own guinea pig, deliberately exposing the vulnerability of his body by choosing to be "off" his medication during the hearing. In an incident he discusses in detail in *Lucky Man*, conservative radio host Rush Limbaugh accused him of deliberately exaggerating his dyskinesias in a TV performance in order to manipulate his audience (Fox, *Always Looking Up* 131). For his TV appearance, then, Fox chose to be "off" his medication for a testimony in which he tries to convince the U.S. senate to allot more funding to PD research:

> My timing was so good, it was Swiss. The metaphorical "mole" had been whacked; the tremors and stiffness should have been neutralized for the next hour or two, but a blast of dyskinesias soon hit my brain and body. An easy technical explanation, like "overmedicated," would actually be a misnomer. . . . For the rest of the shoot I would be in the literal sway of levodopa's side effects: the rocking, dipping and diving of dyskinesias. (*Always Looking Up* 122)

At the core of Limbaugh's strident criticism of Fox's actions, then, was the accusation that Fox had actually "faked" or at least exaggerated some of the symptoms; an allegation, however, which Fox was able to disprove.

As Lemke has illustrated, moreover, the notion of a "biopolitics from below" has also meant that patient communities themselves explicitly engage in discussions about the ethics of biomedical research as it pertains to their own condition. According to Lemke, "A third area of this involvement by self-help groups and patients' associations consists in their participation in ethics committees and parliamentary counseling as well as the development of guidelines for the regulation of the use of technological procedures" (128; my trans.). It is in this context that it is highly significant that Fox should have intervened directly into debates about stem cell research and the ethics of such research. As he notes in *Lucky Man*, "Since my testimony in Washington, I have often been called upon to represent the P.D. community in the media, most notably during the national debate about embryonic stem cell research that monopolized the news during much of the summer of 2001" (249).

What emerges in this context is more than a mere dialogue between life writing and life sciences in discursive terms. Rather, what is at stake here is the use of a specific narrative by a specific patient – here, the use of autobiography and political activism by Michael J. Fox in order to achieve funding for stem cell research. In this sense, then, what is at stake is not only Fox's writing his autobiography and making his diagnosis public, but also the ways in which he has set out to strategically control the ways in which this narrative circulates in a public and a political arena. Setting out to use his own life writing narrative, then, Fox turns life writing into a means for political activism. Moreover, Fox himself is quick to stress the fact that the ability to lobby for an increase in funding for stem cell research and the possibility of founding his own organization is itself a sign of privilege. As he elaborates in *Lucky Man*,

> In the last couple of years, I've gone from talking to my agent on a cellular phone to discussing cellular biology with some of the world's leading scientists. It's a whole different world. If I'm with my peers in the entertainment business, I can at least fake being one of the smarter people in the room. In a group of neuroscientists, I just try to listen carefully and take a lot of notes. (248)

What emerges here, in line with Lemke's description of biopolitics from below, is a sense in which patient communities – and celebrity spokespersons like Fox in particular – enter the (neuro)scientific debate around new forms of treatment. What is more, since funding for such research is often short, patient initiatives such as the foundation founded by Fox himself may in fact be able to influence future research.

The downside of this form of activism, Lemke has cautioned, may lie in the way in which it may privilege some patient groups over others. Those communities which do not include a celebrity as their main spokesperson, in other words, may be marginalized in this very process. Moreover, Lemke emphasizes that both concepts of genetic citizenship and biopolitics from below may in fact be counterproductive since they call for benefits to be extended to some patient groups and genetically different communities, rather than stressing the need of health care for all. This may hold true for both a biopolitics from below and for calls for genetic citizenship. Lemke observes,

> The rights and claims demanded by associations of those concerned are articulated less in the name of general health care and universal rights, than on the basis of a specific genetic profile, which is usually shared by

> only a few individuals. This makes the political articulation of rights more difficult, since the emphasis lies on genetic difference rather than on a common biological identity. (129; my trans.)

This idea as well as the concept of "genetic citizenship" will be taken up again in more detail in Chapter 7.

What is at stake in what I am reading as Michael J. Fox's "biopolitics from below," then, is a deliberate instrumentalization of the haunting of his own body as a Hollywood celebrity living with Parkinson's Disease. Precisely by using this form of "ghosting," to use Marvin Carlson's term (Carlson 2), Fox deliberately employs and highlights the way in which his body will be perceived both as the award-winning actor and a person diagnosed with Parkinson's Disease. The concept of a "biopolitics from below" is thus perhaps misleading, or at least, it is rendered more complicated by Fox's strategic use of his own body. Fox uses his celebrity status, in a form of "biopolitics from above" in which the celebrity comes to stand in for the PD community, in order not only to gain more visibility for Parkinson's Disease, but also to successfully lobby for funding. As some critics have noted, however, this politics may further marginalize those patient communities who do not have a powerful celebrity as their spokesperson. They, too, may want their Michael J. Fox. Thus, as Kristin Barker has recently suggested, the fibromyalgia patient community has lamented the fact that they do not have a celebrity spokesperson of their own (n. pag.).

6.5 "A Hole in the Head": Life Sciences *as* Life Writing

At the same time, as in the dialogue between life sciences and life writing which informed the decision – by both the patient and the surgeon – to go through with Fox's brain surgery, what Fox appeals to is life writing at its most powerful. He wants to push stem cell research, he argues, because of the life which this research may make possible for persons living with Parkinson's Disease, including himself. Quite simply, he informs the jury, he wants to be able to dance at his youngest daughter's wedding. What this implies, then, is also the power of life writing as a rationale for changing decision-making processes in the life sciences.

It is for this very reason, the ability to retain the sympathy and the respect of his audience despite or because of the way in which he made public his own vulnerability, that Fox describes himself in his first autobiography as a "lucky man" (*Lucky Man* 5). It is through his diagnosis he recalls that he finally overcame his alcoholism and began to take charge of his own life. As Fox writes in his first autobiography, *Lucky Man*, "What [the doctor who first diagnosed his illness] did not tell me – what no one could – is that these last ten years of coming to terms with my disease would turn out to be the best ten years of my life – not in spite of my illness, but because of it" (5).

Crucially, Fox makes clear that any success in the treatment of PD depends on a constructive dialogue between life writing and life science: having researched possibilities of slowing down the process through which his PD symptoms grew worse, Fox eventually decided to have brain surgery. The doctor's willingness to go through with the operation, however, depended on the patient's rationale for wanting an operation in the first place.

There is thus a juncture in the autobiography where Fox's narrative, *Lucky Man*, turns on its head the potential dichotomy between life sciences and life writing. When the trembling in his left side has exacerbated, Fox considers having brain surgery. The way in which he describes this process of decision-making may itself be significant for an analysis concerned with the interfaces between life sciences and life writing: First, Fox is well aware that it is his wealth that enables him to consider this form of brain surgery to begin with, and to consult the specialists who may be able to perform such an operation. As he interviews Bruce Cook, the surgeon who will eventually agree to operate on his brain, however, Fox is well aware that it is not the patient interviewing the surgeon to whom he will, quite literally, entrust his life, but vice versa: "'"As far as Parkinson's tremors go,' Dr. Cook told me recently, 'yours were very severe; most don't get to be so bad. I try to talk people out of surgery if it doesn't make sense for them. Their goal in having the operation has to be a reasonable one.' I hadn't been interviewing him, I realize now; he had been interviewing me" (*Lucky Man* 202). It is the surgeon who is interviewing the patient, trying to decide whether or not he will ultimately agree to perform the operation. Significantly, the surgeon's decision is based on just what it is that we describe as "quality of life", and it rests on a definition of this quality, which seems more akin to life writing than to life science. Ultimately, what convinces the surgeon is not Fox's invoking of his career as an actor, his professional performance which is made impossible by his body's quite literally "acting up," but the reference to a moment from everyday life which is only seemingly trivial: the evening routine when, at night, Fox likes to read to his children, sitting at their bedside:

> "It was something else you said to me," he said. "You talked about Sam. About how difficult it had become to do something as simple as read a book to him. That you couldn't keep the book steady or turn the pages by yourself, and he would have to hold it for you. . . . A lot of people can be on TV but only one person can be your kid's father. When you described it to me in those terms, it made sense. I was ready to go ahead with the procedure." (*Lucky Man* 204-205)

It is in this moment that life writing – here, the oral narrative told by a man who defines himself not so much through his acting than through the life he shares with his wife and children, which informs a decision based in the life sciences. The point which Fox makes here, and which the surgeon insists on, is not only the medical technology available to us at the beginning of the twenty-first century, but the decisions we will have to make on whether to use this technology or not. It is this decision-making, the narrative informs us, which is the challenge of human life in the era of biomedical technology. In this maze of biomedical possibilities and their consequences, Fox's text insists, life writing may be our only way of navigating, of finding directions in, this maze.[1]

What does this mean, then, in more general terms? What Fox describes here in his autobiography is the very process of decision-making which can be described as a co-authorship between doctor and patient. There are many implications to this passage. First, it suggests that a co-construction of knowledge, and of the therapy which is eventually employed, depends on a co-authorship between doctor and patient. While this co-authorship has been taken for granted in fields such as psychosomatic medicine, it may also be addressed, as Fox's account shows, in the field of brain surgery. What this passage also shows is that there

[1] I am indebted to Alfred Hornung for this idea, which was the nucleus of the interdisciplinary research training group "Life Sciences – Life Writing: Boundary Experiences of Human Life between Biomedical Explanation and Lived Experience" which would later develop based on his vision.

does not need to be a dichotomy between a highly developed, technologically advanced medical practice and an attention paid to narrative. As I have tried to outline in the introduction as well as in a number of other instances, Charon cautions that an increasing emphasis on biomedical technologies may lead to a decrease in "narrative knowledge" (*Narrative Medicine* 9). Yet, what Fox's account of the decision-making process illustrates is that this dichotomy is by no means automatic. Rather, this instance points to the necessity of bridging the gap between a highly efficient, state-of-the-art biomedical practice and what Charon would call the power of narrative medicine.

In her work on narrative medicine, Charon turns the act of collaborative reading and writing into medical practice. While Charon is concerned with a specific practice of medicine as well as the didactics of medicine, I would argue that her work resonates across a variety of fields within medicine as well. In a recently published essay, she and Eric R. Marcus describe a specific consultation and the process of co-authorship between herself and her patient: "After I finished writing my note, I turned the monitor toward her and asked her to read it and tell me what I had gotten wrong or what she thought did not belong in a chart that could be read by other clinicians. I then gave her the keyboard and asked her to complete the story of our visit" (Charon and Marcus 282). I would argue that such a process of co-authorship may also be seen as being at the core of Fox's conversation with his surgeon. What is especially noteworthy here is the dialogue which takes place between life writing and life science, a dialogue which is far from dichotomous. Moreover, the "poles" of life sciences and life writing are not "embodied" by the brain surgeon, Dr. Cook, and the actor, respectively; rather, both Fox and Cook base their decision-making on a dialogue between life sciences and life writing. This, moreover, may be an instance of narrative medicine in Rita Charon's concept of the term: The surgeon agrees to go through with the operation only after listening to the patient's narrative, and by taking into account all elements from this narrative, also and especially those elements seemingly unrelated to the patient's illness. The surgeon is well aware that the act of surgery will re-write Fox's life, just as he informs the patient of the risks involved in this operation; and he stresses the fact that this decision can only be made through a form of co-authorship between the patient and the surgeon. The surgeon will avail the patient of his skill only if he too, sees the operation as being justified. This moment, as it is described in Fox's autobiography, I believe, is almost a utopian one: it captures the ways in which decisions can be made only through a co-authorship between the medical practitioner and the patient. At the core of Charon's notion of co-authorship is the sense that medical practice, too, can be seen as a narrative, or at least to include narrative elements. (To reduce medical practice only to narrative practice, one might argue, may be counterproductive.) Reflexivity, Charon argues, is not only to recognize the ways in which one's "findings" are shaped by or conveyed in narrative, but also to reflect on the specific "culture" in which this narrative is set and, to some extent, made possible. Charon and Marcus point out, "The reflexive practitioner takes account of multiple contradictory perspectives, sees himself or herself from outside the self, critiques not only his/her actions but his/her stance, and acknowledges the co-creating role he or she plays in the study of the object as it unfolds" (284). According to Charon, the relevance of what she calls "reflexivity" has already been stressed by the field of psychotherapy; yet, it may not have been discussed by other fields within medicine to the same extent. It is for this reason, I believe, that the conversation between Michael J. Fox and his brain surgeon may be especially significant in this context. According to Charon and Marcus,

> A core dimension of the creative process is reflexivity, conceptualized as the capacity of an individual to observe the self with the same methods with which that individual studies phenomena. The concept of reflexivity is most often used by social scientists, oral historians, or psychotherapists to suggest that the clinician or scientist or anthropologist must recognize the role that he or she plays in the phenomenon under study. (283)

To return to Fox's narrative, the point which the surgeon makes is not only that the life sciences can reshape and rewrite human lives at the beginning of the twenty-first century, but that we must carefully weigh the consequences ensuing from these rewritings. The challenge, that both Fox's text and the surgeon's narrative record is to accord to life writing a key role in this process of decision-making. Moreover, this dialogic account in which both the surgeon and Fox assume co-authorship over a life lived with Parkinson's Disease upsets any facile dichotomy between the vulnerability of the patient and the aloofness of the surgeon. The surgeon too, is vulnerable in the sense that he is, and must be, aware of his own fallibility; he, too, cannot perform the operation unaware of the consequences it might have. It is this fallibility of medical practice, performed by human hands, which Fox's narrative captures through the analogy between rocket science and brain surgery. In *Lucky Man*, Fox recalls the moment in which his wife and his mother talked to his brain surgeon in order to assess the risk that his operation would involve:

> "Why do *you* think it is…," I asked Dr. Cook, partly to break the tension, but also because I really wanted to know, "that brain surgery, above all else – even rocket science – gets singled out as the most challenging of human feats, the one demanding the utmost of human intelligence?" To my surprise, Dr. Cook actually considered my question for a beat, took a swallow of diet soda, and then offered an answer: "No margin for error." (208)

The surgeon, too, is well aware that there is "no margin for error" in the surgery he will perform; and precisely because so much is at stake, he will base his decision on whether or not to go through with the operation only on the power of life writing.

The hole in the head which Fox's narrative playfully invokes with a reference to popular culture, namely to a 2003 song by the "Sugababes," at once attests to the power of the life sciences at the beginning of the twenty-first century. At the same time, it deliberately invokes the playfulness of the "hole in the head" which, in Fox's case, is precisely not metaphorical. It is through irony, moreover, that Fox's narrative makes the result of the operation bearable, driving home not so much the fallibility of the life sciences but the ways in which they may not be able to predict each and every outcome of their operations. The operation, Fox writes, is successful; the incision works precisely the way it is supposed to. The power of the life sciences, as Fox describes them in a narrative which is much more than a patient account, lies in the fact that – inconceivable to lay persons – an incision can be made in a person's brain while the patient is fully conscious, and able to communicate with the surgeon during the operation: "I remember – this must have been a couple hours into the operation – Dr. Cook asking me to count to ten out loud. Somewhere between two and four, though, the voice I heard counting sounded as though it was coming from somebody else. . . . And then I remember someone (Dr. Cook?) asking me to put my hand in a position that would cause it to tremor" (*Lucky Man* 209). The operation, Fox recalls in his autobiography, was successful; when he was once again fully conscious, the left side of his body had stopped trembling. Not so, however, his right side. As he ends the chapter in his autobiography devoted to his decision to go through with brain surgery to control the effects of his Parkinson's Disease, Fox notes:

> I was focused on my hand. I stared at it, and waited. Inside of five minutes my fingers began to flutter. It was subtle, no one else would ever have noticed, but it was there. It was just like at the beginning, just like before, with one very big difference: this wasn't my left had I was looking at. There was no question that the operation had been a success; my left side was as still as the sheltered blue bay in front of me. The problem now was with my right – the tremor had moved into the right side of my body. (*Lucky Man* 210)

The moment described here in Fox's autobiographical account of his illness is one of the central moments in Charon's account of narrative medicine: It is the moment in which, even though they have co-written the narrative of therapy, doctor and patient are left to wonder at the unpredictability of the disease itself, the impossibility of fully assuming authorship over the narrative of illness. The hardest part, Fox notes at the end of this chapter, is to resign oneself to the fact that there will be instances in which one cannot assume authorship over one's own life. What Fox's narrative draws attention to is the dichotomy between the control of contingency and the loss of such control. Arguably, modern biomedicine sets out to control all forms of contingency, from the beginning to the end of life. It is in this sense that brain surgery has enabled Fox to stop the tremor on his left side; yet, this control of the contingency of PD eventually turns out to be only temporary: "I picked up some shells for the kids and stuffed them into the pockets of my shorts, and somewhere along the way, as I had almost every day since I'd stopped drinking six years earlier, I said this prayer: *God grant me the serenity to accept the things I cannot change / Courage to change the things I can / And the wisdom to know the difference*" (*Lucky Man* 211; emphasis in original).

6.6 The "Haunting" of Autobiography

What, then, is the relationship between Fox's first autobiography, *Lucky Man*, and his second autobiographical narrative, *Always Looking Up*? I believe that this deliberate re-reading, in *Always Looking Up*, of his first autobiography by the man who wrote it, is to expose the very politics of haunting: If in his "HeartBeat: mb" performance, Baryshnikov deliberately creates a body palimpsest between the present-day dancer and the younger self which his present performance is ghosted by, to use Marvin Carlson's term, Fox does the same in *Lucky Man*: He describes, seven years after the publication of his first autobiography, the fact that the symptoms he thought terrible then seem laughable now from his present vantage point and gives the deterioration of his symptoms:

> In the opening pages of *Lucky Man*, I described a morning in Florida nineteen years ago when I woke up with a hangover and a twitching left pinky finger. In the intervening years, my life has seen many changes. Most mornings, for example, I awake to find my left pinkie finger perfectly still – it's the rest of my body that's shaking uncontrollably. Technically, my body is only fully at peace when my mind is completely at rest – that is, asleep. (Fox, *Always Looking Up* 1-2).

As in Baryshnikov's HeartBeat: mb performance, Fox turns himself into a "vulnerable subject" (Couser, *Vulnerable Subjects* xii) in describing to the audience the painfulness of his everyday routine. If Baryshnikov exposes his body to the audience's gaze by making this body translucent, by providing an interior image of the beating of his own heart, Fox's act of self-depiction is quite similar here. He describes the moment of looking into the mirror in the morning, describing to his audience/readership just what he sees, with no sugarcoating or concealment of the severity of his condition. Even holding a toothbrush, he writes, can be quite a feat:

> Grasping the toothpaste is nothing compared to the effort it takes to coordinate the two-handed task of wrangling the toothbrush and strangling out a line of paste onto the bristles. By now, my right hand has started up again, rotating at the wrist in a circular motion, perfect for what I am about to do. My left hand guides my right hand up to my mouth, and once the back of the Oral-B touches the inside of my upper lip, I let go. It's like releasing the tension on a slingshot and compares most favora-

> ble to the most powerful state-of-the-art electric toothbrush on the market. (Fox, *Always Looking Up* 3)

With characteristic self-irony, he exposes the vulnerability of his body to the audience's gaze, and imagines this audience holding its breath. The politics of haunting which Fox's two autobiographies engage are thus twofold: In his first autobiography, *Lucky Man*, he superimposed on his present day body, already visibly affected by Parkinson's Disease, his younger self, the main actor of *Spin City* and a star comedian who never had to worry about his body spoiling the punch lines. In his second autobiography, *Always Looking Up*, on the other hand, his self-image is haunted by a body already affected by Parkinson's Disease but functional to an extent that his present-day body is not. Why, then, should he have subtitled his second autobiography "The adventures of an incurable optimist" (Fox, *Always Looking Up* dust jacket n. pag.)? As his narrative opens, Fox himself answers this very question:

> At the turn from our bedroom into the hallway, there is an old full-length mirror in a wooden frame. I can't help but catch a glimpse of myself as a pass. Turning fully toward the glass, I consider what I see. This reflected version of myself, wet, shaking, rumpled, pinched, and slightly stooped, would be alarming were it not for the self-satisfied expression pasted across my face. I would ask the obvious question, "What are you smiling about?", but I already know the answer: "It just gets better from here." (*Always Looking Up* 3-4)

Yet, the very cover image of both autobiographies, and the photographs supplied inside the narratives, belie this image of vulnerability. With his face half-hidden by his hand, and smiling shyly into the camera, or in images of himself being kissed on the cheek by his wife, Fox's persona, even and especially in his autobiographies, dares the audience to equate illness with a lack of attractiveness: Fox, the Hollywood film star who has reinvented himself in representing to the public his life with Parkinson's, is fully aware that his shaking notwithstanding, he is still "pretty damn cute" (Fox, *Lucky Man* 237). In this self-assurance, which implicitly also addresses the relationship between sex and disability, Fox's narrative, and his visual self-representation, parallels that of Mikhail Baryshnikov, the aging virtuoso dancer: Baryshnikov, too, knows that he will be sexy even in a wheelchair. Yet, the engaging, by both stars, of the ways in which their bodies will be haunted for the audiences by their previous selves and the rise of these selves to stardom, is not without problems: For what this self-assurance, born of the moment of haunting implies is that sexual attractiveness and disability continue to be at opposite ends of the spectrum of physical desirability: Both men, the narrative they create in their self-representations implies, might not be (as) attractiveness if it were not for the haunting of their bodies in the audience's mind. Had the audience encountered Fox only in his present state of health and had it never known his previous self, unaffected by illness, the outcome would not quite have been the same. Even so, however, the effect of engaging the politics – and the physical aesthetics of haunting – may send a powerful message to an audience trapped in master-narratives of normalcy: namely the simple assertion that illness or disability and sexual attractiveness may not be incompatible. As Navarro notes,

> Jillian Weise, 25, a teacher and doctoral student at the University of Cincinnati, released a poetry book this year to undermine what she called "the stereotype of the disabled as asexual" and "to try to get away from the idea of the disabled as freak." She titled it "The Amputee's Guide to Sex" and filled it with deeply personal verses. "You trace the scar along my spine, and I imagine what it must feel like," reads one poem. ("Clearly, Frankly" n. pag.)

Reading *Lucky Man* now, Fox writes in *Always Looking Up*, is like watching a re-run of *Spin City*; as his own audience, Fox looks at this younger, still healthier self. To embrace his PD diagnosis, he makes clear, is not to judge or despair over the nature of this ghosting. It is in this instance, as in many others, that Fox takes courage from Muhammad Ali, his fellow Parkinson's patient:

> When I see the old footage of my new friend, fighting, dancing, clowning, I feel sad and angry for him. I wondered if he did, too. Was it difficult for him to see a younger, healthier, and stronger version of Ali? . . . Sometimes when channel surfing, I am ambushed by the image of a younger, healthier me. Usually, I just carry on clicking, giving it no more thought than I would an infomercial. There are times though, I confess, when I will pause and set the remote on the coffee table for a minute or two – sometimes longer. (*Always Looking Up* 68)

There is a pitfall, then, in applying Marvin Carlson's idea of ghosting to a reading of Parkinson's Disease as it is carefully scripted into the autobiography of Michael J. Fox. For what Carlson describes, after all, is "just" theater; it is the haunting or ghosting of the actor's present-day performance by his earlier self, his actor presence in previous roles. What does it mean, then, to include not just the actor-presence but the actor's body into this equation? Surely to do so may run the risk of trivializing the experience of illness. As Fox emphatically writes, Parkinson's is not a *role*. And yet, staging his Parkinson's Disease or rather, representing its significance to an audience acquainted only with normalcy, is part of his newly found mission: In this transition, Fox, too, had to come to terms with the personae making up his present-day self.

And yet, there is something powerful, for instance in Mikhail Baryshnikov's inscribing not just the ghost of his previous performances into dance, but also to include the ghosts of the younger embodiment of the dancer into the performance itself: the heart beat thus evokes not only the dancer's exertion and his body in the present, but also the previous bodies which, implicitly, are evoked in and by the performance: the heartbeat in "HeartBeat: mb" echoes the younger dancer's heart which, in this posture, would not have beat quite as fast. It is this sense of echoing, also, which Michael J. Fox brings to his two autobiographies.

It is in the sense of multiple contexts and multiple frameworks being brought to bear on one and the same narrative that the title of Fox's second autobiography, *Always Looking Up*, is deliberately ambiguous. What is at stake, then, is a careful orchestration of theme and background music, and of multiple themes. I am interested, then, in the way in which Fox's second autobiography, *Always Looking Up*, can be read not only as illness narrative but also in terms of a variety of other genres: interreligious romance, celebrity autobiography, or actor's memoir. It is this double or triple framing which his autobiographies – and his second autobiography in particular – engages. For why would his son, born two years before Fox's diagnosis, be named Sam Fox, even though his faith was not Jewish? What Fox evokes in *Always Looking Up* is the irony of coincidence which, of course, through this framing comes to seem much more than coincidence. He describes in detail the naming of his son:

> "Oh wait," Tracy said. "Sam Fox?"
>
> "Yeah, Sam Fox," I said. I was ready to commit.
>
> All of a sudden Tracy started to laugh uncontrollably. "Sam Fox?" she said, still giggling. "It's just so… so Jewish."
>
> "Now I love it," I said.
>
> Tracy is from a Jewish family, and though I hadn't converted, we were married under a *chuppah*. Over the ten years between my arrival in Los Angeles in 1979 and this moment in the hospital with my bride and newborn son, I had become happily immersed in the community and culture of American Reform Judaism. My friends, my associates, and now my family were for the most part Jews. (Fox, *Always Looking Up* 183)

Fox describes, in his autobiography which is shaped by but can by no means be reduced to PD diagnosis, his own genealogy as an actor, and as a person. What emerges from his re-reading of his own life in *Always Looking Up*, is a sense of cultural inwardness, of empathy and an alternative form of cultural kinship. His socialization in Hollywood, Fox, the Irish-Canadian actor writes, was a Jewish one: "I don't know if I fully realized it at first, but a lot of the acquaintances I made upon arriving in Los Angeles and insinuating myself into the entertainment industry were Jewish people – my agents, my managers, and many of the directors, producers, and actors I worked with, as well" (*Always Looking Up* 194). It is by virtue of this immersion in a Jewish-inflected Hollywood community of comedians and producers, Fox muses in retrospect, that his sense of comedy and of acting, has come to be curiously Jewish: "The producer/director Garry Marshall gave me his theory regarding my success in comedy: 'You've got Jewish timing,' he said, 'and a *goyishe punim*.' That is to say, I can deliver a joke in a style that has its roots in Yiddish treater, but I look like the typical 'boy next door'" (*Always Looking Up* 195). It is in this sense, then, that Fox, curiously enough, could be said to have become "Jewish" even before he married Tracy Pollan, a Jewish-American actress in 1988. As Fox himself describes the irony: "In 1985, in an interview with *People* magazine, I was asked if I planned to marry one day. 'Oh yes, definitely,' I said. 'I'm going to marry a Jewish girl.' When the reporter asked me why, I said something along the lines of 'Because I won't have to make any decisions, and I can eat Chinese food on Sundays.' I was half-right – sometimes we have Indian" (*Always Looking Up* 195).

It is in this sense, then, that *Always Looking Up*, as an autobiography, has nothing to do with illness in the first place; or rather, it can also and simultaneously be read as an interreligious romance. By having his son circumcised, Fox writes, he sought to provide him with – or facilitate his access to – a particular sort of genealogy (*Always Looking Up* 183). In an irony which Fox is quick to highlight, his own name could be read as Jewish in the first place: "My surname 'Fox,' common in the Lancastershire area from which my Church of England grandfather emigrated to Canada . . ., I also understood, was a common 'Ellis Islandization' of a number of surnames common among Ashkenazi Jews of Eastern Europe" (*Always Looking Up* 183).

By the same token, I will argue in the next chapter that in Jason Kingsley and Mitchell Levitz's co-written autobiography, *Count Us In*, only one of the chapters explicitly deals with the authors' having Down Syndrome; other chapters deal with the experience of adolescence, the relevance of their Jewish faith to their upbringing, or their plans for their future careers. Where autobiography can be seen to be the "Trojan horse" included, inconspicuously, into the rubric of illness narrative or patient account, is precisely in this complexity. Autobiography, by its very nature, exceeds the narrowness of patient narrative. An author, to put it differently, is always more than a patient. In fact, the very assuming of authorship could be seen to sabotage a medical paradigm in which a given autobiography – *Lucky Man* or *Count Us In* – could otherwise be subsumed. It is hence significant for my purposes here that in the published version of these accounts, publishers often try to "re-medicalize" these autobiographical accounts, as I have suggested in reference to Oliver Sacks' forewords to both Tito Mukhopadhyay's and Temple Grandin's texts. The aim of this study, then, is to deliberately suspend the connection between autobiography and illness/disability narrative, even as I acknowledge the connections between the two.

There is a gap in medical humanities, then, and this is precisely the "excess" that performance studies can bring to medical humanities. For there is a tendency, as critics within and outside the field of medical humanities have argued, to take a patient narrative at face value, to discount or dismiss, in other words, the degree to which this narrative, too, is *staged*. In an interview with Michael J. Fox, George Stroumboulopoulos addresses the question of authenticity: Now that Fox has gone public about his PD diagnosis, he may as well play who he is on the screen as well ("Michael J. Fox on George Stroumboulopoulos"). This, of course, discounts the idea of performance in and of itself; the sense that this performance of a character with Parkinson's Disease by someone who is a PD patient is not a performance, or is a performance to a different degree. What is revealed if we read the interview against the grain through Fox's own life writing, however, is the sense that Fox is not only a patient but he is, first and foremost, a comedian, a comedian using the *material* that his body provides him with. As Fox said in conversation with David Letterman on the Late Show on April 15, 2015:

> LETTERMAN: April is Awareness Month, Parkinson's Disease Awareness Month? That what it is?
>
> FOX [*deliberately drawing attention to the ways in which his body has been twitching throughout the interview*]: I'm fully aware of it. [*The audience laughs*]. It's rocked in with me. ("Michael J. Fox – Letterman")

What is at stake in this example, then, is not the simple act of "coping" with illness through laughter, or through publicly accepting one's diagnosis; it is the idea of performing the way in which one's body is materially changing, and thus drawing attention to the excess[2] implicit in each performance. In many different ways, Michael J. Fox's memoir, *Lucky Man*, takes up many of the issues I have discussed so far. Especially with regard to Tito Mukhopadhyay's *The Mind Tree*, I have asked not only what is to be gained, but also what might be lost from reading Mukhopadhyay's text within a framework of medical humanities. It is this single-purpose reading, I believe, which Fox's memoir resists, even as it explicitly takes as its starting point Fox's PD diagnosis. What is at stake in Fox's memoir is precisely Carlson's idea of the ghosting of the actor by his previous performance; yet, in Fox's account, what emerges is not just the ghosting of a present-day performance by previous on-screen appearances – the ghosting, for instance, of Fox's starring in *Spin City* by his award-winning performance in *Back to the Future*, but also

[2] I am indebted to Anita Wohlmann for this idea of performance with regard to Michael J. Fox's appearance on *The Good Wife* (2009-2016).

the ghosting – in reverse chronological order – of the able-bodied performer by the traces of his own illness. For Fox, it is the idea of "growing up small" which has made for the fact that, from his adolescence onwards, he had been confronted with the stubborn refusal of his body to conform to the norm. His biological frame, as he puts it, stubbornly refused to match his chronological age. From the very beginning of his life, then, there was a confusion of temporalities. It is this confusion of temporalities, as Fox observes with the self-mockery which is characteristic of his memoir, which caused one of the agents to speak of disability. Fox recalls an interview with an agent early on in his career:

> My composure was tested during one particularly memorable interview. The agent in the chair across from me seemed distinctly underwhelmed at the prospect of representing me. An awkwardness hung over the office like a methane cloud. For some reason, she couldn't look me in the eye – her gaze kept drifting down to my feet. Finally, she summoned up the nerve to say what was on her mind. . . . "Listen, Michael, you've got a great look and you're very funny and charming. . . . It's just that I don't understand why [my assistant] didn't mention … that is, I wasn't prepared … well, I wasn't aware that you had a disability." And with that her eyes went back down to my feet. . . . Now we were both staring at my feet. Those weren't orthopedic shoes. . . . [They] were boots – . . . the very height of 1970s cool, in my considered opinion. Embarrassed, I managed to laugh it off while assuring her that my only handicap was being a few inches too short – and, I realized in a sickening flash, several years behind the California fashion curve. (*Lucky Man* 65-66)

Yet, as Fox is keen to observe, it was the stubborn fact of his body – or rather, his height failing to keep up with his chronological age which catapulted him into media success. It was owing to this curious asynchronicity that he was cast as Marty McFly, the teenaged protagonist of *Back to the Future* at a time when Fox the actor was twenty-four years old.

In his memoir *Lucky Man*, a title which deliberately contrast with the Parkinson's diagnosis, which gave rise to the writing of the book in the first place, Fox is quick to point to the irony of asynchronicity which has marked his life: In *Back to the Future*, the beginning of his film career which instantly catapulted him into stardom, it was his body's failing to keep time, its lagging behind the actor's chronological age which proved to be a blessing. It was this same body, however, which ten years later proved to be ahead of his time in Fox's being diagnosed with Young Onset Parkinson's Disease. As Fox writes in his first autobiography, "Young Onset Parkinson's (the appearance of symptoms in people under forty), the diagnosing physician had explained, is rare. These patients make up less than ten per cent of the overall Parkinson's population. This, I'd learn later, made me one of only a hundred thousand or so North Americans in my predicament. Just this once, though, I got no satisfaction of beating the odds" (*Lucky Man* 143).

I believe that in many different ways Fox's memoir *Lucky Man* can be read not from beginning to end but also from end to beginning: In the beginning and at the end of his book Fox explores the different ways in which his own body might be read: as the body of an actor ghosted, in Carlson's sense, by his previous acting personae; *and* as the body of an actor who happens to have Parkinson's Disease. The telos of Fox's narrative is precisely the point of convergence and the dissimilarity between these two forms of ghosting: The end of his career, as Fox puts it, would have been the reduction, by the audience's sympathetic and well-meaning gaze, of the actor to his illness. For Fox, the way in which to emplot and incorporate his illness into story of his life, the telos of his career and his personal life, lay in finally being "off" in front of the camera, in no longer having to hide his symptoms.

I am interested, then, in which sense/what way *Lucky Man*, is much more than a story of illness, and the ways in which – through the very structure of his narrative – it flaunts and insists on its own belonging to multiple genres: celebrity autobiography, Canadian life writing, working class narrative, *and* illness narrative. *Lucky Man* is thus characterized by a curious layering of personae and temporalities: Fox, the narrator, looks back on his younger, able-bodied self with the knowledge of the ways in which his body – the body which enacted its asynchronous temporality in *Back to the Future* – was marked, in the present of writing, by another of asynchronicity: by developing a disease which normally affects persons much older in age. Fox's narrative hence revolves around the notion of vulnerability, and of exposure.

I have argued in this chapter that Fox's autobiographies *Lucky Man* and *Always Looking Up* can be read along various registers, thus by far exceeding their subsuming under the category of a "patient account." In trying to create a dialogue between Fox's literary/textual politics on the one hand and Mikhail Baryshnikov's dance performance, I have inquired into what possibilities the artist/author/performer may have for inscribing the changing material condition of his body into his art. Both Baryshnikov and Fox thus point to what may be termed an aesthetic excess at the core of life writing in both literature and modern dance. It is this aesthetic excess, in turn, which sabotages the reading of Fox's autobiographies as mere patient accounts. It is here that the idea of "medical humanities in American Studies" may gain yet another twist. For Baryshnikov's performance can be discussed and taught, in an academic setting, both in theater and performance studies and in medical humanities. By the same token, Fox's autobiographies contribute to life writing research as much as they may offer illness narratives about persons living with PD. I have tried to propose in this chapter that unless they take into account the material condition of the author's body, humanities readings of life writing texts such as Fox's will fall short of their potential. In other words, unless the humanities re-import the interpretations offered by medical humanities, they may be missing out on an important dimension of life writing narratives. By the same token, unless medical humanities import narratives such as Fox's only as patient accounts, dismissing the aesthetic excess that these narratives have to offer – an excess which turns them into literary narratives –, they may reduce the complexity of a life lived with, but by no means defined by a neurological condition. It is in this sense that, in this chapter, I have read Fox's autobiographies through Rita Charon's method of narrative medicine. This, too, may be a form of re-import: Developed as a tool to change medical practice, narrative medicine may also serve as a means of opening up another layer of meaning in life writing texts. In this sense, too, it can be imported or re-imported into humanities research. Finally, in both this chapter and the one that follows, I want to inquire into the relevance and the currency of "citizenship" in the discussion of both illness and disability. In inscribing themselves into the debate around the question of what constitutes "full citizenship," life writing texts may call for an inclusion of disability into the citizenry of the nation; yet, such inclusion may also come at a price.

7 Writing the Citizen: Growing Up with Down Syndrome in *Raising Henry* and *Count Us In*

7.1 Towards a Co-Production of Knowledge: Life Sciences and Life Writing

The aim of this paper is to argue that knowledge of the human body and the potential of a human life unfolding from this body is being produced not only through biomedicine, but also through life writing and life writing research.[1] Even as medical discussions have recently started including quality of life research to a higher extent, this research may still remain abstract and, to some extent, limited as well. It is at this juncture that life writing research may prove crucial as a field in which alternative knowledge is being produced. The question about the production of knowledge, I believe, is a crucial one. At the beginning of the twenty-first century, who produces knowledge about human life, and by what means? And what is the status accrued to these layers or fields of knowledge? To what extent can they be said to interact and to what degree, conversely, are they commonly held to be incompatible with one another? As Lemke notes, drawing on Foucault's notion of biopolitics, "The second line of reception drawing on Foucault's concept of biopolitics, is interested in the way in which new insights from the life sciences and the development of new technologies enable a new grasp of processes of life, ultimately changing the definition of life itself in a fundamental manner" (121; my trans.). This chapter will look at narratives of living with Down Syndrome as exemplary of such knowledge production. I will investigate two specific life writing texts – *Raising Henry* (2013), Rachel Adams's autobiography of the first three years of raising her son, who was born with Down Syndrome, and Jason Kingsley's and Mitchell Levitz's collaborative autobiography *Count Us In* (2007) –, to look not so much at how Down Syndrome as a medical

[1] For the implications of this distinction, I am indebted to Antje Kley.

diagnosis is depicted in these texts, but at how life writing intersects with or counters such a diagnosis.

What does it mean to grow up with Down Syndrome in the U.S. today? The first simple point to be made here is that medical diagnosis as such may mean nothing in itself; the fact, as Rachel Adams and many other writers and critics have argued, is the question of what this diagnosis means for those on whose lives it is inscribed. Quite literally, Adams argues, the discourse of the life sciences can be understood, made sense of, only through life writing. Adams's seminal narrative, *Raising Henry: A Memoir of Motherhood, Disability, and Discovery* (2013), can be read through many different frameworks at once. First, it is the autobiography of herself as a young mother; in this autobiographical account of mothering, however, Adams at once reflects on her own experience of growing up without a mother, her own mother having passed away when she was very young. At the same time, it is also a mother's biography of her son, of his first three years; as such, it is also a collaborative autobiography.

There is a crucial point to be made here. If life sciences and life writing are understood not independently of each other but as *mutually constitutive*, this perspective at once counters and refutes the power of interpretation (in German, the *Deutungshoheit*) of the life sciences. The point is not only, as Ottmar Ette has argued, that literary (and autobiographical) narratives have a *Lebenswissen,* a knowledge of life which is their own, but also that they are themselves permeated by the discourse of life sciences, a discourse which they incorporate, adapt, and resist. What is at stake in this notion of "permeation" is not quite simply that the life sciences have come to "colonize" our life worlds; it is to say, however, that their "reach" has long since come to extend into our life worlds, and into our own sense of who we are. Yet, as Adams's complex, multi-layered text makes clear, it is up to us to supply this discourse of diagnosis and prediction with the meaning of lived experience. It is here, I believe, that a dialogue between life sciences and life writing can emerge. The point is not that life writing is a mere footnote or a supplement to the life sciences; rather, the point is that one cannot be separated from the other. What is at stake here is also the notion of certainty, as opposed to the contingency of our lives. Adams recalls in her memoir a disturbing visit by her obstetrician after her son Henry was born with Down Syndrome. For one brief moment, the obstetrician's certainty and professional self-assurance has evaporated. Adams recalls,

> On the day I was supposed to leave the hospital my obstetrician, Dr. Lewis, finally appeared. . . . Thinking how much had changed since I last put on those shapeless black maternity pants, I collapsed into tears. She found me sobbing on the bed. My tears were infectious and she began to cry too. "I went back through all of your records," she sniffed. "I wanted to make sure I didn't miss anything so I showed them to my colleagues and everyone agrees there was nothing. There was no sign." (29-30)

What is at stake, we might ask, in this moment of humility, of the doctor's confessing to the patient that the certainties of the medical profession are "captious" ones at best? (Paul et al. 81). What Adams addresses here is the way in which the medical profession may accommodate, or may not make room for, the admission of uncertainty, of the powerlessness of the physician to rule out all contingencies, especially in the arena of reproduction. In this brief moment, the physician can be seen to rewrite, or at least to reread, the story of her own life as an obstetrician. Yet, as Adams notes, in this moment of "human" intervention and acknowledgement there is a curious dichotomy between the doctor's professional self and a self that may be more personal, an off-record self which Adams is at a loss to account for. As Brian Wynne has noted in an essay concerned with the public understanding of science, there is a widespread belief, in the practice of science, "that uncertainties in scientific knowledge [need to be] contained within the private discourse of the scientists and would be misunderstood if disclosed in public" (20). Wynne's account, I believe, can also be applied to the practice of biomedicine. As Adams's recollection of her obstetrician's visit to her hospital room implies, there is a need felt for separating the "private" and the public personae of the scientist or medical practitioner. To reveal the former, it is argued, may have severe consequences for the public understanding of, and trust in, science and scientific practice. At this juncture in her life, however, Adams is all the more dismayed by her obstetrician's inability to reconcile the two selves embedded in her profession. As Adams goes on to say, "At that moment, I hated her intensely. Her demeanor had been robotic throughout both of my pregnancies. Her care was chipper and competent, without the slightest hint of a person beneath. . . . Through my tears, I was curious so see something emerging. For the first time, she seemed human, giving me a glimpse of vulnerability, regret" (34). For Adams, this moment of openness, of vulnerability, is all too brief. When confronted with the question of prognosis, the obstetrician is back to her professional self:

> I told her about [Henry's] weakness, the feeding problems, the hole in his heart. Now she was on familiar terrain. She launched into the same description of the heart that we had already heard from the cardiologist. Her voice was mechanical, as if she had said those words many times before. Jon arrived to help me get home, and the curtain that had lifted to disclose a different view of Dr. Lewis closed permanently. (Adams 34)

What is at stake, then, is what Rita Charon has called the ability to "honor the stories of illness," the scope afforded by the physician to express a certain humility towards the narrative of the patient, a narrative which is, after all, much more than a narrative: it is, quite literally, the story of the patient's life, and her life not only in an ideational, but also in a material sense. Charon writes, "But despite such impressive technical progress, doctors often lack the human capacities to recognize the plights of their patients, to extend empathy toward those who suffer, and to join honestly and courageously with patients in their struggles toward recovery, with chronic illness, and in facing death" (*Narrative Medicine* 3).

What Adams's account of the precarious certainty of the medical professional implies is the call for a space in which both these selves may be able to coexist: What if the obstetrician had been able to incorporate her knowledge of the captiousness of medical certainty (Paul et al., "Captious Certainties") into her way of treating her patient prior to the moment of this patient's giving birth? What if the "personal" and the "professional" selves had not so clearly been at odds with one another? It is this space, also, which Rita Charon's concept of "narrative medicine" calls for and encapsulates: "Along with their growing scientific expertise, doctors need the expertise to listen to their patients, to understand as best as they can the ordeals of illness, to honor the meanings of their patients' narratives of illness, and to be moved by what they behold so that they can act on their patients' behalf" (*Narrative Medicine* 3). It has been argued by many that Charon's approach, in the time of budget cuts and the increasing economization of medical care, remains a utopia.

Yet, the question embedded in Rachel Adams's narrative is whether the absence of "narrative humility" (Charon, *Narrative Medicine* x) can be accounted for only by the logic of budget cuts, or whether, quite on the contrary, it has something to do with the practice of medicine as a profession, and its need for being understood as a practice which can rule out or prevent contingency to the utmost extent.

Disturbingly enough, there is a sequel to Adams's encounter with her obstetrician which Adams is quick to recount as her narrative unfolds. As it will later turn out, the obstetrician was devastated not so much because she felt for Adams and her newborn son in a gesture of what Rita Charon would term the "humility" of listening, but it was rather that she despaired over the imperfection of medical science, an imperfection which had newly been revealed by Adams's son having been born with Down Syndrome to begin with. As Adams eventually comes to realize, "Her tears were real, but not for the reason I had imagined. I thought she was crying because she was sorry for my grief and worry, but it must have been because she was sorry my baby had been born. Like so many other doctors, she believed he was a mistake that should have been prevented, a case of medical science gone wrong" (187-88).

After her son was born, Adams is faced with the uncertainty of what this medical diagnosis of Trisomy 21 may mean for the future life of her son, Henry. It is in this respect that medical guidelines are of no avail. Her roadmap to her son's life with disability,[2] and her own future life as his mother, becomes, not a medical text but a life writing account of parenting a child with Down Syndrome. Adams finds solace in the words of a colleague, Michael Bérubé, whose son Jamie, when Henry is born, is already sixteen years old. She writes, "Many parents of a new baby with Down Syndrome have found solace in Emily Perl Kingsley's essay 'Welcome to Holland.' My road map was Michael Bérubé's book *Life as We Know It*. It taught me that having a child with Down Syndrome was not a tragedy, and that it could, instead, become a route to profound personal and intellectual discovery" (Adams ix). Crucially,

[2] Recent articles on Down Syndrome have preferred to speak of "genetic difference" rather than disability. They have stressed the fact that Down Syndrome constitutes a genetic difference and should hence be sharply distinguished from an illness. While this genetic difference may entail some forms of illness, it is by no means coterminous with them. See Wolf, "Eine Pille."

what emerges here is a network of support, and of support through life writing. Thus, quite simply, life writing can express the uncertainties that the "writing of science" (Lenoir and Gumbrecht n. pag.) and the writing of medicine as life science may not quite be able to provide. What matters at this moment of uncertainty is the necessity to read medical diagnosis through the life unfolding from it. What this implies, also, is the idea of two kinds of knowledge production which may at times intersect, but which often enough are opposed to one another. What Adams is most devastated by after the birth of her son Henry is the foreclosing, by the diagnosis and prediction inherent in medical discourse, of potential life narratives for Henry's future. What matters most to Adams at this juncture in her life is the refusal to categorize her son's life at a moment when this life has only just begun. She refuses to allow for the subsuming of Henry's personality, his uniqueness, under the category of disability:

> This description was so grotesque and clinical. As if the baby could be reduced to a set of predictable features that had nothing to do with his parents' genetic information. It continued, "Down Syndrome sufferers usually have learning difficulties, although the degree of difficulty varies, and many Down Syndrome children are near normal." I was dismayed to see people with Down Syndrome referred to as "suffering" or "afflicted". . . . Were my baby's appearance and personality really so predictable? Wasn't there more to know than the effects of one chromosomal error? (Adams 25-26)

In this sense, *Count Us In*, a collaborative autobiography written by two young men with Down Syndrome, Jason Kingsley and Mitchell Levitz, can be seen as one of the answers to Adams's question. Adams wonders whether the sum total of her newborn son's personality traits can really be predicted by the mere fact of his having Down Syndrome. It is to counter such prediction, the subsuming of a life by a diagnosis that the narrative of *Count Us In* addresses head on: And it addresses it by being, crucially, a dialogue between two young men who happen to be close friends. What *Count Us In* proposes to medical prediction is precisely each of the authors' specific personality: It is in this sense that the structure of *Count Us In* as a collaborative, a dialogic autobiography is so intriguing: In a conversation of two young men growing up with Down Syndrome, what emerges is the idea of personality, of uniqueness, but also of the absence of predictability. As Jason Kingsley writes about his friendship to Mitchell Levitz, "Like my experiences are different from Mitchell and that's how we'll put it in the book. I'm in the middle of high school and Mitchell's been graduated. So our personality changes… We may have different ideas, different dreams" (Kingsley and Levitz 29-30; ellipsis in original). Similarly to *Count Us In*, then, what Adams's memoir of mothering and of her new son's first years does is to oppose prediction to the absence of predictability, to oppose medical discourse through life writing.

Even more importantly, Adams's memoir, *Raising Henry*, and Kingsley and Levitz's collaborative autobiography can be said to be in dialogue in one more respect. Both may address the idea of impossible authorship. When Jason Kingsley and Mitchell Levitz were born, in 1974 and 1971, respectively, doctors predicted to their parents that these two young boys would never be able to learn and to live what has been termed in German a "gelingendes Leben," a full and successful life. In fact, the obstetrician advised Kingsley's parents that their baby son should be "institutionalized at once." As Kingsley writes,

> When I was born, the obstetrician said that I cannot learn, never see my mom and dad and never learn anything and send me to an institution. Which I think was wrong. Today we were talking about if I could see my obstetrician and talk to him, here are the things I would say… I would say, "People with disabilities can learn!" Then I would tell the obstetrician how smart I am. Like learning new languages, going to other foreign nations, going to teen groups and teen parties, going to cast patties, becoming independent, being --- a lighting board operator, an actor, the backstage crew. I would talk about history, math, English, algebra, business math, global studies. One thing I forgot to tell the obstetrician is I plan to get an academic diploma when I pass my RCT's (Kingsley and Levitz 27-28)

It is at this moment that Jason Kingsley suggests that we literally "write back" at life sciences through life writing: What if each medical diagnosis and the knowledge emanating from it were to be re-read through the "diagnosis" of lived experience? What would happen, indeed, if the knowledge generated by the life sciences had to be assessed against and through the prism of life writing? In this discursive relationship between life sciences and life writing, there would no longer be a dichotomy between medical certainty and the uncertainty of life writing. In fact, as Adams's brief encounter with her obstetrician reveals, medical certainty may lie in the habitus of the medical profession; as Brian Wynne has noted, there may simply be no room or framework in which this uncertainty might openly be expressed (20). What would the model of life writing narratives writing back to the life sciences imply? First and foremost, this concept of "writing back" may be problematic in that it would reinforce the idea of the life sciences "colonizing" our lifeworlds; for the power which the life sciences wield over our everyday lives is clearly more complex than mere forms of colonization or "medical imperialism" (Rose 10). Rather, what may be at stake is the idea of knowledge production. At the beginning of a new millennium, who defines human life? Who is to say which life is a life worth living? And on whose certainty may this prediction be premised?

Both *Raising Henry* and *Count Us In* emphasize that the knowledge generated in the life sciences can never be enough; that knowledge about what it means to live with Down Syndrome, or to raise a child with Trisomy 21, is generated to an equal extent through lived experience. It is here that, in a didactic as well as in an institutional sense, medical humanities may be at their most productive: What if, at the time that the obstetrician of Jason Kingsley's mother received his medical training, medical humanities had been mandatory in the education of future obstetricians? What if Emily Perl Kingsley's obstetrician had been able to read narratives by young men and women who had indeed grown up with Down Syndrome? Would he still have suggested to her to have an abortion? To speak only of colonization and dominance here might be to miss the point; what matters is the obstetrician's duty to advise a newborn baby's mother to the best of his or her knowledge. The question is, rather, what this knowledge consists of, and the narratives that it is informed by. Thus, the visit of Adams's obstetrician to her hospital room is both dismaying and potentially empowering: What if there was more room, in the practice of medicine, to accommodate the life writing of physicians, in which they might reveal their uncertainties? What if there was a way for physicians to express, as Rita Charon has suggested, their own humility in the face of contingency, of the contingency of human lives? What is at stake here is the idea that certainty and contingency do not quite exist in a dichotomies relationship to each other; rather, there is a sense in which medical certainty can always only be provisional. Life is always more complicated and more complex than the knowledge which the life sciences are able to generate about them. What is at stake, then, is the possibility of a co-production of knowledge between life sciences and life writing. It is to such a co-production of knowledge, I argue, that both Adams's memorable narrative, *Raising Henry*, and the equally empowering collaborative autobiography *Count Us In* may gesture. The very writing of *Count Us In*, in which the adult authors speak of the fullness of their lives, of their friendships, their love relationships, and their relationship to their parents and grandparents, gives the lie to such a dismissal of the complexity of the lives of persons with Down Syndrome.

Similarly, what emerges from Adams's wondering about the meaning of medical diagnosis for the writing of a life – her son's – is also a profound critique, in the genre of life writing, of the certainties of medical discourse: What is subverted here is the assurance of medical diagnosis as the prognosis of a life lived with Down Syndrome. Who is to say, in other words, what life Henry is going to lead? And who is to say that such a prediction can be made with any certainty? And would this certainty not in itself be presumptuous? Even more crucially, the "road map" (Adams ix) which may guide Henry along the way may not be the literature of medical prediction; it may be the life writing of authors such as Jason Kingsley and Mitchell Levitz.

At the same time, Adams's memoir, *Raising Henry*, raises the question of the choices offered to us in the era of biomedicine. On the grounds of what knowledge, Adams asks, should these choices be made? What Adams is thus concerned with are the choices which new technologies may enable us to make, but also the burden – indeed, the impossibility – of making these choices. Adams emphasizes that it is common practice in the U.S. to advise women to have an abortion once the embryo is diagnosed with Trisomy 21. What are the grounds, then, on which these choices are made? Adams writes about her encounter with Rayna Rapp, an academic like herself who, when confronted with the fact that her baby had Down Syndrome in 1983, chose to have a late term abortion. Adams describes encountering Rapp at a friend's party:

> Even though we had spoken only briefly, I felt we had communicated in a profound and respectful way about the very different choices each of us had made. She had opted not to continue her pregnancy; I had made choices that allowed me to avoid such painful decisions [by choosing not

> to have an amnio]. I knew I appreciated her choices, and I believed she did mine. . . . My chance meeting with Rayna Rapp also left me thinking about the confusing and contradictory messages that surround the notion of reproductive choice in our culture. At the time Rapp decided to have her abortion in 1983, there were far fewer resources for the parents of a child with Down Syndrome. (102-03)

Adam's ending up opposing the discourse of medical prediction is an embracing of the unpredictability of life: No-one, she writes at the end of her narrative, is able to predict what Henry's life will be like; but, for the time being, she is awed that her four-year-old son is starting to read: "'Henry!' I shout. 'You're reading the book!' I feel a rush of love and admiration, swooping down to cover him in kisses, mussing the fuzz of his short hair. I know we have a long way to go. . . . But we all have to start somewhere. I have to marvel at what I'm seeing. My four-year-old son is reading" (Adams 244). The focus of Adams's narrative is thus on her young son Henry himself, his personality, his likes and dislikes. These traits of his personality, her memoir makes clear, have nothing to do at all with his having Down Syndrome; Adams's is the story of a life which has just begun, not a diagnosis. It is in this sense that her memoir is and is not a story of disability; rather, it is a narrative about the unfolding of life in a world which is not determined, but reshaped by the choices made available through biomedicine. What Adams leaves us with is a picture of Henry on his mother's arm, dancing: "In the picture we're dancing. He's slightly out of focus, illuminated by a sunbeam coming in from the window. His expression is pure delight" (1). Through the form of life writing, Rachel Adams thus intervenes – as Jason Kingsley and Mitchell Levitz have done before her – into a discourse which has been highly medicalized, the discourse of living with Down Syndrome.[3] Yet, as I have tried to argue in this chapter, her intervention is twofold: First, through the stories of the first three years of Henry's life, Adams addresses the visibility of a person with Down

[3] This is an idea which recurs in Michael Bérubé's book, *Life As We Know It* (1996), to which I will return in more detail below. Bérubé writes, "When [our son] Jamie finally came home, then, he came home as a thoroughly medicalized child. Not merely "medicated," but medicalized: to talk about him was also to talk about his procedures and prospects in medical terms, and he already had a hefty medical chart to prove it" (41).

Syndrome through a life writing narrative. It is this visibility, and the knowledge gained about living with Down Syndrome through autobiographical narratives such as Michael Bérubé's *Life as We Know It* and Kingsley and Levitz's *Count Us In*, in whose genealogy Adams writes. She notes, "Times had changed [since Rayna Rapp had chosen to have an abortion in 1983]. A person with Down Syndrome can now expect to live more than fifty years, thanks to better health care and a more accommodating social environment. People with Down Syndrome have gained a new visibility, if you know where to look" (Adams 103). At the same time, to read Adams's memoir only as a story of disability would be to miss the point: The point of Adams's autobiography of motherhood is precisely to paint a picture of Henry, her son; to convey to us an image of Henry, dancing in his mother's arms. It is in this image that the solace of autobiography may lie: It is by reading the memoir as a biography of the first years of Henry's life that we do justice to his story, a story which can by no means be reduced to disability.

What genre might Adams's text be classified in, however? So far, I have read in in terms of both an autobiography (of mothering) and a form of writing the life of her son, Henry. To what extent, then, is *Raising Henry* also a biography of a son by his mother? In what way is it a collaborative autobiography, given the fact that Henry's presence is there in his mother's narrative, who is writing her narrative in response to his actions and reactions? At the same time, the collaboration, as Adams notes at the end of her book, is necessarily lopsided since Henry cannot yet represent himself; the aim of the book is thus to create a space which his self-narrative is eventually meant to fill. It is a narrative claiming space for the recognition of a life, and of a life as valuable and meaningful. The concept of life writing, then, may be as enabling as it may, at times, be limiting. Clearly, many different genres – biography, autobiography, diaries, blogs – have been subsumed under one and the same "umbrella" category of "life writing," yet the distinction between these categories have often become blurry precisely through the common rubric of the writing of lives in various constellations. Thus, each reading of Adams's text – the reading of *Raising Henry* as biography, autobiography or collaborative autobiography – will reveal different layers in the text, and will affect the role and the relevance of the speaking subject. At the same time, it could be argued that Tito Mukhopadhyay's autobiography *The Mind Tree* is not only an "autibiography," to use Annette Kern-Stähler's term, but also a son's biography of his mother, whose presence can be felt in every word of the narrative. What emerges in these narratives, then, is also a critique of the autonomous self on whose presence, as many critics have argued, the genre of autobiography has often been predicated. Rather than being based on and conveying an autonomous subject, then, these narratives speak of relationality[4]: the writing of a life affected by illness or disability, these texts reveal, is made possible because of the relationships to the people who make such writing possible. What is at stake, then, is also the process of enabling authorship.

7.2 Disability and Inclusion: Learning from *Sesame Street*

The question with which Rachel Adams's book *Raising Henry* ends, then, is the very same question with which Jason Kingsley and Mitchell Levitz's co-written autobiography *Count Us In* begins: What, Adams wonders, will Henry be when he grows up? It is this question which *Count Us In* can be said to answer, precisely because it is a narrative of what it means to grow up with Down Syndrome. This question, I would like to argue in this chapter, is so intriguing precisely because it addresses the discourse of diagnostics head-on. Medical discourse on Down Syndrome, replete as it is with the prediction of "slow learning" and a lack of capability, would seem to imply that this very question is misguided. The openness of the question – "What do you want to be when you grow up?" – would seem to be constricted by the narrowness of medical prognosis.

The simple but at the same time highly complex suggestion made in Joan Ganz Cooney's foreword to *Count Us In* is that the point is to refuse *not* to ask a basic question of a child with Down Syndrome: What do you want to be when you grow up? The refusal to ask the question, or the habit to think of it as a rhetorical question, at once limits the politics of the possible when it comes to disability. *The point, in other words, is to write a life, not a disabled life*. Cooney notes, "Jason Kingsley and Mitchell Levitz make abundantly clear, to those who still may not know, what people with disabilities want. They want exactly what the rest of us want" (ix-x).

[4] I am indebted to Katja Sarkowsky for this point.

> At the same time, it is here that the two ways of reading a narrative such as Jason Kingsley and Mitchell Levitz's *Count Us In* recur: the book can be read either as a narrative of disability, a book about growing up with Down Syndrome; or it can be read as a book, quite simply, of growing up, written by two young men who happen to have Down Syndrome. Throughout these chapters, it is this question, the question about the dilemma of reading texts which have come to be included through the framework of medical humanities, which recurs. My point is that there is a tension between these two readings, a tension that may, in fact, be productive to the extent that both readings are taken into account, each shedding light on what the other may obfuscate.

In reading *Count Us In*, I am intrigued by the variety of frameworks in which this co-authored autobiographical narrative can be said to participate: the framework of learning and of inclusion; the framework of citizenship and of economic and political participation. In the prior context of inclusion, the children's educational program *Sesame Street* figures prominently; when he was only fifteen months old, Jason Kingsley appeared on the show, for which his mother Emily was one of the writers. Yet, as I will try to show as this chapter progresses, the point to be made here is not only that Kingsley's appearance on *Sesame Street* was about the program's agenda for including children with disabilities; it was also an important step in Kingsley's life which, I will argue as this chapter progresses, has nothing to do with disability. His appearance on *Sesame Street*, then, was also the beginning, as *Count Us In* makes clear, of his future film career. As a young man, Jason Kingsley would come to star alongside Lee Majors in a "mainstream" production (Kingsley and Levitz 22). What is at stake here, then, is to look beyond disability, and to look beyond inclusion. If *Count Us In* is read as an autobiography in the full sense of the term, then, Kingsley's early TV appearance is also the beginning of his future professional life.

What does it mean, then, for Jason Kingsley to appear on Sesame Street? And as who does he appear on this children's educational program? The publication of *Count Us In* is remarkable on a number of levels. First, it stands in direct opposition to both Temple Grandin's *Thinking in Pictures* and Tito Mukhopadhyay's *The Mind Tree* or, in its German translation, *Der Tag, an dem ich meine Stimme fand*, because the foreword to *Count Us In* was not written by a neurologist, but by a screen writer: Joan Ganz Cooney. What, then, does it mean for an illness narrative to be introduced in a foreword by the creator of Sesame Street? What may be at stake here is in fact the practice, in the framing of a particular narrative, of both legitimation and authentication. As I have argued with regard to Tito Mukhopadhyay, this authentication can be accomplished in medical terms – as in the foreword by Oliver Sacks –, or, as is the case in *Count Us In*, it can be performed by a screen writer. Each of these practices of authentication and legitimation has profound implications, I would argue, for the ways in which we read these narratives.

In Cooney's description of the inclusion of children with Down Syndrome on *Sesame Street*, one line in particular may be programmatic for both a politics of reading and the idea of "doing justice" (Nussbaum, *Frontiers of Justice* x): Jason Kingsley, the son of one of the writers of *Sesame Street*, Emily Perl Kingsley, came to be included, Cooney writes, as part of the regular cast of children on *Sesame Street*, as was his friend Mitchell Levitz. Cooney writes,

> At first, we did separate segments with a curriculum and activities for children with special needs. But we learned very quickly that these children didn't need a different format. So our next step was to demonstrate that they did not need to be segregated in special educational programs but could be part of a regular elementary school class: We showed Big Bird going to school for the first time. One of his classmates was Mitchell. The show opened our 1981 season, and we designed a poster showing Big Bird's class, with Mitchell in the front row. (viii-ix)

What does it mean, then, for medical humanities to learn from *Sesame Street*? What would it mean to take *Sesame Street* seriously not just as a children's program, but a program that lays bare the mechanisms of exclusion that may be embedded in a country's education system as such? In his television debut, Jason Kingsley appears as himself: as Jason Kingsley, *not* as a person with Down Syndrome.

> MONSTER: L.
>
> JASON KINGSLEY: O. … V. … E.
>
> MONSTER: What did that say?
>
> JASON KINGSLEY: LOVE!

MONSTER: Give me a hug! [*hugs him.*] ("Sesame Street")

What this simple passage addresses is the very question of inclusion, and the question whether children with Down Syndrome should be included in the "mainstream" or as part of a special needs program. Kingsley's inclusion on *Sesame Street*, then, implies the refusal of segregation. On *Sesame Street*, Kingsley is a child on TV who teaches other children how to spell; he is not a child with Down Syndrome but a child who can spell who also happens to have Down Syndrome. The question of disability, however, is not addressed, neither by the Cookie Monster nor by the narrative framework of the show itself. As Kingsley recalls his earliest TV appearance in *Count Us In*, pointing to a photograph of himself as a young boy, "This is on *Sesame Street*, when the Cookie Monster was showing everyone that I knew how to read" (Kingsley and Levitz 116). As Cooney goes on to note, "Thanks in part to Jason and Emily, *Sesame Street* soon began to include children with Down Syndrome: when Jason was only fifteen months old, he made his television debut sitting on Buffy Saint Marie's lap. When he was six, we showed him counting in Spanish" (viii).

What would it mean, then, for the doctor to watch *Sesame Street*, or to read the life writing of a child he predicted to be incapable of such authorship? The aim of a critical dialogue between life sciences and life writing can never be a "bedeviling" of medical diagnosis, or of prediction. Rather, it must highlight and call for possible forms of overlap, contexts in which medical science takes into account, not only in quality of life research, life writing narratives such as Jason Kingsley's co-authored autobiography, *Count Us In*.

The point made by the *Sesame Street* writers, then, was not just that Kingsley could spell (in English), but that he could also do so in *Spanish*. It is the playfulness and the normalcy included in this approach which at once sets the tone for including disability minus the measured tone of violins described by Michael J. Fox in his criticism of American television. Why, Cooney implies, should American television not learn from Baby Bird and the Cookie Monster? What matters in this form of "doing justice" (Nussbaum, *Frontiers of Justice* x), then, is the very politics of routine. As Cooney goes on to observe, "Thanks to [Emily and Jason], '*Sesame Street*' became the only show that routinely featured children with disabilities – without focusing on their disabilities'" (ix). *Sesame Street* featured these children, then, as children, not as children with disabilities.

It is at this juncture that medical humanities may benefit from humanities research to an extent which may so far have been neglected: For what would it mean to include in the framework of medical humanities not just Kingsley and Levitz's *Count Us In* but also episodes from *Sesame Street*? The "import" of life writing narratives, then, is as important as the framework in which the import takes place. Minus *Sesame Street*, Jason Kingsley's narrative is imported only as patient narrative, or as the narrative of a person with disability. With *Sesame Street*, what is revealed for and beyond quality of life research, is the way in which Kingsley leads a full, creative and productive life. It is this "productiveness" which has profound implications for the concept of citizenship and for what Nussbaum has called "mutual advantage": Twenty years after the first episode on which he starred in *Sesame Street*, Jason Kingsley has indeed gone on to become an actor, and he has gone on to become a "tax-paying citizen." For this very idea of the "tax-paying citizen," or rather the non-tax-paying person who is denied the benefits of citizenship, is the scare crow which has informed the debate on disability, as I will elaborate below.

Like Rachel Adams's memoir of motherhood, *Count Us In* starts with medical prediction: with the life which Emily Perl Kingsley's obstetrician predicted for her son when he had only just been born. As Joan Ganz Cooney recalls in her foreword to *Count Us In*, when Jason Kingsley was born, doctors suggested to his parents that he should be "institutionalized" (viii). As she goes on to note, "Although he was only a few hours old, doctors were telling Emily and her husband, Charles, that Jason would never be capable of anything, physical or intellectual, and that he ought to be institutionalized. Even so, Emily and Charles were planning to bring Jason home and would try to bring him up themselves" (Cooney vii-viii). What emerges here is both the idea of the prediction, by medical doctors, of a particular form of temporality or rather, of belatedness. Like Tito Mukhopadhyay at the age of thee, Jason Kingsley – although "only a few hours old" (Cooney viii) – is already frozen in the temporality predicted for a person born with Down Syndrome. He is, as Tito Mukhopadhyay has put it, outside of time in the sense that he is said to inhabit a different form of temporality. As Mukhopadhyay writes in *Beyond the Silence*,

All the world was a busy place
And I was an idle kind
Disqualified in the human race
A different form of mind. (103)

As in Mukhopadhyay's case, then, temporality and prediction become a sentence – in the juridical sense metaphorized by social and medical practice – which condemns the young patient and his family to invisibility. Kingsley's life begins, then, with his parents' refusal to hide him from view. It is through this refusal, incidentally, that he will go on to make television history at 15 months of age. Crucially, moreover, this dire prognosis – the prophecy that Kingsley would never be able to learn – is being refuted not in the mother's words, but in Kingsley's own writing: In the passage I have quoted at the beginning of this chapter (Kingsley and Levitz 27), Jason Kingsley casually informs the obstetrician, as an imaginary reader of his memoir, about his knowledge of math, and his ability to reason even with an obstetrician. As Kingsley wrote in an autobiographical essay when he was twenty, "I have a disability called Down Syndrome. My bad obstetrician said that I would never learn and send me into a institution and never see me again. No way José! Mom and Dad brought me home and taught me things" (Kingsley and Levitz 21). For the obstetrician, it would have been impossible to conceive of this baby's ever being able to graduate from high school, or starring in a mainstream TV production as an adolescent.

Throughout this book, then, I am interested not only in what the concept of "life writing" does to acts of writing – through what stories, through what channels a "life" (and, more importantly, a "successful" life or a *gelingendes Leben*) is being told – but also with the question of what life writing does to our politics of *reading*, especially in the humanities. I have been concerned with the ways in which bringing a certain lens to bear on the reading of a life writing text narrative expand as well as limit the potential this text has to answer questions which, in philosophy, have been framed as encapsulating a "successful life" and, in medical research, have been discussed in quality of life research. If I have argued above that *Count Us In* can be read as the passing, by Jason Kingsley and Mitchell Levitz, of a citizenship test, then I am also interested in what happens if we read *Count Us In* not from beginning to end but from the end of the narrative to its beginning. What if the same collaborative autobiography were being read through its postscript? Twelve years after the initial publication of the book, then, Kingsley and Levitz, as well as their mothers, Barbara and Emily, talk about how the boys' lives have turned out; how many of their dreams and aspirations have and have not come true by the time the postscript and the subsequent afterword were written. The fact that there is both a postscript and an afterword, incidentally, at once points to the complex notion of temporality or rather, of temporalities, at the heart of this stunning collaborative autobiography. Crucially, *Count Us In* both engages and subverts the idea of teleology inherent in the concept of autobiography. For an autobiography also presupposes a telos, the achieving, often enough, of becoming fully aware of one's own personality and of realizing, to the fullest, the potential of one's life. Crucially, as both Jason Kingsley's and Mitchell Levitz's autobiographical narrative and the narrative biography of their lives by their mothers make clear, they have long surpassed the temporality which had been prophesied for them, and the capabilities associated with such temporality. As their mothers put it in the postscript, "Throughout Mitchell and Jason's early years, we were told to anticipate that their development would slow down, plateau, and eventually stop. On the contrary, we have observed that, like everyone else, people with Down Syndrome continue to grow and learn throughout their lifetime, and to benefit from new opportunities and experiences" (Kingsley and Levitz 181). Yet, as the postscript as well as the afterword make clear, not all their plans have come true twelve years after the publication of *Count Us In*; some plans were procrastinated, some goals still seemed out of reach. For Levitz, being able to drive constitutes an important step towards living an independent life. In a diary entry from July 1990 which is included in *Count Us In*, he writes, "I think I would like to drive so that I could run my own business and to get [what] I need when I'm independent. I do feel driving is important to me so I can have a chance to explore my needs… Driving may be hard, but I have a feeling that I may succeed at a certain age and I would try and see if it works out or not. If it doesn't work out, I would try another kind of transportation" (Kingsley and Levitz 145).

Thus, one issue that the authors' narrative returns to time and again is the desire to drive, and to buy their own cars. Mobility, throughout the narrative, is also associated with the ability to move from place to place freely, without having to rely either on public transport or the help of a relative. Yet, by the time the postscript to *Count Us In* was written, this goal has proved impossible to achieve for both writers. As Levitz eventually acknowledges, "There will be other methods of transportation. I don't think I will ever get those skills. It's difficult for me to face, but I'm learning to accept the fact that I may not be able to do some things that my sisters are doing. Which is a main fact which I will understand" (Kingsley and Levitz 160).

Yet, precisely because the lives which are being written in *Count Us In* are more than "disabled" lives, because the authors challenge us to define, redefine and reconsider the concept of "the good life," the afterword reminds us that in any life, and in any life writing, the achievement of all the goals once prospected at the outset of the autobiographical narrative is both improbable and utopian. The narrative ends by drawing attention not to the end product, the utilitarian principle of a "successful" life, but to the process of living. The prediction of a flawed or slowed-down temporality – the "verdict" of having Down Syndrome – is countered, in *Count Us In*, by the (re)definition of *any* life as processual. In this sense, *Count Us In*, as an alternative autobiography, exposes the telos or ending of "traditional" autobiography as the pose it is, stressing the staging of any life narrated through autobiography.

In keeping with the dictum of autobiography, however, and despite the – rightful – suspension of teleology, *Count Us In* conforms to the idea of the exemplary quality of the lives that are being retold, in keeping with American autobiographies since Benjamin Franklin. By the time the postscript is being published, both Jason Kingsley and Mitchell Levitz have become advocates for their community, have become model representatives of the community for which and out of which they write. If the Franklinian model of autobiography understands the individual as the pars pro toto of the nation, as the ideal or model citizen (Madsen 180), such an exemplary quality is by no means missing from *Count Us In*.

The fact that when Mitchell Levitz graduated from high school, a flag should have been flown in front of Congress, then, marks the long way which the debate on Down Syndrome has come. The flag grants political and social recognition, on a national level, to a person who had once been written out of the civic fabric by medical diagnosis. As Levitz notes in conversation with Jason Kingsley's mother Emily, a flag was flown at the Capitol when he graduated from high school, the first person with Down Syndrome to do so:

> MITCHELL LEVITZ: Harry Greenberg gave the introduction and gave a speech and read a letter from Congressman Fish. He read a letter to recognize myself for the achievements which I had done. In honor of that, at the Capitol they will raise a flag in honor of my graduation. Then I will be receiving the flag.
>
> EMILY PERL KINGSLEY: Did you know that Jason has a flag just like that? It was flown over the U.S. Capitol in honor of his appearance on "The Fall Guy." It's hanging in his room. (Kingsley and Levitz 52)

What informs Jason Kingsley and Mitchell Levitz's life writing, then, is a politics of recognition in a sense related to but not entirely synonymous with Taylor's "politics of recognition" (Taylor, "The Politics of Recognition"). What is at stake in appearing on talk shows, with being recognized by a national ritual of acknowledgment, with sending out picture postcards of the first time that Jason Kingsley voted in the presidential election? As Kingsley recalls, "At age seven I went on the show called 'A.M. Philadelphia' in Pennsylvania. It was a talk show . . . I counted in twelve foreign languages and sign languages" (Kingsley and Levitz 22). These steps, as *Count Us In* make clear, are so significant because they are an enforcement, a cashing of check given to persons with Down Syndrome by the Americans with Disability Act. What is portrayed as absurd in the Bollywood film *My Name Is Khan* – Khan's misguided desire to speak to the American president in person – is depicted as a reality and a dream come true in the case of Jason Kingsley and Mitchell Levitz. They, the narrative makes clear, will eventually speak to Congress in order to describe their situation, to talk about the quality of the lives they are leading and the need for financial, social, cultural and emotional support to achieve and to maintain this quality of life. The point is that they have been given the right to make their political will known: by voting in the presidential election, by talking to congress. What is at stake is the right of political participation, which is one of the most fundamental rights associated with full-fledged citizenship.

What does it mean, then, for legislation to be implemented into social practice? And who enforces such implementation? Crucially, then, *Count Us In* starts not just as a neurologist's "authentication" of a patient's narrative but with an explicit reference to "doing justice" (Nussbaum, *Frontiers of Justice* x) in both a legal and a socio-cultural sense. According to Cooney, "The 1990s Americans with Disability Act prohibits discrimination against individuals with disabilities. It has often been described as the most weeping non-discrimination legislation since the Civil Rights Act of 1964. . . . Long overdue, this legislation will help greatly to make independent living for many more people with Down Syndrome and other disabilities a reality instead of a dream" (ix). What Cooney emphasizes, then, is the way in which medical prediction and social justice theory may work in tandem to trap persons with disability in a vicious cycle: In Jason Kingsley's case, the doctor's prediction, if it had been heeded by his parents, would have condemned Kingsley to being "institutionalized" and to being "educated" at best, in a segregated school. This educational disadvantage, then, would have prevented him from becoming a "tax-paying citizen," whose "unproductivity" in economic terms would have precluded his access to full citizenship. The vicious cycle would have been complete. The writing of his life, and his living it, on the other hand, has disproved not only medical prediction but some theories of social justice as well. Thus, as Martha Nussbaum has argued, theories of justice must be measured against the lives they make possible, as well as the lives they may have failed to take into account. As Cooney goes on to note,

> And yet we as a society still have a long way to go. We are exceedingly careless in this country about working potential; we are persistently reluctant to invest in people at the front end of life in order to achieve a multiplicity of benefits in the long term. For example, we tend to forget that with enriched opportunities and high expectations many children with Down Syndrome grow up to become responsible tax-paying citizens who contribute to their communities in many ways. Jason, now a senior in high school, is looking into higher education and career opportunities, while Mitchell is working and paying taxes and has just moved into his own house. (x)

The link which Cooney evokes between the Civil Rights Act and the 1990 Americans with Disability Act is hence crucial in a number of ways. Crucially, even if the "separate but equal" doctrine had already been turned down in 1954 in Brown v. Board of Education of Topeka, the civil rights struggle called for the enforcement of such legislation.

Moreover, the argument advanced in Brown v. Board of Education was that the present, segregated school system came not just at an immense social but also economic cost (Cheng, *The Melancholy of Race*). Such reasoning, however, as Cooney notes, is strikingly absent from present-day discussions of disability. At the same time, what emerges here is an idea which I have already discussed with regard to the critique, by Lydia Brown and many others, of Temple Grandin's work. Cooney calls for the inclusion of persons with Down Syndrome on the basis of their social and economic productivity, thus, like Grandin, focusing on "high-functioning" individuals like her son. What such reasoning neglects or even runs the risk of dismissing, then, is the idea of what Thomas Couser has called the "cultural value" of disability (*Vulnerable Subjects* 122): From a perspective questioning the concept of economic usefulness as form of normativity, we would argue that a full life and a life worth living must by no means be subsumed under the notion of economic usefulness.

These, then, may at once be the limits of medical humanities: What if a patient narrative is only read as the account of an experience of illness, but not of social discrimination? If it is read only as a call for patient rights, not as a petition for legal and social rights as well? What, on the other hand, if this patient narrative were read not just as a demand for adequate medical care but a call for citizenship to its fullest extent? Where Cooney's foreword to *Count Us In* is programmatic, then, is both in its taking seriously the life writing narrative which it prefaces and in the refusal to step outside the confines of narrative as a concept. Life writing, she implies, is only the first step towards social justice. *Count Us In*, she argues, can never be read just as a medical narrative but must be seen as life writing to the fullest extent; and our understanding of it must necessarily exceed the concept of both narrative and medical humanities. What, then, does this discussion imply for the logic of citizenship at the beginning of the twenty-first century? As *Count Us In* implies, inclusion can take many shapes: it can refer to the field of education, the question of whether or not individuals with disability should be included in "mainstream" classrooms; it can encompass the presence of "disabled" persons in media and popular culture; or it can involve the questions of social, political and economic participation. These forms of participation, moreover, are circumscribed, to a large extent, by the legal parameters that make such participation possible.

It is in this sense that *Count Us In* is programmatic for a politics of inclusion *beyond* medical humanities. For *Count Us In* can be read on multiple levels. First, it can be seen as a patient narrative or rather, a narrative about disability[5]; it is here that the account would sit most squarely with the politics of medical humanities. Second, as I will elaborate in more detail below, it can also be read as a narrative demanding not only patient rights but civic rights, performing a citizenship test of sorts. In this latter sense, it is also a form of life writing, about what may constitute a "full life" or, in German, a "gelingendes Leben." Karin Knorr-Cetina has addressed the debate around new forms of lived reality on the one hand and the notion of the "good life" on the other hand. Knorr-Cetina argues that at the intersection between the life sciences and the humanities, a new concept of "life" itself may be in the process of emerging. As she writes in an article in *Bios und Zoe*, "In my opinion, this concentration on the individual lays the ground for the emergence of a new concept of life, which can be regarded as a link between humanities and life sciences" (Knorr-Cetina 60; my trans.). At the same time, Knorr-Cetina goes on to note that an increasing focus on a potential redefinition of the "human" in the era of biomedicine also entails the discussion of the rights and privileges, but also the duties and requirements to which these "different lives" are subject. The discussion of what Knorr-Cetina calls a "culture of life" (*Kultur des Lebens*) at the intersection between the life sciences and the humanities thus necessarily needs to take into account the concept of the "posthuman." She notes,

> Yet, developments of this kind beg the question about the rights and duties of these future posthuman or transhuman beings. What ethics will they subscribe to? Will those individuals who possess a greater number of prosthetic limbs and mechanical-electronic organs have fewer rights as individuals made from cell structures? Why, however, should the fact that someone is made from organic material serve as a criterion for dis-

[5] As Rachel Adams makes clear in *Raising Henry*, Down Syndrome is not an illness, but a disability; to conflate narratives of disability with "patient narratives" is hence often misleading. According to Adams, "There are many genetic disabilities – Down Syndrome among them – that often have relatively little impact on a person's quality of life. People with Down Syndrome aren't sick; they are disabled" (118).

> tinguishing between humans and non-humans? (Knorr-Cetina 65; my trans.)

Crucially, the nexus between posthumanism, disability, and social justice is also at the core of Martha Nussbaum's study *Frontiers of Justice*. What is at stake here is thus an opening up of the concept of the human; it is now argued that those who, on account of their disability or genetic difference, for instance, have traditionally defined as "differently human" need to be acknowledged as fully human, and by consequence, need to have access to full citizenship rights. At the same time, this claiming of rights, as Knorr-Cetina implies, will go along with the speculations about the ethics to which these newly included subject and potential citizens will subscribe. In this context, the notions of capability, ethics and inclusion are intertwined in a variety of ways. As I will try to argue in this chapter, these are questions which lie at the heart of Jason Kingsley's and Mitchell Levitz's co-written autobiography, *Count Us In*.

It is in this sense, also, that the dialogic form is especially important. For what does it imply that this autobiographical account should be written not just as a first person account or testimony, but as a form of address and of dialogic engagement? There are multiple dialogues in *Count Us In*. First and foremost, there is the dialogue between two friends, Jason Kingsley and Mitchell Levitz, about their friendship. Kingsley recalls the day his friend Levitz graduated from high school: "I felt proud of my friend Mitchell, gave the standing ovation for the three awards [a community service award, the dean's award, and a commendation from the state assembly]" (Kingsley and Levitz 51). Having Down Syndrome, growing up with Down Syndrome, is one aspect of this friendship, but the friendship by far exceeds this similarity. As Levitz tells Kingsley, "Between you and me, we have a lot of differences in what we do and we have a lot in common. But we shouldn't base it on our disability" (Kingsley and Levitz 33).

It is the reference to personality, to each of the author's uniqueness that at once situates the account squarely in the domain of autobiography. It is here, also that humanities and medical humanities can be seen to *clash*: For what the text insists on is that it contains the biography of a friendship, the autobiography of two young men who also happen to be disabled. Yet, their disability is only one characteristic among many. Significantly, "Having " is only one chapter out of thirteen. It is in this sense that throughout this study, I am concerned not only with the narratives which – through the framework of medical humanities – we may come to include into our reading, but also with the ways in which we read these narratives in the first place. Ultimately, my claim that we need to take the genre of autobiography seriously – and to read autobiography as being much more than an illness or disability narrative – is similar to Rita Charon's reminder that we need to "honor the stories of illness" (*Narrative Medicine* x). Ultimately what this may also imply is that we see the stories beyond the illness, to refuse to let the illness part of the story subsume the story as a whole. It is in seeing disability as only one chapter in their book that we may "honor," or do justice to, the autobiography that is *Count Us In*.

Moreover, the dialogic form of *Count Us In* ensures that we do not only have Kingsley and Levitz's opinion on existential subjects such as genealogy or the death of a loved one, but we also have, for instance, their parents' and grandfathers' accounts. As Levitz's grandfather tells him,

> I have to say to you that one of the happiest days of my life was the day you were born. I felt so excited and so exhilarated to have a grandson that it really meant an awful lot to me. And since that time we have had such a great relationship all through the years, from the time that you started to walk to the time you started school, all the way through… Do you remember the time we did American history? (Kingsley and Levitz 106)

What is central about *Count Us In*, then, is the explicit dialogue which it opens up between life writing on the one hand and quality of life research on the other. What Emily Perl Kingsley and Barbara Levitz, the boys' mothers, call for is an explicit dialogue to take place between these two different fields. Life writing and life science, in other words, must constantly be in dialogue with each other. As Emily and Barbara put it, "We have learned the folly of attempting to predict a person's quality of life based on his or her label or condition. These boys have succeeded because they were given opportunities and allowed to take risks, and because we refused to let anyone write them off" (Kingsley and Levitz 5).

What, then, would be the link between *Count Us In* and the 2014 online phenomenon of the "ice bucket challenge" drawing attention to the lives of people living with ALS? In both cases, what is at stake is a twofold attempt to make visible not just a certain type of illness, but the life which is affected by it, and the quality of this life. As Levitz notes in a conversation with his grandfather,

> GRANDPA LEVITZ: You've gone to seminars and spoken about your feelings about having a disability and how you're coping with it and you're kind of advising people that they can cope with it, too. And you're also fighting in the legislature – you went to the Senate in Washington to speak about it –
>
> MITCHELL LEVITZ: To testify, which is more interesting. (Kingsley and Levitz 110)

It is the same goal, then, that triggers the telling of Kingsley's and Levitz's narrative. In this sense, as Thomas Couser has argued, life writing can also be seen as a form of "quality-of-life writing" (*Vulnerable Subjects* ix). As Couser puts it,

> The first connection that interests me is that contemporary life writing, at least in North America, often deals with conditions that raise questions concerning quality of life. The term "quality of life" is intended to distinguish individuals' sense of the worth of their existence from mere quantity, that is, the duration of their lives. . . . A good example of both auto/biography and what I call quality-of-life writing is *Elegy for Iris* (1999), John Bayley's memoir of his life with the late philosopher and novelist Iris Murdoch. (*Vulnerable Subjects* ix)

As Couser notes, life writing narrative can thus engage quality of life research in the life sciences head-on. Yet, I would simultaneously argue that quality of life research, and testifying about their own condition for quality of life research is only one of many frameworks that *Count Us In* engages as a narrative: For the pitfall which is hence inherent in medical humanities as a framework – or a disability studies framework of *Count Us In* – is that quality of life research is directed at persons with impairments, not at humanity as such. As Emily Perl Kingsley and Barbara Levitz put it, quality of life research affects all of us equally, and is hence moored as much in autobiography studies and humanities research as it may be anchored in medical humanities.

7.3 "Fit for Citizenship": Collaborative Autobiography as Citizenship Test

As Nicholas Rose has suggested in *The Politics of Life Itself* (2007), the bestowal of the full rights of citizenship to persons with disability is among the key challenges to social justice at the beginning of the twenty-first century:

> We are seeing the emergence of new ideas of what human beings are, what they should do, and what they can hope for. Novel conceptions of "biological citizenship" have taken shape that recode the duties, rights, and expectations of human beings in relation to their sickness, and also to their life itself, reorganize the relations between individuals and their biomedical authorities, and reshape the ways in which human beings relate to themselves as "somatic individuals." This is linked to the rise of what I term "somatic ethics" – ethics not in the sense of moral principles, but rather as the values for the conduct of a life – that accords a central place to corporeal, bodily existence. (6)

In this chapter, then, I am concerned with the ways in which *Count Us In* can be said to write the citizen into being, and to write into citizenship a person with Down Syndrome. The politics of citizenship, of civic and moral "fitness," as Natalia Molina has put it, are at the core of Kingsley and Levitz's narrative. I would thus like to argue that the citizenship debate at the beginning of the twentieth century may have profound implications for the discussion of "biological citizenship" a century later. Then as now, what is at stake is the way in which "civic fitness" is defined, and who is said to be incompatible with such civic requirements.

My point in this chapter is that two forms of citizenship may in fact be at work in Levitz and Kingsley's co-authored autobiography. First, the book, by serving as a mouthpiece for those living with Down Syndrome, advocates what Rose has termed "biological citizenship"; this form of citizenship, in turn, can be closely related to "genetic citizenship." This form of reasoning, and this form of rights discourse, draws attention to the fact that persons with Down Syndrome have been denied full access to citizenship on account of a chromosomal difference; what is at stake is hence a form of genetic discrimination. Conversely, they proceed to call for full citizenship on account of genetic difference. The work of Paul Rabinow has been crucial in describing such processes of community building, which Rabinow sees as a form of empowerment (Rabinow and Rose, "Biopower Today"). What is crucial here is that what has been termed the "medical model of disability" is turned on its head. While persons with genetic difference had been marginalized and pathologized on account of their condition, they now proceed to appropriate biomedical knowledge about their genetic condition. According to Lemke, "It is assumed that technological innovations and scientific systems of classification provide the material preconditions for new forms of collectivity, patterns of representation and identity politics. In this context, knowledge about particular physical qualities and genetic characteristics determines the relationship of individuals to themselves and to others in a decisive manner" (126-27; my trans.). Thus, these subjects refuse to be biomedicalized, and go on to enlist biomedical knowledge in calling for a specific form of citizenship. As Lemke goes on to note,

> According to Rabinow, self-help groups and patients' associations are no longer passive objects of medical care or research interests in this context; rather, the experience of illness provides a new point of departure for a field of manifold social activities. . . . The dissemination of scientific and medical knowledge does not only lead to new forms of community formation and collective identity, but it also results in the claiming of rights on the basis of biological particularities and entails forms of political activism hitherto unknown. (127; my trans.)

In this context, *Count Us In* as a co-authored autobiography of two writers living with Down Syndrome, then, can be seen both as a form of life writing and a call for specific rights in a context in which, in the sense described by Lemke on the basis of the work of Paul Rabinow, biomedical knowledge has been appropriated by patient communities. As I will argue as this chapter progresses, *Count Us In* as a collaborative autobiography can be read both as a form of political activism and as a literary text that, in the form of autobiography, exceeds such activism.

At the same time, I will suggest below that *Count Us In* can be read both as embedded in notions of genetic citizenship and as being in dialogue with more other, longer-standing discourses of citizenship. In this latter sense, my aim in this chapter is to argue that *Count Us In* can in fact be seen as a citizenship test of sorts. For what is at stake in a citizenship test? What does it mean to test "civic fitness," as Natalia Molina has put it in a different context (x)? There are two pillars at least to "civic fitness," as *Count Us In* makes quite clear; citizenship and civic rights are as much about rights as they are about duties. Of this, too, *Count Us In* makes no secret. It is this framework of civic fitness, I would argue, that is being established by the parents' questions to their son's narrative. Through these questions, it might be argued, *Count Us In* becomes not only a co-authored autobiography written as the dialogue between Jason Kingsley and his friend Mitchell Levitz, but it also becomes the dialogue between two mothers and their sons, and, to a lesser extent, a dialogue between two fathers and their sons. In this sense, Kingsley's and Levitz's parents, even as they are mere co-authors of their sons' narrative, also establish a framework within which this narrative can be *read*.

Crucially, however, it is a framework which by far exceeds disability; instead, it cuts to the core of what it means to be worthy of (American) citizenship. It is here that *Count Us In* both converges with Tito Mukhopadhyay's *The Mind Tree* even as it exceeds its parameters. As Oliver Sacks muses about Mukhopadhyay's writing in his comment on the dust jacket of *The Mind Tree*, there is wonder, for the non-disabled reader, in the fact that an autistic mind is "scarcely capable of introspection" (n. pag.). It is this introspection, the workings of a creative mind which simultaneously marks this mind as "human," which also emerges in Jason Kingsley and Mitchell Levitz's narrative. Like Sacks, we may wonder at the ironies which emerge from Kingsley and Levitz's narrative, ironies which show the authors' awareness of the expectations of their readers, readers who, like Sacks, may see Down Syndrome or disability as being synonymous with the absence, indeed, the impossibility, of irony. As Jason Kingsley puts it at one point in the narrative, addressing the need he sees for readers to engage with *Count Us In*: "The commercials. The commercials should know about Down Syndrome, too. People with Down Syndrome and sometimes people without Down Syndrome should be in the commercials. And they will read: . . . 'Buckle up with Down Syndrome – it's the law!' . . . 'Get Down Syndrome – don't leave home without it!'" (Kingsley and Levitz 11). Yet, it is significant that the framework into which this narrative is embedded never quite stops at the invocation of wonder. Rather, it goes on to "cash in" on these politics of wonder by demanding, quite specifically, a set of rights. To wonder at a disabled person's artistic and creative expression (music, art, writing), the narrative implies, may be not that far removed from the politics of what Rachel Adams has called "freakishness" (x), from the politics of voyeurism involved in a non-disabled public gazing (if no longer quite staring at) a disabled person's *mind. Count Us In*, then, refuses to rest or content itself with the politics of wonder. Instead, it urges a mainstream public to come out of its bewildered, if well-intentioned stupor to include persons with (mental) disability into the civic fabric. In this call, quite simply, it can also be seen as a call for full citizenship for persons with Down Syndrome.

It is in this sense in the narrative of *Count Us In* that Jason Kingsley and Mitchell Levitz can be said to both take and pass a citizenship test. Why else would their account of their lives with Down Syndrome contain the sections "Beliefs, Traditions, Loss and Grief" (119-25), and "Politics and World Affairs"? (126-41). As Mitchell Levitz casually notes, "I have a strong interest in politics, government and world affairs" (Kingsley and Levitz 20). The same differentiation and knowledge of world affairs is evident in his friend Kingsley's comment: "We are worried about the people who are starving in Africa. We are worried about the war in Russia. We are worried about the poverty in South America. We are worried about the problems of the students in China" (Kingsley and Levitz 131). From the perspective of narrative strategy, it is all the more powerful that the call for citizenship rights which, I argue, is at the core of *Count Us In* is only an implicit one: What we get to know as *Count Us In* unfolds is the political opinions, the values and beliefs of two young men, to whom it would be impossible to deny civic participation. *Count Us In* thus writes the citizen without explicitly calling for a citizenship test; even as the entire narrative can in fact be said to be a passing of this test in its demonstrating Jason Kingsley's and Mitchell Levitz's civic and moral fitness.

I am thus reading Kingsley and Levitz's co-written autobiography as an application, by two authors with mental impairment, for full access to U.S. citizenship. *Count Us In* can hence be seen as a form of naturalization. As in the nineteenth-century racial prerequisite cases described by Ian Haney López and Matthew Frye Jacobson, then, applicants have to prove their "fitness for self-government" (Jacobson 68). Where in the case of immigrant petitioners for naturalization during the nineteenth century, both race and culture were marshaled in order to gauge the degree of a claimant's assimilability, what emerges in the case of people with Down Syndrome is the intersection between "rationality" (Nussbaum, *Frontiers of Justice* 98) as mental fitness and a form of cultural knowledge. It was this same cultural knowledge – as proof of their potential Americanness – which nineteenth-century immigrants had to prove in order to gain assimilation. As Jacobson has noted about the petition by a Syrian applicant for naturalization, Tom Ellis, "in identifying Ellis as [white], the judge . . . could have been referring to any of a number of things . . . – Ellis's social bearing, his proficiency in English, his dress, his manner, his style, his demeanour" (239). As Jacobson illustrates, Ellis's "naturalizability" hence hinged not only on his skin color, but also on his social, cultural and linguistic "proficiency." It is this same proficiency, I would suggest, which Jason Kingsley and Mitchell Levitz set out to demonstrate in their collaborative autobiography. *Count Us In* can thus be read as a petition for both the naturalization and normalization of people with Down Syndrome. As in the racial prerequisite cases, these claimants, in order to gain access to the civic body, cannot subvert or question the assumptions of normativity, but they must seek to confirm them.

The fact that *Count Us In* should engage the framework of citizenship tests implies that there is an *unspoken* citizenship test when it comes to including persons with (mental) disabilities in the U.S.. As Rachel Adams makes clear in *Raising Henry*, personhood and its connection to citizenship rights has often tended to exclude persons with genetic disability. According to Adams, "We live in a society that equates personhood with self-possession, autonomy, and the ability to reason. Those who lack such qualities have often been excluded from the rights and responsibilities of citizenship, and even deemed to be less than human" (107). I would thus like to argue that *Count Us In* can be read as a form of citizenship test, pointing, if implicitly so, to the connection that, throughout U.S. citizenship and naturalization history, has been made between civic (and "moral") fitness and the right to become naturalized or to exercise the rights (and responsibility) associated with full citizenship. At one point, Jason Kingsley addresses the question of citizenship right on: "And disabled and Down Syndrome people can also be good citizens of the world. They may have problems, but they may have contributions to contribute for the rest of the world to be proud of" (Kingsley and Levitz 132).

This citizenship test, what is more, is never formally offered; paradoxically, for these marginalized/"disabled" subjects, the right to *take* a citizenship test would already be a step ahead. *Count Us In* can thus be said to write into being not just the citizen with Down Syndrome, but it can also be said to grant to this person the right to take a citizenship test in the first place: The book, I argue, is the citizenship which in the U.S., persons with Down Syndrome are not (yet) allowed to take. The logic of a citizenship test, then, is itself controversial; yet, it may be argued that in a society where some communities only have restricted access to the full amount of citizenship rights, it constitutes a step forward.

The debate around citizenship and naturalization has thus mostly been related to the issue of immigration, not disability. Nonetheless I would argue that the two debates cannot be separated from one another, based as they are on the rights and duties connected to holding U.S. citizenship. According to the INS website to which I will return below, one of the duties associated with the right to holding citizenship is the paying of taxes. It is this concept, then, – the ability to live an independent life, to hold a job, and to pay taxes – which looms so large in both Martha Nussbaum's account of her nephew Arthur as well as Michael Bérubé's son Jamie. Unless a theory of citizenship takes persons with mental impairments into account, Nussbaum argues, it will fail to live up to its promise:

> Children and adults with mental impairments are citizens. Any decent society must address their needs for care, education, self-respect, activity, and friendships. Social contract theories, however, imagine the contracting agents who design the basic structure of society as "free, equal, and independent," the citizens whose interest they represent as "fully cooperative members of society over a complete life." They also often imagine them as characterized by a rather idealized rationality. Such approaches do not do well, even with severe cases of physical impairment and disability. It is clear, however, that such theories must handle severe mental impairments and related disabilities as an afterthought, after the basic institutions of society are already designed. Thus, in effect, people with mental impairments are not among those for whom and in reci-

> procity with whom society's basic institutions are structured. (Nussbaum, *Frontiers of Justice* 98)

I am trying to argue in this chapter, then, that *Count Us In* addresses precisely the idea of the "afterthought" of theories of citizenship: In their collaborative autobiography, Jason Kingsley and Mitchell Levitz set out to prove that they are indeed "free, equal, and independent," and that they are "fully cooperative members of society." This narrative proof of their civic fitness, however, cuts both ways, in an instance which I have already observed with regard to criticism leveled against the work of Temple Grandin. Persons with mental impairment who do not possess Kingsley's and Levitz's mental abilities, on the other hand, may be marginalized by their very attempt to claim citizenship on the basis of civic fitness. Like Temple Grandin in her attempt to prove her full humanity through the use of irony – through not only mastering, but bending meaning –, Kingsley and Levitz inscribe themselves into the basic assumptions of civic fitness without, however, questioning the concept of civic fitness as such.

In line with Martha Nussbaum's argument about social justice, then, *Count Us In* may be said to implicitly address the idea that theories of social justice must not remain abstract, but must be assessed against the specific lives they make possible. She writes, "Theories of social justice should be abstract. They should, that is, have a generality and theoretical power that enables them to reach beyond the potential conflicts of their time, even if they have their origin in such conflicts" (Nussbaum, *Frontiers of Justice* 1). What is at stake is hence the relationship of the specific example – as a "test case" for theories of social justice – and the abstraction or universal applicability which must necessarily remain distant from and may never be reduced to the example. At the same time, however, Nussbaum goes on to say that "theories of social justice must also be responsive to the world and its most urgent problems" (*Frontiers of Justice* 1). These are, she writes, disability, the problem of theories of social justice to go beyond the framework of the nation-state (thus disregarding those who fall outside the logic of "nationality," and animal rights. All of these concerns are closely tied to the concept of citizenship, of who should or should not be given the rights usually attributed to citizenship as both a concept and a set of (legal) rights. According to Nussbaum,

> [today] there are three unresolved problems of social justice whose neglect in existing theories seems particularly problematic. . . . First, there is the problem of doing justice to people with physical and mental impairments. These people are people, but they have not as yet been included in existing societies, as citizens on a basis of equality with other citizens. The problem of extending education, health care, political rights and liberties, and equal citizenship more generally to such people seems to be a problem of justice, and an urgent one. . . . [Solving] this problem requires a new way of thinking about who the citizen is and a new analysis of the purpose of social cooperation (one not focused on mutual advantage), and because it also requires emphasizing the importance of care as a primary social good . . .. (*Frontiers of Justice* 1-2)

The key concept here is the idea of "mutual advantage" (Nussbaum, *Frontiers of Justice* 2). What is at stake, Nussbaum asks, in extending citizenship rights to people with disabilities? What, for instance, does the right to vote imply, and what would it mean for concepts of narrative, of authorship, and of self-articulation?

In each section of their narrative, then, Kingsley and Levitz set out to prove another aspect of their independence, and hence their compatibility with the requirements for citizenship. It is thus far from accidental that a large section of *Count Us In* is devoted to Kingsley's and Levitz's respective career plans. As Levitz writes, "[I am] planning on college, planning on being independent. I've been looking at colleges like New York Institute of Technology. . . . [After college], I probably would get a job working in a government office and to learn the same skills and do what I'm doing now in Assemblyman George Pataki's office in Peekskill" (Kingsley and Levitz 162). These plans, I would argue, are crucial both within a framework of life writing – closely related as they are to what it means to live a "full" life – *and* to the notion of citizenship. Crucially, then, *Count Us In,* as both a citizenship/naturalization test and a form of life writing, ticks off, one by one, the question which Kingsley and Levitz would be required to answer, did they have the right to *take* the citizenship test in the first place. As a PBS news article has recently pointed out, however, there is as yet no clear policy about whether or not persons with disability have the right to vote:

> At a time when election officials are struggling to convince more Americans to vote, advocates for the disabled say thousands of people

> with autism spectrum disorder, cerebral palsy and other intellectual or developmental disabilities have been systematically denied that basic right in the nation's largest county. A Voting Rights Act complaint submitted Thursday to the U.S. Justice Department in Los Angeles goes to a politically delicate subject that states have grappled with over the years: Where is the line to disqualify someone from the voting booth because of a cognitive or developmental impairment? The complaint by the Disability and Abuse Project argues that intellectual and developmental disabilities, including conditions such as Down Syndrome, are not automatic barriers to participating in elections. It seeks a sweeping review of voting eligibility in Los Angeles County in such cases, arguing that thousands of people with those disabilities have lost the right to vote during the last decade. (Blood n. pag.)

Crucially, the newscast explicitly addresses the question whether there should be a test determining the "fitness" of individuals with disability for exercising the right to vote. Rather than requiring such a test, the newscast argues, what is significant is the expression of the desire to vote, and hence to participate in the political process: "'If somebody can articulate in whatever way … that they want to vote, that they have an interest in voting, that's the only test that should be applied nationwide,' Thomas F. Coleman, the group's legal director, said at a news conference outside the federal courthouse, echoing a recommendation from the American Bar Association" (Blood n. pag.).

Moreover, voting rights for persons with disability differ locally, as well as from state to state: "All but about a dozen states have some type of law limiting voting rights for individuals based on competence. But how those laws are enforced varies widely, advocates say" (Blood n. pag.). Crucially, as the newscast notes, persons with physical disability have long contested their exclusion from franchise; the bar to voting has been harder to contest, however, for people with mental disability: "For years, advocates brought attention to the obstacles to voting faced by the physically disabled. More recently, the focus has shifted to the mentally or developmentally disabled, who advocates say have long been stigmatized in the voting process" (Blood n. pag.).

Count Us In makes no reference to what Mitchell Levitz had to do to be allowed to vote; it starts by recording the act of voting, with a picture of Levitz standing at the voting machine. As the PBS newscast notes, in many states, disabled persons wanting to vote were made to take literacy tests: "The complaint says judges in Los Angeles Superior Court use literacy tests to determine if adults in limited conservatorships should have voting rights, a violation of the federal Voting Rights Act" (Blood n. pag.).

What *Count Us In* does, then, is to show, unasked, that Jason Kingsley and Mitchell Levitz can do much more than pass a literacy test; given the chance, they would also pass the naturalization test. My point is that the uncanny match between the questions contained in the citizenship test and Kingsley's and Levitz's autobiographical account are far from accidental. Rather, they point to what is the implicit telos of the book: to call for civic inclusion for people with mental disabilities. Crucially, in the passage quoted above, the PBS newscast refers specifically to persons with autism and with Down Syndrome. My point is, then, that the discussion of texts like *Count Us In* needs to be related not only to medical humanities and life writing research as critical frameworks, but also to a legal rights debate. It is this debate, I would argue, which the sections included in *Count Us In* sets out to trigger: "Politics and World Affairs," "Becoming Independent," and "Our Future Plans."

What then, are the parameters of the citizenship and naturalization tests? My argument in this chapter is that *Count Us In* addresses these parameters one by one, and it addresses them in an implicit declaration of the "civic fitness" of two young men with Down Syndrome. What, then, is the definition of citizenship in the U.S.? As the "Citizens' Almanac" puts it, "U.S. citizens have important rights and responsibilities" (U.S. Citizenship and Immigration Services 2). Among the responsibility of a citizen, of course, is the duty to "pay income and other taxes honestly, and on time, to federal, state and local authorities" (U.S. Citizenship and Immigration Services 7). Crucially, it could be argued that questions about income, the ability to budget one's salary and to pay one's mortgage have nothing to do with an autobiography unless, as I propose in this chapter, the autobiography implicitly contains a citizenship test. The parameters of civic fitness which *Count Us In* addresses, then, strongly overlap with the questions also asked in a citizenship tests, and with the aspects which have been key to the debates about citizenship and personhood. At first sight, it may seem strange for the narrative to take up the question whether either Kingsley or Levitz might consider joining the army. As Levitz asks his friend at one point in the narrative: "Jason, in the future, are you planning on being in the armed forces?" (Kingsley and Levitz 129). The point which I am trying to make in this chapter is not that the collaborative autobiography *Count Us In* explicitly poses as a citizenship or naturalization test. Rather, I am suggesting that, consciously or not, both the questions and the answers contained in the autobiography are in dialogue with the categories, which the naturalization tests require as proof of an applicant's "civic fitness." As official sources state a citizen's duty is also the responsibility to "*[d]efend the country if the need should arise.* The Armed Forces of the United States, the Military, is currently an all-volunteer force. However, should the need arise in times of war, it is important that all citizens join together and assist the Nation where they are able" (U.S. Citizenship and Immigration Services; emphasis in original). It is the context of the history of civic duties, then, that the discussion of Kingsley's joining the army in case of war can be seen in. As both a life writing narrative and a call for civic inclusion – by the narrative's implicit answering of the questions contained in the naturalization test – *Count Us In* is thus both highly nuanced and highly sophisticated. At the time that the dialogue between Jason Kingsley, Mitchell Levitz and their parents takes place, there is the Gulf War. As Levitz tells Kingsley,

> Jason, there are things you have to remember. What you're saying about – if this war did end up here in the United States, there will be many damages. More importantly, this will affect the economy. The economy is where all the money is stored to help the citizens and to budge our moies for safety. Because right now we are in a recession. With this in mind, and the cost of Operation Desert Storm, it will mean more problems, more cutbacks. (Kingsley and Levitz 128)

Emily Perl Kingsley's asking her son whether he thinks the war with Iraq is justified, then, "tests" both her son's knowledge of current politics and his sense of civic duty. On both levels, her son passes the test, as does his friend Mitchell Levitz. What is at stake here, then, is the interconnection between life writing on the one hand and the discourse of citizenship on the other.

If I have argued above with regard to Rachel Adams's book *Raising Henry* that life writing narratives can be seen as producing knowledge in their own right, this is true not only of the production of "biomedical" knowledge produced in narratives about living with disability, but it is also true of the production of civic knowledge. It is here, I believe, that

Count Us In constitutes a crucial intervention. If, as I will suggest below, the question of "biological citizenship" is one of the key questions of the twenty-first century, then most discussions are confined to raising the question, the ethical issue inherent in the bestowal of biological citizenship. What *Count Us In* does, on the other hand, is that it goes on to put the theory of calling for rights for "disabled" subjects into practice by first drawing up and then passing its own citizenship test. The parameters of the discourse of citizenship and what Natalia Molina has called "civic fitness," (x) I would propose, are crafted into the very logic of *Count Us In*. The knowledge produced through life writing, then, can be civic as much as it can be biomedical.

The rights conferred to persons holding U.S. citizenship, then, include both the right to vote and the right to "run for elective office" (U.S. Citizenship and Immigration Services 4). Both these rights are emphasized, and discussed, throughout the life writing narrative of *Count Us In*. Crucially, there is no mention, in official sources of disability with regard to voting. The right to vote is granted to naturalized or natural-born US citizens who are at least 18 years of age and who have not been declarted "mentally incompetent" ("Citizenship Rights and Responsibilities" n. pag.). The de-facto restrictions on voting rights, for people with mental impairment, have hence hinged on the assumption of "mental incompetence." It is this assumption, I would suggest, that through their wide-ranging discussion of politics, morality, religion, and culture, Jason Kingsley and Mitchell Levitz seek to disprove. The topics of this collaborative autobiography, then, may be triggered through the questions asked by their mothers, which provide the framework for the autobiography, a framework which often remains unseen. It may be their mothers' framing of their questions, and the answers provided by Kingsley and Levitz, which are based on the logic of a naturalization test. This multiple framing, of course, makes the authorship of *Count Us In* as a collaborative autobiography highly complex, and perhaps in some sense controversial. Yet, I would argue that even if their mothers frame the parameters of their sons' account of their lives, the sons' authorship nonetheless remains unquestionable.

Crucially, even if the Americans with Disabilities Act prohibits discrimination with regard to work or housing, there is no mention of voting restrictions. Similarly, the right to stand for public office makes no mention of disability; this is as true of the presidential eligibility as it is of other public offices. As Article II, Section 1, Clause 5 of the U.S. Constitution states,

> No Person except a natural born Citizen, or a Citizen of the United States, at the time of the Adoption of this Constitution, shall be eligible to the Office of President; neither shall any Person be eligible to that Office who shall not have attained to the Age of thirty five Years, and been fourteen Years a Resident within the United States. ("Presidential Eligibillity" n. pag.)

The fact that *Count Us In* should "tick off," one by one, the requirements for "civic fitness" (Molina x) which, historically, have also been asked of immigrants applying for naturalization, then, points to a lacuna in citizenship legislation. As Rachel Adams as well as Martha Nussbaum has noted, the debate about personhood and citizenship has been slow to address the rights of persons especially with mental or genetic disabilities. It is in this sense that *Count Us In* is highly complex as an autobiographical narrative: It is a narrative that is at once a testimony to the civic fitness of its authors, and the long version of a citizenship test which the authors have not officially been allowed to take. It may thus be curious that the text addresses the rights debate only implicitly; it starts out with the first time Jason Kingsley voted in a presidential election, without detailing the problems which often surround such voting rights for persons with disability. It is from the recognition of the land mark of voting rights, however, that the difficulties in ensuring this right can be inferred. Kingsley writes about a photograph of himself which has been included in *Count Us In*, "In 1992 this is me voting for the presidential elections. I voted for the winner Mr. Clinton. This is the first time I voted in any election" (Kingsley and Levitz 118). What is crucial here is that even as this passage refers only to the fact that Kingsley voted in the presidential elections, the narrative of *Count Us In* – precisely as a narrative citizenship test – can be seen as written proof of the fact that Jason Kingsley and Mitchell Levitz know how to *exercise* this right to vote. Why else should the narrative dwell in so much detail on Kingsley and Levitz's commenting on the presidential debates leading up to Clinton's election? In Kingsley's comment, there is the sense of being an informed citizen which has been central to the debate on citizenship rights, not only with regard to disability: "And now I am coming up to eighteen. Let me tell you what my future goal of being eighteen is.

Being eighteen I have to be eligible to vote. This is a Presidential Election. I am voting for my President. Who? Clinton? vs. Bush. Or Ross Perot. I haven't decided who I'm going to vote for. I have to listen to the campaign" (Kingsley and Levitz 25).

One of the aims which *Count Us In* as a co-authored narrative can be said to achieve is that it writes into normalcy the political participation of two men with Down Syndrome. It is the casualness with which the narrative documents this political participation which makes it all the more powerful: *Count Us In*, after all, is just a discussion between two young men about presidential politics. As Levitz tells his friend Kingsley, "Now, let's go into the specifics, regarding the debates. I believe that Bill Clinton is not telling the truth. If he raises taxes in Arkansas, he may raise taxes to American taxpayers" (Kingsley and Levitz 133).

7.4 Running for Presidency: The Limits of Inclusion

Perhaps uncannily, in the texts that I am discussing in this study – the "mainstream" film *My Name Is Khan*, Martha Nussbaum's philosophical account of her nephew in *Frontiers of Justice*, and the collaborative autobiography *Count Us In* – the same idea recurs: the desire, on the part of the "disabled" subject, to speak to the American president. In each of these instances, this desire is at once judged to be a failure of political judgment, a failure to comply with the requirements of American citizenship: the minute the "disabled" subject wants to speak to the president directly, or worse, wants to run for president, he has simultaneously failed the citizenship test.

In all of these texts, diverse as they may be – *My Name Is Khan*, *Frontiers of Justice*, and *Count Us In* – the same scene occurs to spiral the demand for inclusion beyond reach: In *My Name Is Khan*, Khan is imprisoned due to his misguided attempt of wanting to speak to the American president directly. In *Frontiers of Justice*, Nussbaum recalls how her nephew chose to express his political opinion by constantly referring to President Bush simply as the "resident" (Nussbaum 206). To make matters worse, in the course of *Count Us In*, Levitz announces at one point that he may want to run for presidency himself. As he tells Kingsley matter-of-factly, "I would like to run for president of the United States…" (Kingsley and Levitz 164). In all these instances, what emerges is the ability – or rather, the failure – on the part of these autistic/disabled subjects to understand the concept of *representative* democracy. It is this failure to comprehend one of the most central aspects of the American democratic system, then, which at once serves to exclude them from citizenship. How, these narratives ask, would a person be allowed to vote if he does not understand that it is impossible to speak to the president directly? In the contemporary U.S. as much as in American history, civic competence looms large in the debates about who should and should not have the right to become an American citizen. Moreover, historically, there were naturalization tests – the so-called "racial prerequisite cases" (Haney Lopez x), for those immigrants who were deemed to be on the brink of whiteness and hence of legal inclusion. In these naturalization tests, too, the immigrants petitioning for the right to be naturalized had to prove their knowledge of the workings of American democracy. This knowledge, in turn, is also true of the U.S. naturalization test; civic fitness is hence assessed through questions such as "What is an amendment?," "What do the first ten amendments do"? or "Who is one of your state's senators now?" (U.S. Citizenship and Immigration Services n. pag.) It is for this reason, I suggest in this chapter, that – prompted by their mothers' questions – *Count Us In* proves the authors' in-depth knowledge of the U.S. political system.

It is this competence, I would argue, which is also at issue in these accounts of disability that I am discussing in this study. The minute he announces that he wants to run for president, then, Kingsley has failed the citizenship test. And yet, why would he be said to have failed? Historically, there was a time when, not so long ago, it would have seemed outrageous for an African American candidate to even run for presidency, let alone win the election. With Barack Obama, the first black American president was elected only in 2009. Yet, there seems to be a vast difference between disability, especially mental disability, and racial difference. If race, as Haney Lopez has argued, is a social and not a biological category, disability is rooted in biology to an extent, arguably, which does not apply to race. And yet, the Americans with Disability Act (ADA) has been compared and directly related to the Civil Rights Acts. For Barbara Levitz and Emily Perl Kingsley, the idea behind the book *Count Us In* is to achieve for disability what has already been achieved for race: the right for disability to be recognized as a social, not a biological category. Given this similarity, then, it may not be so outrageous for Mitchell Levitz to want to run for president in the first place. Conversely, the degree to which we think this desire to be absurd marks the difference which we still see between race and mental disability,and the extent to which, with regard to mental disability, biology seems to trump social categorization. How, some would ask, can we allow civic participation – the right to vote, let alone to hold a political office – to someone who seems cognitively unable to understand the principle of representative democracy?

Like his friend Jason Kingsley, then, Mitchell Levitz has *mastered* the citizenship test the minute he no longer wants to run for president of the United States; and, in much more nuanced a manner, he has understood the difference between "politics" and "policy":

> Even though people agree or disagree on different issues, all people are entitled to their own opinions. That is what I have learned about why being involved in government and policy is significant. There is a big difference between politics and policy. If a person gets involved in politics, they need to be able to be elected to *represent* people in their district. With policy, people can be in the background by creating laws and programs that will help and support people with disabilities. This is why I chose to be involved in policy work instead of politics. (Kingsley and Levitz 192-93; itablics mine)

Given this insight, contained in the afterword as a corrective to his initial autobiographical account, Levitz now smiles at the fact that he once wanted to run for president, thus passing his citizenship test or the citizenship test which the dominant, non-disabled culture draws up for him. And yet, the narrative of *Count Us In* cautions us to think twice about what we deem absurd in the first place.

At the same time, it must be noted that when Mitchell Levitz was given an award for graduating from high school, Assemblyman George Pataki addressed this very question: Why would it be absurd to imagine a person with Down Syndrome run for political office? This question implies the limits of inclusion:

> "He was born with Down Syndrome and often that is something that results in the child being placed away from the mainstream and not involved academically and socially in the usual activities of childhood. And through the exemplary efforts of his mother and father, Barbara and

> Jack Levitz, and through his own extraordinary efforts, he has led an exemplary life. [He] is working as an intern in my district, coming and helping me with constituent programs. We expect to see him graduate from high school next year and run against one of us some year. I wish you would recognize his courage and dedication. Seated behind me, Mitchell Levitz." (Kingsley and Levitz 18)

What is crucial here is that Pataki should be referring to the idea that Mitchell Levitz, too, may one day want to run for political office. Unlike in *My Name Is Khan*, however, this is not a joke at the expense of the disabled subject who has not yet understood the concept of representative democracy; rather, it is a way of envisioning the horizon of political inclusion which also comprises the right to hold office.

Yet, the main argument of *Count Us In* rests on the idea of opportunity and the concept of learning: As both Jason Kingsley and Mitchell Levitz emphasize, they are slower at learning what their classmates have already mastered; yet, even if knowledge comes with a time lag, they are nonetheless confident that they will eventually "catch up." It is this sense of slow but steady learning, of acquiring competence through hard work, that may also apply to the idea of running for presidency. If at one point in the narrative, Levitz failed the (implicit) citizenship test by imagining that he would one day want to run for president, he implicitly corrects this mistake by proving his nuanced knowledge of politics later on. Years later, he corrects this view by saying, "Major importance is to help people with disabilities. . . . Being an advocate, speaking out, talking to other people with disabilities" (Kingsley and Levitz 172). It is this nuanced comprehension of the political process which marks his entry into the "mainstream," and which makes for the fact that, given the right to take it, he may in fact *pass* the citizenship test. Similarly, Levitz has understood the concept of representative democracy, no longer wanting to hold a political office, he wants to work as a congressman's aide. As his mother reminds him, on Clinton's committee of advisors there are a number of persons with disability. Moreover, both Kingsley and Levitz understand their book – their life writing account of what it means to live with Down Syndrome – as an expression of their political will. It is their book that they want to send to the president. As Kingsley puts it, "Probably after the book comes out, I was thinking Clinton might read the book" (Kingsley and Levitz 116). By wanting to send their book to the president as a testimony about disability and their own quality of life, as well as a guideline for decision-making, then, Jason Kingsley and Mitchell Levitz *prove* their knowledge of the workings of American democracy.

It is at this juncture that, unlike Khan, and, to a lesser degree, unlike Martha Nussbaum's nephew Arthur, Jason Kingsley and Mitchell Levitz choose a form of political expression which is *appropriate*. It is in this sense that *Count Us In* is a form not only of life writing but also of political and legal testimony. It is a testimony, to use Natalia Molina's term in a different context, to their own "civic fitness" (x). It is this testimony that the text – *Count Us In* in its published form – records in both narrative and picture. There is, included in the narrative, a photograph of the first time Mitchell Levitz was allowed to vote in the presidential election. This, then, is the telos which Nussbaum also envisions for Arthur: "If the course of his education goes well, Arthur might hold a job that is commensurate with his high intelligence, and thus be 'productive' in the economic sense . . ." (*Frontiers of Justice* 128).

Count Us In as a narrative, then, is highly astute in petitioning for citizenship for persons with Down Syndrome: As we read Kingsley's and Levitz's discussion as to who, in the presidential election of 1996, should become the American president, it is hard to remember their disability, or the consequences it has been said to have for their ability to comprehend the civic process. As they debate the role of environmental justice in the presidential campaign, it is impossible to deny to these young men civic fitness. As he tells Levitz, Kingsley supports Al Gore as Bill Clinton's running mate because of his commitment to the environment:

> I like Gore better. He's a partner to Clinton and he's more focused on many issues that help Clinton to learn about the world.... He is about the environment. If Clinton and Gore sit down together to tell him about the environment. Because we need both parts. One is how people would change the environment. That's one mixture of Gore and Clinton. Or Clinton might say "What kind of community or kind of environment would we put people into a specially good government?" (Kingsley and Levitz 137)

At this juncture, too, the concept of medical humanities, let alone of illness narrative unravels as the sole frame of reference in which to read *Count Us In*: What, in other words, would a discussion of environmental justice have to do in a patient narrative, an account of disability? The framework of the narrative thus deliberately sabotages the concept of appropriateness. It is in this sense that *Count Us In* is an autobiography to the fullest extent, an autobiography which refuses to be only a patient narrative. It is here that medical humanities may in fact clash with humanities readings of one and the same text. If medical humanities have a close affinity to life writing, as I have argued above, if they enable us to read some autobiographies as patient accounts whose inclusion may have an impact on medical practice, talking about environmental justice or the right candidate for American presidency would seem profoundly out of place in this context. If, on the other hand, *Count Us In* were read not only in a medical but also in a civic framework, a framework aimed not at medical treatment but civic inclusion, such passages would no longer be out of place. By the same token, if a text like *Count Us In* were taught in an American Studies classroom, which course syllabus would it be part of? I have argued above that Tito Mukhopadhyay's book *The Mind Tree*, may figure in any discussion of (postcolonial) autobiography, even a context far removed from disability studies. Ultimately, I am thus calling for an ethics of reading, an ethics of reading which fuses medical humanities with the humanities even as it recognizes the differences between the two. By the same token, *Count Us In* may be incorporated not only within a framework of disability, but also of environmental justice. The degree to which we think of a chapter on environmental justice as being misplaced in the autobiography of two persons with Down Syndrome marks our degree to step out of the confines of medical humanities, useful as they may be in myriads of different contexts.

What marks *Count Us In* as a collaborative life writing narrative not only of the boys' lives but also of their parents', is the refusal not to "aim high." As Barbara Levitz and Emily Perl Kingsley state right at the beginning of the narrative – a narrative authored by six different persons, the boys, their parents, and their grandfathers – there was a widespread belief, as the boys were growing up, that children with Down Syndrome should not be taught "academics"; that teaching them academics would be a pointless and useless endeavor. Minus academics, then, how would Jason Kingsley and Mitchell Levitz ever have become enabled to understand the concept of representative democracy, and the complexity of the political process? By the same token, and seen from a particular utilitarian perspective, it would have been pointless for Kingsley's grandfather to teach him physics:

> JASON KINGSLEY: And then later we had science experiments like magnets, like the north pole and south pole. Our first experiment was how to make a compass.... When ships want to know where to go, they use a magnet with a small bowl of water an a-
>
> GRANDPA KINGSLEY: A needle. We had two magnets –
>
> JASON KINGSLEY: And you told me like poles would repel and opposite poles would attract. . . . We also had our box called Physics. Oh yeah, and my measuring experiments. (Kingsley and Levitz 112)

It was their refusal to abide by this advice which may in fact have paved the boys' path towards citizenship. At the same time, it may be useful to note that what may be at issue here, too, may be the concept of the social meaning attached to a biological quality. In American history, there was a time when it was argued that it would be useless for African Americans to attend university; as Booker T. Washington famously argued in his debate with W.E.B. Du Bois, such academic education would be useless since African Americans would never be allowed to work in academic positions in the first place. This was a line of argument to which Du Bois famously replied, "I sit with Shakespeare and he winces not" (Du Bois 139). What an entire century later emerges in an autobiography written by two young men with Down Syndrome, then, is nothing less than their right or desire to sit with Shakespeare. It is in this sense that Jason Kingsley's musing on Shakespeare's idea of human beings as mere players on the stage that is life is far from accidental, but can in fact be seen to be programmatic of the narrative as a whole: "Shakespeare said, 'All the world's a stage and the people are merely players' and any special place or time is the backstage crew. Our perceptions are cameras to look at the actors who play the characters so real" (Kingsley and Levitz 63). If in his foreword to Tito Mukhopadhyay's narrative, neurologist Oliver Sacks is amazed at the fact that an "autistic mind" should be capable of introspection, Jason Kingsley's narrative gives the lie to those who would have believed that a person with Down Syndrome was incapable of comprehending, let alone musing about, Shakespeare's philosophy of life. In *Count Us In*, Jason Kingsley and Mitchell Levitz indeed sit with Shakespeare, and he winces not. Historically, as Natalia Molina and many others have noted, the racial prerequisite cases were cases in which immigrants had to prove not just their civic fitness, but their moral aptitude for becoming naturalized American citizens. Crucially, then, morality was key to the parameters of "fitness for self-government" (Jacobson 68). As Ian Haney López has observed, petitioners were asked if they believed in monogamy.[6] In such a context of moral as civic fitness, what does it imply that Levitz's discussion with Kingsley repeatedly returns to the question of Kingsley's faithfulness to his girlfriend, Tami? Speaking of Kingsley's long-distance relationship to Tami, Levitz asks his friend about his commitment to Tami:

> MITCHELL LEVITZ: Do you feel having a girl closer to you, would that change your feelings for Tami?
>
> JASON KINGSLEY: It would not change my feelings for Tami in the world. You can live with only one true love, who you are going to get married with. But if you have a semi-girlfriend, which means that you need someone to warm your heart and make you feel special… it's happy and good all over and have being normal. . . .
>
> MITCHELL LEVITZ: Would Tami be jealous? . . .
>
> JASON KINGSLEY: She doesn't mind. Unless there's sexual stuff. (Kingsley and Levitz 78)

If, as I am trying to argue in this chapter, the book *Count Us In* implicitly imports the categories required by a naturalization test, it addresses civic as well as moral assumptions. As Levitz reminds Kingsley, entering a relationship, let alone marrying one's girlfriend, also means taking on responsibility. This responsibility, Levitz emphasizes, is moral and emotional as much as it is economic:

[6] In *Ex parte Shahid*, for instance, a petitioner's case was turned down not only because of his inability to speak English, but also because of his suspect moral values. According to López, the court noted that Shahid "writes his name in Arabic, cannot read or write in English, and speaks and understands English very imperfectly. . . . His answers to the questions of whether he is a polygamist or a disbeliever in organized government were in the affirmative, and he could not be made to understand in English the purport of the questions asked" (72).

> I think once I get married to a woman, then I would take a very serious commitment, that [sic] the responsibilities, take care of my wife, take care of my children. In my marriage, if a woman that I chose to have sex with, if she agrees and is ready to take the commitment, to take the step in our relationship, then I would be ready and I would have sex with her. Then I would probably decide, if she was taking birth control pills. (Kingsley and Levitz 91)

Crucially, this passage can clearly be understood in relation to the question whether a person with Down Syndrome will ever be able to lead an independent life, to have a life and a family of his own. If the earning of citizenship rights also rests on moral responsibility, Mitchell Levitz clearly passes the test. As Michael Bérubé, whose narrative I will discuss in more detail below, has emphasized, moreover, the question of reproductive rights has historically been key for persons with disability, many of whom were forced to undergo sterilization at the beginning of the twentieth century.

The question of reproduction, the right to raise a family, in turn, is key to what it means to live a "full life." As Jason Kingsley puts it, "I don't think I could live a full life without children" (Kingsley and Levitz 92). The central point which *Count Us In* addresses, then, is the question of a disabled individual's living an independent life. In this aspect, too, *Count Us In* can be inserted into a genealogy of previous autobiographies, most of which involve an individual's struggle for personal autonomy. It is this sense of rebellion against what he views as his parents' dominance over his life that Jason Kingsley addresses. This juncture, I would argue, is more than mere generational conflict; it is at the core of what it means to assume authorship over one's own life. It is against his parents' "dominance" over his life that Kingsley drafts his own "declaration of independence" (Kingsley and Levitz 152). As he writes in 1992,

> Dear friends, adults, teachers, and parents,
>
> This is Jason Kingsley. I am utterly alone and stressfully upset.
>
> I will tell you why. I know I am learning about school and life, but I have a difficulty to learn things. Now I understand a lot of stuff. Can you let me be on my own and in the future. You will have to let go of me. I'm not a kid and a teenager. Seventeen years I'm dying to be a man.

> "Get off my back please!" Even though I am deciding things now, I want to be myself alone. It's not easy but this is the way it is. I'm sorry to make you upset but let me to be free.
>
> Thank you,
>
> Jason Kingsley (Kingsley and Levitz 152)

Crucially, both Martha Nussbaum and Michael Bérubé have stressed that the Western discourse of (human) rights has centered on individual autonomy. The passage cited above, Jason Kingsley's personal declaration of independence, then, can be read on multiple levels. First, it is a letter written by a "disabled" subject asking his teachers and parents to grant him more independence in living his life. Second and even more importantly, however, it addresses the question of individual autonomy head-on, and is thus once again interwoven with the discourse of citizenship and of civic rights.

Thus, this declaration can be read on a number of levels all of which are interrelated. First, Kingsley's letter quite straightforwardly answers one of the questions which immigrant petitioners for American citizenship have to answer in their naturalization test: "What did the Declaration of Independence do? " Secondly, he connects his knowledge of American history and of American political history to his own claim for a full, independent life. The point is not that Kingsley testifies, for quality of life researchers, about what, in his opinion, constitutes a good life; rather, he subtly and with much irony demonstrates his desire to take charge of his own life: With an irony which at the same time demonstrates his nuanced knowledge of American history and politics, he drafts his own declaration of independence.

7.5 Reading Autobiography as Resumé

What, however, if Jason Kingsley's and Mitchell Levitz's life narrative were read not just from beginning to end, but from end to beginning? Even more importantly, what if it were being read not only as an autobiography, much less a disability narrative, but as a *resumé*? I am concerned here with the very concept of (in)appropriateness. Why would it seem absurd to think of this autobiography not just as (the answers to) a citizenship test, but as a resumé submitted by a person with Down Syndrome for a regular job? At the end of the postscript, Mitchell Levitz is in the process of applying for a job, working on his resumé.

Crucially, the book *Count Us In*, too, can be read as a resumé for both of its authors individually. What *Count Us In* both records and proves is not only its authors' civic fitness – a fitness, I have argued, which informs their answers to the questions of an implicit citizenship test – but also their economic fitness. As I have suggested above, both of these instances – proving civic and proving economic aptitude – are closely interconnected, as citizenship has historically been denied to those deemed to be "unproductive" or morally "unfit" subjects. Yet, there is a difference between mentioning or noting in passing, as I have done above, that Mitchell Levitz had just moved into his own house by the time that *Count Us In* was published, and discussing in detail what Levitz does for a living. As Levitz states at the end of his co-authored narrative, "Now I own my own townhouse and I work for both the Westchester Institute of Human Development, a University Center on Developmental Disabilities, and also for the Self-Advocacy Association of New York State. I work on disability projects and do training" (Kingsley and Levitz 192).

To read the narrative through the resumé of its author is thus to take seriously a complex politics of reading. As I have noted above, to re-import the framework of medical humanities back into the humanities may challenge us to reconsider some of the methodologies we have dismissed as "obsolete." As in the concept of ethnic writing, the "death of the author" (Barthes 1967) may prove problematic for reading a narrative by a disabled author. Yet, even if we were to concede that there may be some relevance of an author's life and social location to his or her writing, to read an autobiographical and thus a literary narrative through the website of its author may be making matters worse: it may imply not only reading the author's life back into the narrative but worse, to dwell on his biography as a clue to the author's "intention." My aim, however, is by no means to engage in or resurrect the concept of "intentional fallacy"; rather, my goal is to inquire about the materialities of the lives which are being written about in autobiographies such as *Count Us In*. This is not to say that *Count Us In*, like all autobiographies, is not also autofictional, and that the narrative of an author with Down Syndrome is not also a staged narrative, or that the author's website is less staged than his narrative.

Yet, to look at the author's website, I propose, may trigger a different framework of reading, a reading which, I will argue below, is direly missing in a recent article about teenagers with Down Syndrome attending German high schools in what I am reading as a half-hearted attempt at inclusion. To suggest that an autobiography may simultaneously be read as a resumé, and to look at the author's website, may in fact be confronting stereotypes head-on, to lay to rest the assumption that to be born with Down Syndrome will preclude the possibility of ever *having* a website, let alone one authored by oneself. For the obstetricians who prophesied to Jason Kingsley and Mitchell Levitz a different, a "retarded" temporality, to think that they would one day have their own website would have seemed absurd. It is in this sense, then, that it is no means by accident that *Count Us In* should refer to the fact that at the time the postscript is written, Mitchell Levitz is just in the process of updating his resumé, and will proceed to join the faculty of the Westchester Institute of Human Development. The autobiographical narrative thus substantiates the resumé, and vice versa: the skills that the resumé lists are being confirmed by the narrative. As Barbara Levitz notes, "It is gratifying for me that Mitchell and I have become colleagues in our work as professionals in the disability field during the last few years" (Kingsley and Levitz 197).

In this chapter, then, I have been trying to ask what would happen if we read *Count Us In* not as a narrative about growing up with Down Syndrome, but as a text whose purpose may be multifold. First, if we take Mitchell Levitz's part of the narrative, the text can also be read as a resumé; secondly, it can also be seen as a way for two young men with Down Syndrome to call for the rights to fully fledged citizenship. If we start with the prior possibility of reading, the idea of reading *Count Us In* as a resume, the text can be seen as the long version of the resumé of a young man, academically trained, who is on the job market. Reading *Count Us In* in these terms, then, may have nothing at all to do with disability, and the fact that the applicant happens to have Down Syndrome may be secondary to the skills which he has to offer, none of which have anything to do with medical diagnosis.

What is at stake in this reading of a life writing text as the job application resumé of its authors (or rather, one of its authors), is also to read *Count Us In* not from front to back but from back to front: Since *Count Us In* is a narrative about growing up with Down Syndrome, to read the text as one of the author's resumé is to start out from the education which he has gained, an education which he now draws from in his resumé. As he writes, "I need to put together a resumé and a letter of application. And references, which I definitely have" (Kingsley and Levitz 177). Here too, it may seem crucial that Levitz has his CV online. As he describes his work on his website with the Global Down Syndrom Foundation,

> Mitchell Levitz has been a spokesperson on behalf of individuals with developmental disabilities and has served extensively on councils, boards, taskforces and conference planning groups in New York State, Ohio and nationally. He has been actively engaged in addressing school and university groups as well keynote and workshop presentations for national, statewide and regional conferences all across the country. More than 13 years ago, he joined the staff and faculty of the Westchester Institute for Human Development – a University Center of Excellence in Developmental Disabilities affiliated with New York Medical College, and serves as the Self-Advocacy Coordinator. He teaches graduate students, coordinates a self-advocacy group, develops health training materials and curriculum based on self-determination, and work [sic] on a variety of other grant projects. He especially enjoys serving in a leadership role with the Council of Community Advocacy (COCA) of the Association of University Centers on Disabilities (AUCD) as well as the AUCD Project Advisory Committee. He continues to participate in numerous self-advocacy leadership teams, conferences and forums. ("Mitchell Levitz" n. pag.)

Cynically speaking, from an ableist perspective, for Mitchell Levitz to *have* a resumé in the first place would argue against a narrow predefinition of what limited career path society has in store for people like Mitchell Levitz. The question which *Count Us In* asks, with the boys' narratives being echoed in their mothers', is: If Levitz and Kingsley were to sit with William Shakespeare, would Shakespeare wince? The fact that the ADA has been compared to the Civil Rights Act, then, is crucial for my purposes here: The rights which we may now take for granted with regard to race may still have a long way towards implementation with regard to disability.

The idea of reading a narrative as a resumé, then, is also significant as it engages the concept of color-blindness or rather, of "ability-blindness," a concept which has been critical to me in a number of contexts discussed in this study. As I have argued above, the idea of "color-blindness" as Morrison has described it can be related to different strategies of reading when it comes to disability. When we read Levitz's resumé, then, we do not see his picture, in a marked difference between German and U.S. American standards for job applications, for instance. What we see are the written words on the page; words which, in the resumé as well as in the written autobiographical account that is *Count Us In*, are unaffected by the fact that Levitz sometimes stammers (Kingsley and Levitz 196). The idea of what I would call "ability-blindness" is crucial here, as is the concept of color-blindness in the sense investigated by Morrison, an idea which I have discussed in Chapter 6. Morrison writes in *Playing in the Dark* that she experimented, in her earlier fiction work, with writing a text that was not color-coded. Yet, she writes, it soon turned out that such a text was impossible to write, so deeply were "color" and "color-consciousness" (Appiah and Gutman 1996) embedded in the U.S. American social fabric. Moreover, proponents of Critical Race Studies have stressed the fact that color-blindness may be a universalist fiction, or a fiction of universality, which may in fact mask the universality of whiteness, a whiteness which is usually taken as representative of a social norm at the expense of the conveying of "ethnic" subjectivities. Yet, as Anthony Appiah and Amy Gutman have argued, color-blindness may nonetheless remain a telos in the strife for social justice; hence, no-one would dispute the fact that it is a step ahead for the inclusion of ethnic minorities *or* people with disabilities that there are no photographs on a resumé. Thus, I would argue that autobiographical narratives such as *Count Us In* engage the concept of ability-blindness as a concept, precisely because they insist on the word on the written page. To be sure, this notion of ability-blindness, too, may be troubled by the fact that it presupposes, as the prerequisite for social inclusion and acceptance, the eloquence of the writing subject. As Barbara Gibbs Levitz has noted, people often praise her son's eloquence, an eloquence which, it is implied, stands in direct contrast to his disability:

> In recent years, he has developed an unexpected grasp of complex vocabulary. After speaking with Mitchell, many people remark about his language skills and his ability to communicate his ideas so articulately. This is despite the fact that he sometimes stammers, getting stuck on the first letter-sound of a word. He deals with this problem by quickly fig-

> uring out another, appropriate replacement word. (Kingsley and Levitz 196)

Yet, even as it would be problematic not to note the fact that the path to sameness is paved, in Levitz's case, through both class and education, there is nonetheless a sense in which the power of life writing may lie in its ability for its author to speak to us in disembodied form; his difference no longer being visible or audible.[7]

What does it mean, then, not to simply see the continuity between autobiography and resumé, between life writing and job-hunting, but also to read Levitz's autobiography through his research on human rights? Crucially, what is at stake here is the difference between theory and practice, between "writing about" one's condition and theorizing it. At the heart of the citizenship test which is *Count Us In* is the question whether Jason Kingsley and Mitchell Levitz are able to understand what it means to live with disability, to not only express their experience but to reflect on it. Yet, both of these levels are ultimately related to the idea of lived experience, with life writing, as I argue throughout these chapters, "talking back" at the life sciences. I would like to argue, however, that Mitchell Levitz's life writing research means more than such self-expression; it is the ability to step out of life writing into a form of research which by far transcends his own life. Crucially, I have argued in Chapter 4 that Temple Grandin has made a life for herself by studying, and becoming an expert in, animal studies. As she herself states in *Thinking in Pictures*, there are two sides to her career: In one part of her life, she is an animal scientist; in another, an advocate for people with autism.

What is significant about reading *Count Us In* as the extended resumé of its authors, then, is that it at once engages and subverts the idea of leading a "productive" life. As Martha Nussbaum has argued with regard to her nephew, Arthur, such utilitarian thinking is itself unproductive, and may be severely limiting for ideas of social justice and the politics of inclusion. Nonetheless, *Count Us In* complicates this notion – the absence or the lack of a need for a resumé – by drawing attention to the fact that what is at stake is not the idea of leading a life that is pro-

[7] On the politics of "sound as aesthetic practice," see Sabine Kim's study *Acoustic Entanglements: Sound and Aesthetic Practice* (2017).

ductive for the general public, but the sense that finding a line of work that is fulfilling is also an essential part of a "gelingendes Leben."

Throughout this chapter, then, I have experimented with notions of reading, with employing different "lenses" or paradigms with which to read one and the same text. Reading *Count Us In* within the framework of medical humanities may be useful, then, for expanding the notion of patient experience; as Kingsley and Levitz expressly state at the outset of their narrative, one of the "intended readers" for their book is the obstetrician who told Jason Kingsley's mother that her son would never be able to lead a successful life. By including autobiographies and other forms of life writing to draw attention to the patient's experience, then, medical practice may come to change, particularly in the temporalities it predicts for subjects with disability. This is a point made throughout both Tito Mukhopadhyay's life writing and the narrative of *Count Us In*. At the same time, medical humanities and the notion of ability-blindness seem to be mutually exclusive; a resumé, in other words, would have no place in medical humanities. And yet, as I am trying to argue here, the true potential of medical humanities may be realized only to the extent to which it is able to read the same narrative as both a patience narrative and a resumé; if it can conceive of, even insist on imagining, the patient's life after s/he has left the doctor's office. In other words, to apply Appiah's and Gutman's argument about race to the context of disability, color-blindness only works in conjunction with color-consciousness. It may be crucial to keep in mind precisely the intersection, then, between the concepts of ability-blindness and ability-consciousness.

There is a teleology to this chapter, and one that is closely modeled on the narrative choreography of Jason Kingsley and Mitchell Levitz's narrative. If I have started this chapter by seeing in life writing an alternative form of knowledge production, it is important to ask in what ways such alternative knowledge is being incorporated and into what frameworks it is included. In the afterword to *Count Us In*, Mitchell Levitz writes, "Our book is recommended reading for schools, colleges, and universities" (Kingsley and Levitz 193). Clearly enough, this is a sense in which life writing may have a profound impact, and in which life writing may shape the ways in which we come to interact with persons who have a given disability. What Levitz does not say but what may easily be included here is that the book may in time become required reading not just in schools, colleges and classrooms but also in medical education. To the extent that medical humanities are being included in medical education, *Count Us In* may in time become standard reading, and knowledge production about persons born with Down Syndrome would no longer solely be a domain of biomedicine. Even more importantly, the book may thus change the way in which obstetricians advise women whose children are born with Down Syndrome, and the lives which medical practitioners can help envision for the parents and siblings of children with Down Syndrome. What would it have meant, Jason Kingsley and Mitchell Levitz implicitly ask, if the obstetrician who once told Kingsley's mother that her son should be "institutionalized" had had access to a life writing narrative such as *Count Us In*? What advice would he have given her then? It is in this sense that this chapter seeks to come full circle, from the ending of *Count Us In* to Rachel Adams' recent autobiography of mothering her second son, *Raising Henry*. Sadly, what Adams describes is an obstetrician not so far removed from the perspective which had once been taken by the obstetrician of Emily Perl Kingsley twenty years earlier. Obviously enough, Kingsley's obstetrician did not take into account life writing narratives such as *Count Us In* in the advice she gave to her patients, believing instead in the "perfectibility" of the medical profession, a profession often hinging on genetics as a key discipline. At the same time, the knowledge that Adams turns to when she is in need of guidance for decision-making is no longer medical expertise; rather, she turns to life writing narratives as alternative sources of knowledge. In trying to imagine the life that her newborn son Henry could be leading, Adams turns to narratives such as *Count Us In.* This, then, is the potential of life writing, and the potential of life writing being an alternative source of knowledge, even and especially in the era of biomedicine.

7.6 Decision-Making in the Era of Biomedicine: Michael Bérubé's *Life As We Know It*

What is at stake, then, is an idea far more complex than mere application of life writing narratives to medical education. What framing the debate through the parameters of knowledge production does, I would argue, is to address the entire field of decision-making, and hence to think of humanities research as intervening into the social choices enabled by medical technologies. It is in this context that the question of the "research" on the basis of which choices are being made – the choice whether to carry a pregnancy to term or to abort a fetus with, for instance, Down Syndrome – takes on particular significance: What if, Bérubé asks, these choices were being made not on the grounds of *medical research* but of *life writing research*? I believe that Bérubé addresses a lacuna here which has not explicitly been discussed in studies exploring potential interfaces between medicine/biomedical practice and the humanities. What if the knowledge produced by the humanities through life writing research played a central role not only as supplement to medical discourse or a "tool" used by helpless parents through internet research when faced with a life-altering decision, but as scientific, empirical research in the sense proper? As it stands, both Bérubé's *Life As We Know It* and Levitz and Kingsley's *Count Us In* remind us, decision-making and the medical advice which doctors give to parents rest on the rather accidental question whether or not the doctor has met, or read about, persons with Down Syndrome. An idea which is expressed by Jason Kingsley in *Count Us In* – the act of sending a copy of his book to his mother's obstetrician – would then move to the center of current debates about social choices in the era of the "technological reproducibility" (and technological alterability) of human life. What if, indeed, such a taking into account of the knowledge generated by life writing research were made an aspect that it would be *mandatory* to consider, not only for doctors, but for parents as well?

What started as a pragmatic question – What is the status of medical humanities in American Studies? – may thus have led to a question which may be fundamental not just for American Studies research, but for humanities research in general. What, indeed, will be the status of the humanities in the twenty-first century? I believe that what is crucial to consider here is that the question moves us beyond entrenched debates about whether or not the knowledge produced in the humanities needs to be "applicable" in any palpable sense. Rather, the parameters within which we have so far asked the question may have been, if not entirely flawed, then at least misleading. What may be at stake, then, is whether the humanities set out to intervene into current debates on the "social meaning" of biomedical advances, and the extent to which they are willing to do so. I would like to argue here that life writing research may be one of the arenas which will be paramount to such intervention. It is here, however, that the debate may return full circle to the notion of institutionalization, a notion addressed but not elaborated by calls for the integration of medical humanities into medical training: For what such an intervention requires is precisely that life writing texts such as Bérubé's *Life As We Know It* and Kingsley and Levitz's *Count Us In*, as well as Rachel Adams's *Raising Henry*, be read not only in English Departments, but in medical education, and that they be read in the latter field not as optional footnotes, but as core texts pointing to an arena which by far exceeds, even if it is related to, quality of life research.

The question, then, is not only what is being taught in medical classrooms but also the *status* of what is taught: Adams notes that when she was writing *Raising Henry*, she agreed to give a lecture to medical students: "Our second set of meetings took us into the belly of the beast. We were invited back to the hospital . . ., this time to speak to a group of obstetricians" (120). Yet, this lecture was, of course, optional and not mandatory in these students' education. In this context as in myriads of others, life writing research – and the life writing narrative authored by Adams herself – is a mere footnote to quality of life research, a field which is itself optional in medical education. As Adams goes on to note,

> The glitch I saw in the system of obstetrical training was that the very doctors who devote themselves to helping women achieve a healthy pregnancy often know nothing at all about children. . . . How can an obstetrician be expected to manage the news that a fetus has Down Syndrome or Kleinfelter's [sic] or spina bifida when she's ignorant about what it's like to live with, or parent a child with, those conditions? I remembered Dr. Lewis's feeble attempt to comfort me by saying that a child with Down Syndrome lived in her neighborhood. At the time I wondered bitterly whether that was really the best she could do after all her years of medical training? (121)

Life writing research thus often remains, at best, a footnote to a footnote; it is far from being central to the existential choice which modern medicine enables, but also forces us to make. Yet, it is at this juncture, too, that Bérubé's narrative, *Life As We Know It*, intervenes, by asking a question so chilling that it has often remained unasked in contemporary narratives by parents of children with Down Syndrome: On the grounds of what knowledge did doctors, even towards the second half of the twentieth century, advise parents to have their children "institutionalized"? Just as for Adams, Bérubé's book about raising his son Jamie was a "road map" (ix), Bérubé's own road map was Emily and Charles Kingsley's account of raising their son Jason. The most terrible aspect of the obstetrician's advice, Emily Perl Kingsley recalls, was the doctor's "prediction" that their son would never be able to recognize them as his parents in the first place:

> The obstetrician took my husband aside and told him that this was a child who was never going to accomplish anything. This was a child who, he said, would probably never sit up, stand, walk, talk, or have any meaningful thoughts whatsoever. He would never recognize us as his parents. He would never be able to distinguish us from any other adults who were halfway nice to him. . . . (qtd. in Bérubé 31)

It is for this reason, then, that the obstetrician recommends that Jason Kingsley be institutionalized. What is remarkable in this context, however, is that the Kingsleys refused to let life science – in the sense of the obstetrician's prediction of their newborn son's dismal future – evolve into life writing. In other words, they refused to have their son's life be written by the life sciences and the "medical dogma" ("Dr Oliver Sacks-Narrative and Medicine") of the time. This act of resistance, especially at a time when no alternative knowledge about the lives of children with Down Syndrome who grew up outside of institutions was available, cannot be overestimated; it would pave the way for other parents, like Michael Bérubé, to follow their example. This, then, was Charles Kingsley's retort to the obstetrician's remark about his son's future. As Emily Perl Kingsley recalls,

> This was about as rock-bottom as you can get. The expectations he gave us were nil. After the obstetrician gave Charles this terribly gloomy advice, Charles said one of his most brilliant lines ever. He said to the obstetrician: "Okay, maybe my son will never grow up to be a brain surgeon. Maybe all he'll ever be is an obstetrician!" (qtd. in Bérubé 31)

To Bérubé, the father, it is simply unbearable to imagine what would have happened had parents before him, let alone he himself, followed this medical advice. He goes on to observe,

> [It] was pronounced by the best-trained medical practitioners in the world, who told families of kinds with Down's that their children would

> never be able to walk, talk, dress themselves, or recognize their parents. Best to have the child institutionalized and tell one's friends that the baby died at birth. Only the most stubborn, intransigent, or inspired parents resisted such advice from their trusted experts. (Bérubé 27)

As is by now well-documented in medical research, the ability to bond with and be cared for by their parents has far-reaching consequences for the physical development and well-being of new-born infants. It is this care, Bérubé is well aware, which enabled his young son to become what he is today. What is unthinkable, then, is to imagine a child with the capacities that Jamie has at the time that Bérubé is writing – the capacity to empathize with others, to interact with his parents and siblings – being institutionalized because medical diagnosis believes him incapable of these very qualities: What Bérubé describes with chilling clairvoyance is that the prognosis becomes a self-fulfilling prophecy: The child whom medical practice pronounces to be a "vegetable" becomes a "vegetable" (60) only because of this prognosis. As Bérubé puts it,

> It is entirely possible when prospective parents learn . . . that their child will be born with Down Syndrome, they will interpret this as an objective discontinuity. If they are told by their physician that their child will never learn and never have a meaningful thought, then they are all the more likely to make a decision based on 'probabilities': *Yesterday we thought we were having a "normal" child; today we learn she will be a vegetable.* (60; emphasis original)

Had Jamie been institutionalized, his mother-in-law reminds Bérubé matter-of-factly, he would not have become Jamie: "'Well, Michael, if he were taking up every day in a state mental hospital, he wouldn't *be* this little guy'" (Bérubé 33; emphasis original). What is behind this sober statement, I believe, is an entire iceberg of social choices: a reminder of the lives which were abandoned, destroyed and made unlivable by a medical advice *not* founded on life writing research but on a strikingly improvised mixture of hear-say and conjecture. Even more crucially, if indeed life writing research is to be integrated into medical decision-making, it needs to be taken much more seriously by all medical practitioners, not only by parents who, like Bérubé, have taken on the task of refuting medical prediction. Just as today, medical training includes training future physicians in how to communicate a diagnosis, much is to be gained from training them to integrate into their everyday practice the findings of life writing research. What all these narratives ask – Bérubé's account of his son Jamie, Adams's memoir of the first three years of raising Henry, and Kingsley and Levitz's account of growing up with Down Syndrome – is whether or not the doctors who once counseled parents of a child with Down Syndrome had done their math: Whether indeed they found it necessary to ground this advice not on hear-say (as Adams's obstetrician casually informs her, a girl with Down Syndrome lived down the street from her own house), but on life writing research. In any question located within the realm of medical diagnosis, a doctor not familiar with a given symptom would be quick to read the relevant literature; what happens, however, with information related to the lives made possible or impossible by a certain condition? Where would the physician read up on such questions, questions which are as central to medical practice as is biomedical information? It is here, I believe, that the practice of narrative medicine is related but not entirely synonymous with life writing research. What narrative medicine does is to urge doctors and medical practitioners to reflect on their everyday practices, and through such reflection, to produce their own life-narratives. Moreover, doctors are asked to take seriously, and to engage with, patient narratives as a form of life writing. What, however, if life writing research as a scientific practice were integrated into this approach? If the "medical" literature which doctors had to consult for each case they are being presented with included life writing texts and life writing textbooks? And if it included them as *medical* literature?

What emerges in Bérubé's description of the lives of countless parents who trusted their doctors' advice and had their children institutionalized, is a vicious cycle of medical diagnosis, medical prediction and the politics of institutionalization: In this logic, medical prediction held that children with Down Syndrome would not be able to learn; because they were then sent to live in institutions, however, they were unable to develop to the fullest of their possibilities and capabilities, thus seemingly ending up confirming the physician's prediction.

What is even more chilling in this respect, I believe, is that Bérubé's account indicates that in doctor's – uninformed – suggestion that a child born with Down Syndrome should be "institutionalized," there is also a measure of life writing involved, if one entirely based on hear-say, conjecture and misinformation: As outlined above, the most decisive argument which doctors historically used as "evidence" for their advice of institutionalization is the idea that a child born with Down Syndrome would never grow up to be able to recognize his or her own parents. This, too, could be said to be a form of life writing, if only in the sense that it is writing out a life deemed possible for persons with Down Syndrome. Nonetheless, what is crucial to note here is that an advice is given through explicit reference to the writing – the unfolding – of a given life; the advice here is not medical – as it would be in references to physical impairments or the ability to speak – but it is something much more fundamental: the ability of a child to interact with its parents. What is striking here, I believe, is that the doctor's reference is not simply to the child's mental impairment – the mental inability of the child to recognize its parents – but the way in which this inability is framed. This, I believe, is where medical advice is based on the writing of a life as an impossible one, a life which is not seen to be a life "proper": Even more devastatingly, the prediction is self-serving here because the parents – trusting medical advice because of its socially acknowledged ability to predict the future course of a given life – condemn their child to the state of a "vegetable" by believing the doctor's advice that the child is born in a "vegetable" state to begin with. The diagnosis becomes its own prophecy. Yet, even more significant for my purposes here, this vicious cycle is based on a piece of advice which is itself taken from the realm of life writing, if only in the sense of the doctor's writing *out* a life. The point to be made here, then, is that medicine may never be as free from or independent of life writing even where life writing never explicitly enters the picture. In the instances cited by Bérubé where parents committed their children to institutions, the doctors' advice was often predicated on off-hand references to lives they had witnessed second-hand; yet, tragically, there were no alternative life writing texts available to these parents.

It is far from accidental, then, that the metaphor of being a "vegetable" should return in many of these narratives, from the documentary about Tito Mukhopadhyay's life to the account by Emily Perl Kingsley of the first year of Jason Kingsley's life. What emerges, moreover, is a continuity of knowledge production through the intertextual connections between life writing narratives. From the moment his own son Jamie was born, Michael Bérubé writes, he was confident that Jamie would not grow up to be a "vegetable" because Emily Perl Kingsley had once refused to heed her doctor's advice. Bérubé quotes a memorable passage from Emily Perl Kingsley's narrative:

> In the interest of having maximum stimulation and color and input, we tore down the old, bland, pastel-colored wallpaper we had originally chosen and replaced it with wallpaper that had huge, brilliant, red and purple flowers. I kept saying to him, over and over, 'See the flower, see the flower.' Frankly, I didn't know what else to say. Then one day, when he was about four months old, I said, again, 'See the flower,' and he turned and put his little hand right in the middle of a big red flower. . . . In any case, I went crazy. I jumped up and down and I started to cry and I ran to the phone and I called up Charles and I said, 'This kid can learn! There's something in there! This is not a vegetable!' And that was the first day that, emotionally, I made a commitment to my own child. Up to that point, I was going through the motions. . . . But that was the day when I started to recognize that perhaps my son was a human being. Perhaps he was a person and an individual. (138-39)

It is in this sense that Rachel Adams's remark that when faced with the challenge of deciding on future life plans for her son, her "road map" was Bérubé's *Life As We Know It*, is much more than a remark; it may be central to discussions of the status and relevance of life writing research for decision-making in between biomedicine and social practice. What is at stake in calling for the integration of life writing research into biomedical decision-making, then, is that decisions are not made solely on the basis of medical prognosis, but on the basis of the lives which have already unfolded from such decisions. This idea is related to but not synonymous with the idea that medical practice should also be informed by the social understanding of medical science, the notion that the medical and the social are always-already interrelated. Rather, it is to say that the experts which need to be heard in order for an informed decision to be possible are the persons who have experienced the consequences of said decision. Crucially, as both Kingsley/Levitz and Bérubé argue, medical progress has now, for the first time in human history, enabled these subjects to make their voices heard, and to intervene into discussions about the quality of life of persons with Down Syndrome.

It is in this context, also, that the phrase which Bérubé chooses as the title for his book – "life as we know it" – may be especially significant.

The point is precisely that in the era of biomedicine, life may no longer be as we know it; and life may unfold – or be reshaped – in ways more complex than ever before. This, then, is the challenge posed to all parties involved – to parents of children with impairments, but also to doctors who now have to counsel these parents on how to deal with such impairments. The credo and call to arms which is at the core of Bérubé's book is our ability to deal with, and to cope all its complexity, the idea that life may not quite be as we know it. It is here that the doctor's lack of knowledge may emerge all the more visibly: When faced with a life which may unfold not quite the way "we" know it, what will our prediction, what will our prognosis be? At the same time, as Bérubé makes clear, it would be short-sighted to argue that such a challenge to the question once asked by Erwin Schrödinger, "What is life?" (x) arises only from those lives which are altered by disabilities or impairments. Rather, the point which Bérubé makes is that such contingency may be true of all lives, and we may hence ask the same questions at a much more fundamental level. It is for this reason that in this study, I have chosen to discuss life writing narratives from a wide variety of arenas. What may be at stake here, then, may be the continuities rather than discontinuities between narratives of autism, of Down Syndrome, of Parkinson's Disease, or simply of the way in which the body is transformed through processes of aging. All these narratives point not so much at the contingency arising from a particular condition – a genetic condition, an age-related disease – but the contingency of all human life. If indeed the idea of "life writing" is taken seriously with regard to these very different narratives, what is at stake is the unfolding of a life in the act of narration. It is in this sense that autobiography always-already converges with philosophy.

In the best scenario imaginable, then, life writing cannot only resist the predictions of the life sciences which had emerged without taking life writing into account, but life writing will be able to change the predictions pronounced by the life sciences. Eventually, Jason Kingsley, who the obstetrician had said "would never amount to anything," would write a book, a book about his own life and his friendship with Mitchell Levitz. This, then, is his conclusion: "'I'm glad that we didn't listen to the obstetrician. If we tell the obstetrician about this [our book], he will responded differently to all other families with a baby with a disability . . . . And then he will be a better doctor" (qtd. in Bérubé 32). It is this hope which encapsulates the relevance of life writing, and its use in medical education. What if, Rachel Adams, Michael Bérubé, Jason Kingsley and Mitchell Levitz ask, the reading of life writing were made mandatory in medical education? This, I believe, is more than the call for the inclusion of medical humanities into the curricula of medical schools; it is the idea that life writing can also be seen, and must serve, as a form of life science. As the authors suggest in *Raising Henry*, *Life As We Know It*, and *Count Us In*, the meaning of life, its quality and success, far beyond the economic implications of this latter concept, can only be defined through a dialogue between life sciences and life writing.

What emerges in these texts, then, is not only a network of narratives, but also a network of knowledge production. Each of the texts discussed in this chapter is the "road map" (Adams ix) to the others; what is at stake, however, is much more than mere intertextuality. Rather, what emerges from these forms of authorship and co-authorship is a sense of solidarity, across and beyond disability. In Nussbaum's call for a world in which her nephew Arthur can benefit from the full rights of citizenship, she includes a reference to Jamie Bérubé: "Jamie Bérubé loves B.B. King, Bob Marley, and the Beatles. He can imitate a waiter bringing all his favorite foods, and he has a sly sense of verbal humor" (*Frontiers of Justice* 97). The point made in both Nussbaum's *Frontiers of Justice* and Michael Bérubé's *Life As We Know It*, then, is not only that in terms of social access and political participation, our theories of justice may still have a long way to go; it is also that they imagine and co-author the lives that may eventually be possible for Arthur and Jamie. What these writers do, then, is much more than to establish a link between autism and Down Syndrome, and to note that both need to be seen not in terms of a "disability" that can easily be defined, but in terms of a continuum. While the notion of such a continuum has long been acknowledged with regard to the autism spectrum, Bérubé proposes that it can also be applied to persons with Down Syndrome. In his epilogue, Bérubé refers to a review of one of his early articles about Jamie by Steven Pinker. Pinker writes, "'I take the point of Bérubé's essay to be that there is a greater range of functioning among Down Syndrome children than most people think and that, for both ethical and practical reasons, every Down's child ought to be treated as if he or she were in the upper part of the range'" (qtd. in Bérubé 252). Ironically, Pinker's disagreement with Bérubé's article is not so much about the "spectrum" of disability when it comes to living with Down Syndrome, but about the use of language; Pinker implicitly opposes Bérubé's claim that it makes all the difference in the world whether children like Jamie are referred to as "retarded" or "delayed." The same may be said, of course, of Pinkerton's use of phrases like "Down's child," in which the child comes to be defined – first linguistically and then conceptually – through his genetic disposition.

What is at the core of Bérubé's narrative, then, is the advocacy by a father of his son, just as Martha Nussbaum, in *Frontiers of Justice*, speaks of and for her nephew Arthur. At the same time, the juncture which virtually all of these narratives are concerned with, then, is the journey from co-authorship to authorship: Rachel Adams and Michael Bérubé both gesture towards a time when Henry and Jamie will be able to write their own narratives, to author the narratives of their own lives. Bérubé ends his book about Jamie with the following words: "My job, for now, is to represent my son, to set his place at our collective table. But I know I am merely trying my best to prepare for the day he sets his own place. For I have no sweeter dream than to imagine – aesthetically and ethically and parentally – that Jamie will someday be his own advocate, his own author, his own best representative" (264). In this context, it is all the more remarkable that *Count Us In* should end with a reference to precisely such authorship, such self-advocacy and self-representation. As Mitchell Levitz notes in the postscript, "I did some writing, too, including chapters in two books on disability and human rights" (Kingsley and Levitz 192). At the beginning of the twenty-first century, then, these debates, in both *Count Us In* and *Frontiers of Justice*, are deeply interconnected: What, both studies ask, does it mean to be "human," and what is our definition of humanity which precedes the bestowal of citizenship?

In this chapter, I have read a life writing text through two forms of citizenship discourse. First, I have used the model of "genetic citizenship" described by sociologist Paul Rabinow in order to discuss a specific form of community building or *Vergemeinschaftung*, which can also be said to be at the heart of *Count Us In*. What emerges in this reading, I believe, is an interdisciplinary dialogue between discourses from biomedicine, models created by medical sociology, and life writing research. I have thus been interested in the ways in which a life writing narrative may circulate in a wider terrain, the ways in which it can be included in studies of genetic citizenship, for instance. At the same time, I have argued that in addition to this model of genetic citizenship, *Count Us In* may also be in explicit dialogue with notions of citizenship as "civic fitness." It is in this sense that a double bind may ensue which I have also traced in the work of Temple Grandin in Chapter 4. Even as Kingsley and Levitz may prove their full humanity – and hence the right to full citizenship – by proving their civic fitness with regard to political opinion or sexual morality, they may in fact reinforce notions of civic normalcy and normativity. Seen from this perspective, *Count Us In* may serve as a citizenship test which leaves the parameters of normative understandings of citizenship intact. Finally, the idea of social usefulness and of the compatibility of the disabled subject with normative assumptions of what makes a productive citizen, is ultimately reinscribed by this form of life writing as proof of civic fitness.

Up to this chapter, then, my study has been concerned with forms of individual life writing. Even as *Count Us In* is, of course, a collaborative, co-authored form of autobiography, its emphasis is ultimately on the rights of the individual. It calls for the inclusion of persons living with Down Syndrome by proving their sameness in the terms of the dominant discourse, and thus their full humanity. This discourse of individuality, in turn, is embedded into a notion of genetic citizenship, the idea that full access to citizenship rights must not be denied to persons and communities with genetic difference. Yet, as in the case of Temple Grandin, *Count Us In* ultimately fails to address the privileged position of their authors. Growing up in a Jewish middle-class community, both Jason Kingsley and Mitchell Levitz had access not only to highly efficient medical care, but also to an excellent education. Such possibilities of living up to their full potential, however, may not be available to those who are disenfranchised not only on account of their genetic difference, but also in terms of race, class, or gender.

In their attention to patient narratives, medical humanities, then, may have been centered on the concept of individuality. It is this scope of inquiry that the following chapters seek to interrogate and to broaden. The next chapter will be concerned with collective forms of life writing, as well as with the ways in which social, political and geopolitical disenfranchisement can lead to instances of medical discrimination and the denial, to entire communities and even nations, of the right to health and well-being.

8 *Blue Hawaii*? Adam Horowitz's Film *Nuclear Savage* and Collective Life Writing in the Pacific

The preceding chapters have focused on different forms of life writing, and the inclusion of life writing – as illness narrative or as aging narrative – into the field of medical humanities. These forms of life writing, it must be noted, concerned the writing of individual lives; the coming to terms, through the very aesthetic of a life writing narrative, written or otherwise, to an existential experience of human life such as aging or illness. The following chapters of this study will be concerned with collective forms of life writing.[1] What happens, in other words, if the writing of an individual life is inseparable from the writing of collective lives? How is the framework, how are the parameters of "life writing" as a concept altered in this process of collectivity? "Life writing," then, can be seen not only in the literal sense of writing a life but also as writing down, or rewriting, the answer to the question of what it means to be "human" at a given moment in time. It is in this sense, I believe, that the reach of medical humanities may be substantially broadened to encompass different definitions of the human, definitions which have been shaped, in part, by medical practice. This shift towards both collective forms of life writing and narratives which draw attention to instances of racial and cultural discrimination, moreover, sets out to engage what Thomas Couser has seen as a potential bias in life writing. He writes, "As it happens, those who produce narratives of illness and disability are not diverse in terms of race and class. They tend to be white and middle

[1] In a different version, the ideas addressed in this chapter were published in the volume *Border Stories: Narratives of Peace, Conflict and Communication in the 20th and 21st Centuries*, ed. by Beate Greisel et. al. (2017). I am grateful to Senta Sanders for inviting me to the conference which preceded this volume, and for her suggestions, which went into the reshaping of this chapter.

class. Before they became ill or impaired, many were already professional writers or worked in professions where writing was part of the job" (Couser, *Vulnerable Bodies* 4). With Couser's caveat in mind, I will be concerned in this second part of my study with bodies which are indeed different both in terms of race, class, and social and geographical location. Moreover, my plea is for extending the corpus of life writing beyond written autobiographies, focusing on life writing narratives as they are embedded, for instance, in documentaries or feature films.

The chapters in the last part of this book thus engage the nexus between life sciences and life writing from a perspective which differs from that of the previous chapters: What is at stake in the chapters that follow is the embeddedness of medical practices not only in a historical, but also in a political and an ideological context. By exploring what Alondra Nelson has called "medical discrimination" (xi), as it has affected not only African Americans in the U.S. but also indigenous communities across the globe, I want to investigate the ways in which life writing as a cultural, but also a political practice can be seen as a way of performing justice in the face of such "medical discrimination" (Nelson xi). If for the illnesses or medical conditions discussed in the preceding chapters, no one could be held responsible, such responsibility is strikingly different for those medical conditions which were brought about or exacerbated by political regimes under specific historical conditions. The "cases" I will discuss in the following chapter – the nuclear holocaust in the Pacific and the musealization of indigenous remains in Western museums – engage with the concept of life writing in one fundamental sense: They address the question of which lives, which bodies are defined as "human" in the first place. Once a given body is defined as sub-human, as human of a different order, I will argue with regard to the "nuclear pacific"[2] and the politics of musealizing indigenous bodies, medical and museal practice can justify what would otherwise be unjustifiable. Life writing, on the other hand, can be seen as an antidote to the writing out of lives by museal and by medical practice. Moreover, I am interested in why these "cases" of medical practice having gone ethically awry have not traditionally been considered within the frame-

[2] For a discussion of the concept of the "nuclear Pacific," see, for instance, Elizabeth DeLoughrey, "The Myth of Isolates."

work of medical humanities. Making a case for the inclusion of these cases and these questions within medical humanities, I want to argue that their recontextualization may make us wonder not just about the reach of medicine in reshaping human lives but also about medical definitions of the human. Conversely, to the extent that we exclude these narratives from the realm of medical humanities, arguing instead that they refer more to questions of indigenous rights or environmental justice, we may risk perpetuating the racialist practices that gave rights to these severe human rights violations in the first place.

What is at stake, then, is precisely the link between what Thomas Couser has called "vulnerable subjects" (*Vulnerable Subjects* xii) and what Alondra Nelson terms "vulnerable communities" (x). It could be argued that by focusing on the relevance of patient narratives in the didactics of medicine, laudable as this practice may have been, medical humanities have run the risk of neglecting the communal dimension of illness. This communal dimension, in turn, can be brought about by already existing inequalities – in quite another sense of pre-existing conditions – being translated into inequalities of health. These inequalities, as Alondra Nelson has argued in her groundbreaking study, *Body and Soul: The Black Panther Party and the Fight against Medical Discrimination* (2011), can take two forms in particular. First, they may be seen in an unequal access to health care and, at their worst, lead to "medical apartheid" (Nelson xi). Second, such inequalities can lead to a suspension of human rights and medical ethics when it comes to racialized communities within or outside the U.S.. At the core of a discussion of "medical discrimination," then, needs to be the question of "what lives [are] valued," as Nelson puts it (x), and, I would add for my purposes here, what lives are valued as human lives to begin with. It was the translation of social prejudice into medical practice, Nelson argues, that made possible, for instance, the Tuskegee experiments: "Questionable scientific practices conducted with vulnerable communities that have recently come to light make evident this register of health politics. In 2010 the historian Susan Reverby uncovered the deliberate infection of Guatemalan men and women with syphilis in the late 1940s by a U.S. researcher who was also involved with a notorious study of the disease in Tuskegee, Alabama, that began in the 1930s" (x). The term "medical apartheid," coined by Harriet Washington and cited by Nelson, may be especially significant here since it denotes the relationship between the

(Western) scientist and a subject who is seen as racially inferior to this scientist and is hence powerless to combat the scientist's definition of his or her subjectivity. Nelson speaks of the "vexed, uneven encounters between agents and racialized subjects of biomedicine" which constitute "medical apartheid" (xi). What is crucial for my purposes here is the intersection between a politics of racialization – the dehumanizing or erasure of indigenous subjects as human subjects or, as I will put it here, as humans of a different order – and a subsequent exposure of these racialized subjects to medical experiments which would otherwise have been impossible to conduct on human beings. It is hence crucial to note that Nelson should explicitly link the practice of U.S. scientists in Guatemala and within the U.S. (in Tuskegee). Thus, what is at stake is the pernicious link between an imperial or neo-imperialist politics and what may be termed a politics of internal colonialization.

The next three chapters will also be concerned with a dialogue between life writing and life sciences especially in the context of trauma research. Yet, here again there is a sense in which the individual perspective may be pitted against the communal perspective through the discourse of biomedicine. As I will try to show as this chapter progresses, the discourse of trauma, as it is conveyed through life writing narratives,[3] may lead to the recognition, by the state or the court, that an injustice has been committed; yet, this trauma may be seen as affecting this individual as an individual, not as a member of a community that is already racialized within the social fabric. As Alondra Nelson has argued, it is hence imperative that we link the individualist perspective – the solace of new developments in biomedicine as a cure for an individual's illness or trauma – to a perception of illness or trauma as it may affect an entire community. This illness or trauma, what is more, may result from the fact that this community was subjected to certain biomedical practices only because it was a "racialized" community to begin with. It is in this sense, then, that Nelson cautions against the universalist implications of a discourse on the progress of biomedicine. She writes,

[3] This is an idea which I will discuss in more detail in the next chapter.

> Milestones in health and medicine are conveyed as bearing on the broadest political and social ideals. The recent tenth anniversary of the decoding of the human genome, for example, brought with it the cautious hope for the progression of genetic science from the lab bench to the bedside. This scientific landmark was notably accompanied by then president Bill Clinton's proclamation that this feat had established "our common humanity." (Nelson ix)

As I will try to prove in this chapter, drawing on Adam Horowitz's documentary film *Nuclear Savage*, medical experiments that were conducted for the benefit of "our common humanity" could be conducted only at the expense of lives whose human rights were suspended. While the "event" of nuclear testing in the Pacific has widely been publicized, I am interested in the rationales, within and outside the practice of biomedicine that made this event possible. Moreover, I am interested in the ways in which these rationales can be countered, and in which indigenous or minority communities may provide evidence that may eventually lead to the indictment of the powers or authorities that made such medical experiments possible. Thus, as Nelson argues, what is at stake is not a dismissal of biomedicine as a practice, but a careful scrutinizing in the inequalities of power which may be embedded in this practice. As Nelson goes on to argue through the example of the Black Panther Party's fight against medical racism, "In doing so [trying to shift the power in medicine], these communities did not assert a blanket rejection of medicine. Rather, they laid claim to a critical conception of healthfulness: a right to health equality and freedom from medical discrimination" (xi-xii).

As the historical precedents of the Marshall Islands and the musealization of native remains forcefully illustrate, medical practices do not arise from a void; rather, medical practices, far from being supracultural, may in fact be deeply bound up in the cultural and racial prejudices of their time. It is the time-boundedness as well as the culture-boundedness of medical practice that the following chapters will explore, by focusing on the ways in which indigenous lives have been instrumentalized by specific practices in the life sciences. In this context, my plea is for broadening the scope of medical humanities, and for broadening the scope of life writing. Life writing research and medical humanities, it can be argued, have focused on individual experience rather than the writing of collective lives. Such a focus may in turn contain a certain Eurocentric premise. The concept of "medical discrimination" (Nelson xi), on the other hand, may be seen as a way out of the dichotomy between the individual and the collective: Medical discrimination, as Nelson makes clear, would encompass both the individual dimension and the individual experience of medical discrimination, as well as the collective perspective on questions such as illness or trauma.

What if, I would like to ask in this chapter, the trauma of what has been called the "nuclear pacific" were to be included into the field of medical humanities? In this context, the field of the "history of medicine" would appear in an altogether different light. If in the previous chapters, I have tried to address the question of how changes in medical diagnoses and in medical definitions of certain conditions affected the lives of individuals (persons with Down Syndrome, as Michael Bérubé reminds us, would still have been institutionalized in the twentieth century), the next two chapters will look at the ways in which medical history, the emergence of new fields within medical and life science research such as radiology – were deeply intertwined with the violation of the rights of certain groups. What is the ethical legacy, in other words, of the emergence of these new fields of life science research, and what are the lives that made this research possible, lives which were seen as "expendable" in the progress of medical science? It is this question, then, that Adam Horowitz's 2011 film *Nuclear Savage* can be said to ask.

What are the borders of our postcolonial world, if it is in fact a postcolonial world? What are the conflicts, and what are the settings for this conflict? In this chapter, I would like to argue that *Nuclear Savage* by Jewish American filmmaker Adam Horowitz – which can be said to argue that our world is neither quite postcolonial nor its national borders – the borders of the postcolonial nation-state – can be said to be clearly defined. In this context of both fuzzy postcoloniality and even fuzzier borders, Horowitz asks us a question which is ultimately unanswerable: if you want to make a film about an event so horrific that it defies the power of our imagination, what genre would you use? And if you were to make a documentary film, what if no one were to believe you that this event really took place?

Horowitz's film states a case, and it indicts the U.S. for what he calls crimes against humanity which are so horrendous that they could not possibly have been committed by a democratic nation. In 1953, the U.S.

government conducted a series of nuclear tests on an atoll in the Pacific which came to be known as the Bikini Atoll. In what ensued, government scientists proceeded to study and measure the impact of radiation and nuclear fallout on human bodies and human lives, bodies which happened to be those of what government rhetorics at the time tellingly called "savages." It is for this very reason, the genealogy of calling indigenous peoples "savages" and of going on to subject them to a nuclear holocaust, that Horowitz's film establishes a connection between the practice of nuclear testing and those on whom such testing was conducted: It is this juxtaposition which gives the film its title, *Nuclear Savage*. The ethics and the legal maneuverings which would ensue from this series of nuclear testing hinged on two questions in particular: First, whether the exposure of human bodies to radiation had been deliberate; and second whether or not it mattered that the bodies which had been exposed to radiation happened to be indigenous bodies.

As Horowitz's 2011 documentary film makes clear, it was because of the delicacy of such questions that the government documents describing the so-called "Project 4.1," the study of the effects of radiation on human lives, came to be classified and would not be unsealed until decades later. When they were unsealed, their content was so toxic for the concept of Western democracy that they have since circulated, or rather, failed to circulate in a curious void: The full extent of the horrors of Project 4.1 has not yet been addressed, and has not been made fully public.

8.1 Precarious Lives and States of Emergency

How then, could nuclear testing in the Pacific have taken place? How could it have been compatible with the idea of American democracy? It is in this context that I would like to focus on the work of Judith Butler and the concept of what she calls "precarious lives." As Butler writes in the preface, "The five essays here were all written after September 11, 2001, and in response to the conditions of *heightened vulnerability* and aggression that followed from those events" (*Precarious Life* xiii; emphasis added). In both *Precarious Life: The Powers of Mourning and Violence* (2004) and *Frames of War: When is Life Grievable?* (2009), Butler creates the concept in the wake of 9/11 and a state of emergency in which the torture of "Arab" bodies was held to be constitutional, also since it occurred on territory which was itself curiously extraterritorial, outside and at the same time at the mercy of U.S. legislation. As Butler goes on to say,

> I also consider . . . how certain forms of grief become nationally recognized and amplified, whereas other losses become unthinkable and ungrievable. . . . Some lives are grievable, and others are not; the differential allocation of grievability that decides what kind of subject is and must be grieved, and which kind of subject must not, operates to produce and maintain certain exclusionary conceptions of who is normatively human: what counts as a livable life and a grievable death? (*Precarious Life* xiv-xv)

I believe that Butler's reading of the precariousness of some lives over others can also be applied to a wide variety of other contexts as well. When and under what circumstances, Butler asks, can lives become precarious? In the context which Butler investigates, one form of precariousness gives rise to another: Because in the wake of the terrorist attacks, the U.S. American nation had been reminded of the precariousness, the vulnerability of American lives, it proceeded to retaliate against "Other" bodies whom it believed to be potential perpetrators of the violence from which this vulnerability had arisen in the first place. The sense of the vulnerability of one's own life thus gave rise to violence, defined as *necessary* violence, in order to end the state of precariousness. Butler writes, "And though for some, mourning can only be resolved through violence, it seems clear that violence only brings on more loss, and the failure to heed the claim of precarious life only leads, again and again, to the dry grief of an endless political rage" (*Precarious Life* xix). It was this determination to see one's precariousness not as the rule but the exception in Western lives – a privilege which, Butler makes clear, was itself born of a historical location and was itself a form of privilege –,[4] which led U.S. legislature to define Arab bodies as humans

[4] As Butler goes on to note, "the dislocation from First World privilege, however temporary, offers a chance to start to imagine a world in which that violence might be minimized, in which an inevitable interdependency becomes acknowledged as the basis for global political community" (*Precarious Life* xii-xiii).

of a different order. This, Butler writes, gave rise to a change in the politics of mourning: Because those lives who were of a lesser humanity, a humanity of a different order, the atrocities and losses which affected them did not quite have to register to the same degree; the loss of these lives, Butler reminds us, did not quite have to be mourned.

The conclusion which Butler draws from a historical moment in which some lives were considered precarious while others were not, is that we can only end it by realizing that there must never be a difference between lives that we can mourn and those we cannot. In both *Precarious Life* and in *Frames of War*, then, Butler describes states of emergency; states and conditions under which it was curiously permitted to suspend some human rights in the service of a larger good. It is such a state of emergency, too, which Adam Horowitz's film chronicles: The Cold War, his film argues, was a perpetual state of emergency; Americans lived in fear of the Soviet Union dropping an atomic bomb on the American nation. It was this fear, then, which reminded Americans of the "precariousness," the vulnerability of their lives. This vulnerability, then, led to a state of exception, as it did in the wake of the attacks of 9/11 described in Butler's studies. Given this state of emergency, what was permissible in the study of human lives? It was in this context of a suspension of some legal rights and some human rights – or rather, the suspension of some rights which were not quite said to be human – that Pacific Islanders were seen as surrogates of the American lives threatened by what was seen as an impending nuclear threat by the Soviets. U.S. life scientists at the height of the Cold War needed to come to terms with the state of this precariousness: What, in this scenario of speculation, would happen to human beings if indeed they were exposed to nuclear radiation? Cynically, Horowitz's film makes clear, the precedents of two atomic bombs dropped by the U.S. on Nagasaki and Hiroshima provided some evidence of the effects of nuclear fall-out, but more testing seemed to be necessary. What if the U.S. were to conduct some tests of its own? It was thus that Project 4.1 was born, a study of the effects of nuclear radiation which was originally meant to be conducted on mice. Yet, the life scientists were quick to conjecture that studying mice was never quite the same as studying humans; and thus the framework of Project 4.1 curiously shifted from mice to men. Where, however, could such effects of nuclear fall-out on humans legitimately be tested? The Marshall Islands seemed a fitting location for such human testing; they had been under U.S. jurisdiction since World War II, and they were only somewhat inhabited.

In order for nuclear testing on human beings to be both ethically and legally permissible, then, I would argue with Horowitz that they would have had to have what I would call a "humanity of a different order," a state of not quite being fully human. What are the discourses, however, which set the grounds for this humanity of a different order? What cultural imaginaries was Project 4.1 indebted to, what cultural imaginaries accounted for the curious and curiously unethical shift from mice to men? Horowitz lays the groundwork for what will in fact be an ethical and an aesthetic indictment of U.S. government politics in the Pacific by creating a link between two interconnected trajectories: First, he revokes the politics of what I would call the Pacific Pastoral, and second, he invokes what Native American critic Gerald Vizenor has called the "myth of the vanishing Indian." According to Vizenor, the politics of conquest worked in insidious ways in U.S. history: Because the settlers needed the land for the expansion of what John O'Sullivan in 1845 called the "yearly multiplying millions," Native civilizations were bound for extinction: Each native was doomed to vanish, to be superseded by the superiority of "Western" civilization. The insidiousness of this logic, I would like to argue in this chapter, is that the myth of the vanishing Indian is a global one: From the U.S. to Australia and the South Seas, the conquest of native lands – and the subjugation of Native peoples – was justified through the alleged inferiority of "savage" communities and civilizations. This inferiority, Horowitz's film argues, made possible the nuclear horror in the South Pacific.

8.2 The Myth of the Vanishing Indian and the Terra Nullius Doctrine

Horowitz's first culprit in the allegation of the atemporality or anteriority of the indigenous communities of the South Seas is none other than Paul Gauguin who went to Tahiti to paint naked savages, especially naked savage women, as in his 1902 painting, "The Offering." Yet, like the ethnographer Malinowski before him who had gone to the Trobriand

and admired the native women,[5] Gauguin saw only what he wanted to see: The women's nakedness reflected the painter's wish that they were not, as Butler puts it in another context, of his time, but of another time, a time well before his own, well before the onset of both modernity and alienation. As Butler writes, "it is argued that [the Other] is not of our time, but of another time" (*Precarious Life* xx). And yet, in order for this asynchronicity to be achieved, an act of staging was necessary: quite simply, the women had to be made by the painter to take their clothes off, since for the models to be fully clothed would reveal, not only to the painter but also to his audience, that they were actually of his time, and the time of his audience. The asynchronicity between the primitive and the painter, then, is the wishful thinking of a Western civilization alienated from itself. It is for this very reason that Adam Horowitz, the filmmaker, starts his documentary film with what is in fact a global mapping of indigeneity:

> [voiceover by Adam Horowitz] I had always dreamed of the South Pacific. I had read stories like *Robinson Crusoe, Moby Dick,* and *Mutiny on the Bounty.* Classic stories about white Europeans, who, by getting lost in the South Seas, had learned something about themselves and the world from which they came. My love affair with the Pacific began as a child with art and books and with movies and television. I had bought into the classic myth about the white man in the tropics, bringing progress and civilization. I wanted to live in the exotic postmodern world of *Hawaii Five-O.* Or better yet, to go back in time to follow in the footstep of Captain Cook or at least, the Captain Cook I had seen in the movies. I wanted to be Fletcher Christian. Actually, I wanted to be Clark Gable as

[5] Subsequent research, especially based on Malinowski's diaries, showed that scientific "interest" and sexual desire converged in the case of the seemingly disinterested ethnographic observer. While Malinowski pioneered the method of "participant observation," his work is thus far from uncontroversial. Rather, the diaries, published by his widow after his death, revealed the personal implication of the ethnographer into his observations. The publication of Malinowski's diaries were called a "minor scandal" by James Clifford, who subsequently stressed the necessity of including the ethnographer's subjectivity into his work and of making his or her location visible rather than concealing it, as Malinowski had done. See Clifford, "On Ethnographic Authority."

> Fletcher Christian. But the World I found in the Marshall Islands was not some fantasy Garden of Eden. It was a paradise lost, a paradise turned upside-down. (*Nuclear Savage*)

What then, is the connection between Paul Gauguin and the "myth of the 'vanishing Indian'"?[6] In this context, the vanishing Indian has become a vanishing Pacific islander, or more accurately, a Marshallese. Cynically speaking, there is no ethical issue involved in conducting nuclear tests in the Pacific because the Marshall Islands are not quite inhabited. What then is the logic of this "not quite" of human habitation? It is here that the idea of the naked savages painted by Paul Gauguin and the idea of the vanishing doctrine takes us directly to the so-called terra nullius doctrine. What, then, does terra nullius mean?

In the myth of the "happy, amenable savage," a number of insidious doctrines converge, all of which insisted that indigenous peoples were not of "our" civilization either in terms of temporality nor of humanity. The infamous "terra nullius" doctrine had once held, as in Australian law, that indigenous populations were part of the flora and fauna of the newly discovered land, and hence were not, and perhaps would never be, fully human. I am thus deliberately refusing to think only in national terms, to argue that the "case" of terra nullius in Australia has nothing at all to do with nuclear testing in the Marshall Islands. Instead, I want to employ the perspective of what I would call "comparative indigenous studies" to argue that there may in fact be a trajectory that links the way in which Western governments thought about indigeneity. Looking at the Pacific triangle, I argue that there is a direct link between the doctrine of "terra nullius in Australia" and the idea that the Marshall Islands were not quite inhabited.

What, then, did "terra nullius" mean in Australia? As formulated by the Australian High Court in the Cooper v. Stuart decision (1889), it held that native population did not own the land they lived on and European settlers could hence take possession of this territory. The terra

[6] For a detailed discussion of this concept as it is used in Vizenor's work, see Lee (84).

nullius doctrine thus held that "indigenous peoples have no property rights."[7] As the online description of the Reconciliation Project puts it,

> What made the Doctrine of Discovery so devastating was the application of a related legal concept, the principle of terra nullius. Terra nullius is a legal theory, or more accurately a legal fiction (something which may not be true, but is assumed to be so in order to facilitate particular legal findings) which holds that 'discovered' lands were, or are, empty. As a result of this 'emptiness,' European powers asserted a unilateral right to simply take territories and resources within their jurisdictions. To put it another way, the legal fiction of terra nullius allowed European powers to simply assume that the underlying title to the entire territory belonged to those powers, rather than to the indigenous nations actually living there. (reconciliationproject n. pag.)

And what would terra nullius mean for the rights of the Aboriginal peoples of Australia? It meant, quite simply, that they would not be given human rights until a referendum changed the Australian Constitution in 1967. Crucially, struggles for Civil Rights legislation with regard to indigenous Australians were sparked off by the Warburton Ranges of 1957, which involved issues of malnutrition and the effects of nuclear testing in the desert.[8]

Without human rights, as Australian Noongah writer Kim Scott so powerfully argues in *True Country* (1993), "Aboriginals" could be shot

[7] See Watson 999 (n. 15 footnote). The concept of terra nullius is thus closely tied to the "theory of discovery." See also Dörr, "The Background of the Theory of Discovery."

[8] Struggles for civil rights also involved calls for a change in citizenship legislation, a debate in which the political activism of Albert Namatjira was crucial. At the time, all "full-blood" Aboriginals were regarded as wards of the state; because he was of mixed-race descent, however, Namatjira was an Australian citizen. The minute he associated with his indigenous kinsmen, however, this was seen as a suspicious act; sharing drink with them was defined as illegal and Namatjira was hence breaking the law. As I will argue in more detail in Chapter 9, laws can hence be read through life writing research and through the lives that these laws make possible, or impossible. For a detailed discussion of Namatjira's activism and the Warburton Ranges controversy, see National Museum Australia, "The Warburton Ranges Controversy."

like game, and they could be killed with impunity. Sadly enough, then, it is only a small step from a deer to a guinea pig, and it is not very far from Australia to Rongelap in the Marshall Islands.

8.3 The Pacific Pastoral and Visual Complicity

What, then, is the connection between terra nullius, the myth of the vanishing Indian, and the Pacific Pastoral? It is at this point that Horowitz, in his filmic version of what can in fact be seen as a court case indicting the U.S. government for crimes against humanity, calls his second witness after Paul Gauguin: Elvis Presley. How, then, is Elvis Presley complicit either in the myth of the vanishing Indian or the Pacific Pastoral? How, we may ask, could Elvis's dreamy eyes possibly be imperial? In what way would the happy image of Elvis Presley in a Hawaiian paradise be complicit with the logic of Manifest Destiny? Elvis's version of the Pacific, it could be argued, hinges on the actor's bare chest, which at the same time signifies his figure's casting off the garments of Western civilization. Thus we may want to address the image of nakedness first; like the happy "savages" who are his consorts, Elvis, the American gone native, has taken his shirt off. He, too, is (half) naked, and his color is (almost) that of the native. Once the film *Blue Hawaii* is over, however, Elvis will put his shirt back on; not so the natives. The choreography of many of the scenes featured in the film is also worth noting: The natives, of course, kneel at Elvis's feet, happily accompanying, through their own indigenous chorus, the sounds of Manifest Destiny and an imperial U.S. presence in the Pacific. Hawaii, of course, had become a state of the union only in 1959. For all its seeming innocence, then, there is a complicity both visual and cultural between the 1961 Elvis Presley film *Blue Hawaii* and the Pacific pastoral which, Horowitz's film argues, made nuclear testing in the Pacific possible.

The King's Polynesian adventure *in Blue Hawaii* is complicit, then, in creating and perpetuating the image of the Pacific pastoral. It is these Pacific pastoral aesthetics, then, which Horowitz both evokes and indicts in their complicity with the nuclear horror in the Pacific. The imagery of the pastoral, Horowitz argues, was itself the reason why nuclear testing in the Pacific became possible. For an imperialist gaze and the Manifest Destiny of Western science, the Pacific was imagined as a clean slate, a virgin territory to be imprinted by the narrative of Western progress, and the progress of Western science. It is this timelessness which the aesthetics of Horowitz's filmic narrative resurrects time and again in what is in fact an infinite loop of the key moment of the film: The detonation of Charlie Bravo, an atomic bomb a thousand times bigger than the atomic bomb which nine years earlier, had been dropped on Hiroshima. As the film is quick to add, Hiroshima was seen by government scientists as the first instance in which the effects of nuclear radiation on human subjects could in fact be "tested" in actuality. Through this cynical reasoning, Hiroshima could in fact be seen to become the first test in a series of nuclear testings which involved human subjects; subjects, however, who were curiously ascribed of what I would call a humanity of a different order.

It is here that in Horowitz's visual imagery, the Gothic postcolonial and the Pacific pastoral converge: The horror of the actual image – an atomic bomb exploding against the background of a landscape so beautiful that it can only seem paradoxical – becomes all the more blatant because the setting in which it takes place is so paradisiacal. To be sure, this is the postcolonial Gothic in disguise; it is Gothicism cloaked in images of aesthetic beauty. This, then, is the key moment in Horowitz's film: Even if our subconscious mind registers that what we see is not quite congruous, the aesthetics of the image in fact seem quite beautiful, as if this mushroom cloud was oddly in keeping with the landscape. To make matters worse, Horowitz deliberately underlays this scene of a mock-beautiful cloud in the Pacific with Polynesian music which evokes, not the horrors of nuclear testing but tourism in the Pacific. In this scene, it is almost as if Elvis's soothing music of the atemporality, the timelessness of the Pacific provides the soundtrack of the dropping of a bomb innocently called Charlie Bravo on a seemingly uninhabited Pacific atoll. As the film's voiceover puts it, "Over sixty years ago, an American Air Force bomber followed this exact route to begin a series of atmospheric nuclear tests, conceived with all of the hubris of the American Empire" (*Nuclear Savage*).

What *Nuclear Savage* makes clear is that the scenario of the Pacific pastoral managed, by a time-honored trick which had already been successfully performed in the U.S. itself, to make its inhabitants vanish. In both cases, the allegation of what Gerald Vizenor, in a U.S. indigenous context, has called the "vanishing Indian," however, was only the wishful thinking of an imperialist regime that described itself as democratic. For Western science on the path of nuclear testing, what marred the image of a white mushroom cloud against a clear Pacific sky was the image of the natives stubbornly dotting the landscape, testifying to the fact that these islands *were* in fact inhabited. What Horowitz makes clear, then, is that this stubborn fact of inhabitation, which in the U.S. had threatened to eclipse the very idea of discovery, could only be neutralized by a time-honored trick of imperialist/colonialist imagination: that of terra nullius. What if, white settlers asked not only in Australia but in the settler societies of the U.S., Canada and New Zealand as well, these lands were not quite inhabited? It is this "not quite" of Pacific inhabitation, Horowitz suggests, which makes the mushroom cloud in the Pacific possible. In order for the Pacific pastoral to work, then, terra nullius has to kick in just when the "natives" threaten to raise their heads and give the lie to the Western imperialist looking for yet another adventure in the make of Western progress, this time the progress of Western science through nuclear testing.

The horror which Horowitz's film drives home through the infinite loop and the hula music was that there were two kinds of audiences to this curious image of a mushroom cloud in the Pacific: There was the Western world and the Western scientist looking on at what they saw as a planned experiment; and there were the indigenous Marshall Islanders looking on at a spectacle which would concern them in ways more horrific than they could have ever imagined. No-one, Horowitz's film makes clear, should have witnessed the spectacle of the mushroom cloud at such a close range. The feat which the filmic narrative accomplishes, then, is that it reinserts the Marshall Islander into the picture as a spectator of a scene which he should never have been able to witness from such a close angle. It is this form of spectatorship, the spectatorship of the eye-witness, which contains all the horror of nuclear testing in the Pacific. Horowitz's film juxtaposes documentary footage from the U.S. government and his own filming of testimonials by survivors of the atomic tests who recall the day of nuclear testing:

> U.S. GOVERNMENT FILM: You have a grand stand seat here to one of the most momentous events in the history of science. In less than a minute, you will see the most powerful explosion ever witnessed by human eyes.

LIJON EKNILANG: Yes, I had a dream at the same time as the bright light. I was dreaming that I was in the middle of all the fire. Things fall down from the sky, and when they hit the ground, there was a fire and I was in the middle of all the fire and I never seen anyone and I tried to call everybody but nobody showed up. I become more scared in my dream and when I wake up, I see the light so bright. I was more scared than ever.

U.S. GOVERNMENT FILM: The problem this time is especially occult because this entire area, the Pacific, is subject to radiological fallout. And this area is inhabited by some 20,000 people.

JOHN ANJAIN [*in his native language, translated through subtitles*]: There was a gigantic noise, and a huge gust of wind from the bomb. The wind was very, very hot. It was hotter than fire.

MARSHALLESE WOMAN [*translated from the Marshallese in subtitles*]: The fallout was white powder that burned our skin.

ROKKO LANGINBELIK [*translated in subtitles*]: Our hair started falling out and we all got very sick.

MARSHALLESE WOMAN [*translated in subtitles*]: We were all throwing up like a very bad flu.

ROKKO LANGINBELIK [*translated in subtitles*]: We heard there was weatherman nearby us on Rongerik who told them not to drop the bomb because the wind was blowing this way. They knew what they were doing. They dropped the bomb anyway. They wanted to find out what would happen to us from the bomb. They used us as human experiments.

U.S. GOVERNMENT FILM: As you can imagine, sentiment is running pretty high about now and there is reason for it. If everything goes according to plan, we'll soon see the largest explosion ever set off on the face of the earth.

JEBAN RIKLON [*translated in subtitles*]: Burnt skin peeling off people. Nausea and diarrhea… Vomiting… People's hair falling out…

U.S. GOVERNMENT FILM: For the sake of all of us and for the sake of our country, I know that you join me in wishing this expedition well. [*announcement in the background*]: It is now 30 seconds to zero time. Put on goggles or turn away. Minus 10 seconds, nine, eight…

JEBAN RIKLON [*translated from Marshallese in subtitles*]: That all happened to me at the age of two. I thank God that I'm still alive.

> U.S. GOVERNMENT FILM: ...six, fiver, four, three, two, one…
>
> SUBTITLES: 'BRAVO' Hydrogen Bomb Test March 1, 1954. The Bravo test was 1,000 times larger than the bomb that destroyed Hiroshima. 'Bravo' was the largest nuclear test ever conducted by the United States. (*Nuclear Savage*)

For what the Marshall Islanders were witnessing on March 1, 1954, on another cloudless day in the Pacific, was nothing less than the destruction of their own lives. That destruction, Horowitz's film may be said to argue with Rob Wilson's concept of "slow violence," would be both fast and slow, and it would affect their past, their present and their future at the same time. Where Horowitz's film is so powerful, then, is that it insists on conveying each and every scene of the horror of what would become a nuclear Pacific through the eyes of two audiences simultaneously, one witnessing the spectacle from a safe remove and one looking on a scene that should never have been there for human eye-witnesses to observe. To be an eye-witness of Charlie Bravo was to spell out – or rather, to be *made* to spell out – one's own doom. The power of Horowitz's film, then, is its visual alternation between wide-angle shots and close-ups, each connected to a particular form of spectatorship in the Pacific.

At the same time, *Nuclear Savage* addresses the extent of what we might call visual complicity. Every time we see, in the infinite loop with which the film insists on confronting us, the mushroom cloud explode against a blue sky that our mind insists on ascribing some kind of serenity, we, too, become complicit in not seeing the eye-witness. This, then, is the power of Horowitz's film: he reinserts the eye-witness into the picture, and hence makes us aware of the degree of visual complicity. It is this visual dissonance, the jarring of visual synchronicity, which could not be more complex and could not be more devastating. For the master narrative of nuclear testing in the Pacific, Horowitz's film makes clear, is that of visual remove: of an uninhabited island paradise to be studied as a laboratory experiment of the effects of nuclear fall-out on human lives. Each time we see the mushroom cloud which our mind insists on registering as beautiful, we are complicit in the remove of spectatorship.

8.4 The Pacific as Life Sciences Laboratory

The Pacific, for Project 4.1, became the laboratory of Western science. It was a laboratory made possible, however, only through the imperialist wishful thinking of terra nullius. The point of terra nullius, of course, is not so much the inability to see the indigenous inhabitants but the willful act of blinking and blanking them out of the picture. It is quite simply the act of *un*seeing the native. The visual master narrative of nuclear testing in the Pacific, then, was to enlist a world audience in the politics of visual remove: Spectatorship became impossible, in other words, without becoming complicit in the visual project of Western science. Even as this pseudo-scientific gaze zooms in from the mushroom cloud on the people – people? – who were affected by the fall-out, the gaze remains detached. The camera's gaze becomes that of the physician, a physician detached but sympathetic, now examining the effects of radiation on human skin. Tony de Brum, Minister of Foreign Affairs of the Marshall Islands from 2014 to 2016,[9] is himself a survivor of these horrors:

> HOROWITZ: Tell me, what is Project 4.1? What did you find out?
>
> DE BRUM: For every test series, there is a list of programs. Like, for example 1.1 is blast measurements by photography, 1.2 is pressure studies, then wave studies… Each one gets a number. Crater survey, you know, how big the crater comes out, is 3.2. All of these things. But amongst the programs listed, program 4 was biomedical studies. Now, this document is November 53. . .
>
> RESEARCH ASSISTANT: Pre-'Bravo'
>
> DE BRUM: Pre-'Bravo.' And the title as it was in this program is "Study of Response of Human Beings Exposed to Significant Beta and Gamma Radiation due to Fall-Out from High Yield Weapons." Here, for example, is a picture of John Anjain, the magistrate of Rongelap, with this little placard: Rongelap number 40. That was his guinea pig number. I don't mind saying, he called it that himself the last time I spoke with him. And it's dated March 16, 1954, Project 4.1.

[9] It is notable that Tony de Brum has held this office three different times; his most recent appointment was in 2014.

> U.S. FILM EXCERPT: To the AEC Argon Labs in Chicago last week came seven men, Natives of the Marshall Islands. These are fishing people, savages by our standards. John is mayor of Rongelap, which is 100 miles from Bikini. When the white powder fell, people thought it was snow. It wasn't snow but incinerated carbon, highly radioactive. The Marshallese caught by fall-out got 175 Roentgens of radiation. Most humans are exposed to less than 20 Roentgens in a lifetime. So a cross-section, a delegation was brought to Chicago for testing. The first was John, the mayor of Rongelap Atoll. John, as we said, is a savage, but a happy, amenable savage. His grandfather ran almost naked on his atoll. John reads, knows about God, and is a pretty good mayor.
>
> JOHN ANJAIN [*translated from Marshallese in subtitles*]: That was the beginning of our demise from the hydrogen bomb in 1954.
>
> U.S. GOVERNMENT FILM: When the ritual of the iron room was over for John, it began for the others until, one by one, they had all gone through it. As each finished, he was told it was over and he was given apples and other good things to eat. And the seven men put on the suits and topcoats they had been lent in Hawaii, which they would return in Hawaii on their way back to the islands of Utirik and Majuro in Rongelap Atoll in the middle of the Pacific Ocean where hardly anybody lives. (*Nuclear Savage*)

Here, too, the film insists on countering the allegedly disinterested spectatorship of Western science with another kind of spectatorship. In *Nuclear Savage*, we see the effects of nuclear fall-out not only through the interested but detached gaze of the physician but through the eyes of the eye-witness, who watches his own skin peel off. It is this eye-witness account, the account of a woman who is made to watch her own body disintegrate in the aftermath of Charlie Bravo, which shocks us out of the visual complicity so ingrained in narratives about nuclear testing in the Pacific:

> [*voiceover*] In the Marshall Islands, a program called Project 4.1 was established by the Department of Energy to use Marshallese people as perpetual guinea pigs in these nuclear studies. It was no accident that people were exposed. Recently, with the release of documents, heretofore secret or classified, it is to believe that Marshallese population, different groups at different times, were used for radiation experiments. There were projects and programs conducted by various agencies in the

> United States, which involved exposing people and studying them. (*Nuclear Savage*)

Moreover, in keeping with this shattering of visual remove in which we, too, may be complicit, Horowitz's camera refuses *not* to show the doctor examining the victim of the nuclear fall-out his own government brought about: the camera, in fact, zooms in not only on the patient, but also on the doctor. In a Gothic Pacific version of Malinowski studying the natives, Horowitz's camera insists on a wide angle shot which includes, and implicates, the physician in the picture. There is no such thing, Horowitz makes clear, as the scientist's disinterest in or detachment from what or rather, whom he is studying. It is at this point that *Nuclear Savage* supplies us with a glimpse of the physician's biography: Dr. Robert A. Conard, a government physician, was sent to study the effects of radiation on human lives, and he sympathetically looked on as these lives proceeded to disintegrate under his own hands:

> [*voiceover*] U.S. government scientist and doctor, Robert A. Conard, studied the Rongelap Islanders for over 30 years and was the first doctor to examine the Islanders immediately after the 'Bravo' bomb test fiasco. As if the Islanders initial near fatal exposure to radiation was not enough, three years later, Dr. Conard and other U.S. scientists decided to expand their ongoing experiments to a higher, more sinister level by returning the already badly exposed Islanders to their contaminated Atoll in 1957, three months after John Anjain and the others had been studied and filmed in Chicago. Although living on a clean, uncontaminated island far away from the nuclear test area, in June of 1957 the Islanders were loaded onto a U.S. Navy ship and told they were finally going home and that the Island was now safe. The true intent of U.S. scientists was made abundantly clear in a secret meeting in Washington a year before by U.S. atomic commissioner Merril Eisenbud when he made the following statement on July 14, 1956: "That island is by far the most contaminated place on earth and it will be interesting to get a measure of human uptake when people live in a contaminated environment. While it is true that those people do not live the way Westerners do . . . , it is nevertheless also true that these people are more like us than mice." And, in a scientific study of the fall-out victims published in March of 1957, three months before their return to Rongelap, Dr. Conard and his colleagues wrote: "The habitation of these people on the island will afford most valuable ecological radiation data on human beings. The vari-

> ous radio isotopes present can be traced from the soil to the food chain and into the human being." The Rongelapese would remain on the Atoll for another 28 years. They lived on land and ate food contaminated with radiation and for all that time, were studied by U.S. government scientists to determine the effects of radiation from nuclear bombs on human beings. (*Nuclear Savage*)

It is here once again, that Horowitz's camera doubles the gaze: what the camera gives us is not only the image of the doctor studying what can only be seen as a human specimen; but it is the simultaneous image of the specimen himself looking at his own hand. Through this latter form of spectatorship, the spectatorship of the eye-witness watching his own body fall part, Horowitz's camera and his filmic narrative make clear that there can be no such thing as a human specimen. Pace terra nullius, these islands *were* inhabited or else eye-witness accounts would not have been possible in the first place.

It is at this point that Horowitz's narrative insists, not just on countering scientific visual detachment with the close-up of eye-witness accounts, but also on superimposing, through historical wide-angle, one history on top of another: It is curious, the Jewish American director observes, that American judges indicted German physicians at the Nuremberg trial for crimes against humanity, and found them guilty of using human subjects for medical experiments. Can there be degrees of acceptance, Horowitz's film asks, in which the use of human guinea pigs may be permissible in some contexts even as it is illegal in another?

8.5 Postcolonialism and Environmental Justice: Greenpeace off the Coast of Rongelap

How, then, did the people of Rongelap survive the atrocities of the horrors inflicted on them by U.S. government? What, moreover, is the role of Greenpeace in this context? First, the people of Rongelap or Rongelapese refused to believe in the predictions of the life scientists, the same life scientists whose search for medical progress had turned them into human guinea pigs in the first place. They distrusted the evidence that the life scientists had provided, and trusted instead in the evidence provided by their own eyes and that of their children, whose lives had been virtually destroyed by nuclear testing. The question that

Horowitz's film asks in this context is a crucial one: Who, what form of cognizance or jurisdiction could the Rongelapese appeal to in their plight? How could they defy the orders of the life scientists, and the U.S. government for which these life scientists worked? The people at Rongelap, then, chose to rewrite their lives by refusing to believe in the predictions of the life sciences. They survived because they believed in the evidence of what they saw, the suffering of their children and their own suffering, in spite of the evidence that the scientists provided. In the end, they appealed to Greenpeace to end their suffering; and they were eventually evacuated by the *Rainbow Warrior*. This, I believe, is a signature moment not only for justice, but for justice in all its facets. First, it is a moment which marks the survivance of the indigenous community of Rongelap; it is the refusal, to use Vizenor's words, of the native to vanish. The life sciences, in this context of Gothic neocolonialism, become but a sinister handmaiden of Manifest Destiny. In this form of Pacific survivance, the native refuses to vanish and boards the *Rainbow Warrior* instead. Second, the moment of the Rongelapese boarding the *Rainbow Warrior* testifies to the solace of supranational, non-partisan organizations like Greenpeace. As Greenpeace states on its website, "Greenpeace is an independent campaigning organization, which uses non-violent, creative confrontation to expose global environmental problems, and to force the solutions which are essential to a green and peaceful future." Thirdly, this moment of evacuation, in which both Greenpeace and the Rongelapese know that the certainty of the scientists that the island is no longer contaminated is sinister cynicism, marks a powerful convergence of ecocriticism and postcolonial or in this case indigenous justice. For the total destruction entailed by nuclear testing in the Pacific is a destruction both of the land and the lives of those who inhabited this land. In its proud defiance of national jurisdiction, the *Rainbow Warrior* was known, already in 1985, for its fight not only for environmental justice, but for human justice as well. As Graham Huggan and Helen Tiffin have argued in their study of *Postcolonial Ecocriticism* (2006), in myriads of different instances, it is futile to try to disentangle postcolonial justice and environmental justice in the first place. It is this impossibility of disentangling environmental rights and indigenous rights that this scene forcefully illustrates, a scene in which the Rongelapese are evacuated from their own island by the Greenpeace ship *Rainbow Warrior*.

8.6 Towards an Alternative Politics of Mourning: John Anjain

The film resists the pernicious myth of terra nullius, then, by engaging in a form of life writing that is at the same time a form of witnessing and a form of mourning. For as I have tried to argue above by applying Judith Butler's study of the politics of mourning to the "case" of the Marshall Islands, the unequal politics of mourning may also serve to exacerbate the effects of the terra nullius doctrine in the Marshall Islands. No one really mourns the death of a deer, we are not quite that sad about roadkill. What the film has to engage in in order to resist the politics of both terra nullius and the absence of mourning is to enact an alternative politics of mourning. The conclusion which Butler draws from a historical moment in which some lives are considered precarious while others are not, is that we can only end it by realizing that there must never be a difference between lives that we can mourn and those we cannot. In their own testimonies, brought only to the court of documentary film, the victims of nuclear testing are given names, histories, and genealogies. They testify as survivors of nuclear testing in the Pacific, of a series of nuclear tests in which they themselves were the guinea pigs. The feat which Horowitz's film accomplishes, then, is that he lets the guinea pigs testify about the atrocities inflicted on them, and that he reveals the savageness of an alleged civilization that would turn human beings into guinea pigs. Horowitz turns the patient file into a life writing narrative: he confronts us with fathers mourning the deaths of their children, and of the illness of their grandchildren:

> JOHN ANJAIN [*translated from Marshallese in subtitles*]: I got thyroid cancer myself. I had to go to the hospital in New York for an operation to remove it. My daughter Dorothy got thyroid cancer. Two of my sons, George and Zicriat, also had cancer. And my son Lekoj died of Leukemia. And one of my grandsons got thyroid cancer as well. (*Nuclear Savage*)

This scene is powerful for a number of reasons. John Anjain speaks to us as a survivor, and he speaks to us as the former magistrate of Rongelap. How, the film asks us, could the American government have turned magistrates into savages? Wouldn't the very fact that Rongelap had a mayor, and magistrate, been evidence enough of their civilization? Like Gauguin, the white gaze of the U.S. government undressed the savage in order to make him a savage in the first place; for only if he were indeed a savage he could be turned into a guinea pig. By testifying as a former magistrate of Rongelap, then, John Anjain reveals to us who the real savage was in the wake of nuclear testing. But John Anjain's testimony is powerful on yet another level: He speaks to us not only as a magistrate, but also as a survivor of the nuclear testing of which he himself was a guinea pig; but he also speaks to us as a father who mourns the death of his son at the hands of the U.S. government and its pernicious nuclear testing in the South Seas. By witnessing the mourning of a father for his son and his grandson, the film enacts what I would call a politics of alternative mourning, and hence restores the humanity of a people turned into "virtual guinea pigs" by nuclear testing. In this act of witnessing, we can escape our own visual complicity: we, too, mourn the lives thus lost in the Pacific. It is in this form of alternative mourning that the humanity of the victims is restored.

Yet, what the film also drives home with both empathy and bitterness is that the only court to which John Anjain can appeal for the crimes against humanity committed by the U.S. in the Marshall Islands is the court of documentary film. Legally, there was no question that the U.S. had the right to conduct nuclear tests in the Marshall Islands, which they had already colonized during the Second World War. This territory, clearly enough, was there for the asking. It is in this sense that the film, in the absence of another form of jurisdiction in the Marshall Islands, becomes the only court available for the restoring of justice, and for mourning the lives thus lost to nuclear testing in the South Seas.

8.7 The Mourning of Brothers: The Mayor of Rongelap

In its alternative politics of mourning, then, the film listens to the fathers mourning the deaths of their children and grandchildren; but it also listens to the brothers who would never know the siblings who died long before they were born. In this alternative politics of mourning and of witnessing, Horowitz's film restores the genealogies of the Rongelapese, genealogies which nuclear testing in the Pacific had virtually destroyed. Horowitz's film *Nuclear Savage* lets the fathers mourn the deaths of their children, and the brothers grieve for the siblings they would never know. By restoring this genealogy, moreover, a genealogy linking the living to those who died in the wake of nuclear testing, the film conveys the atrocious scope of nuclear testing, and the ongoing legacy of nuclear horror in the Pacific. James Matayoshi speaks to us not only as Mayor of Rongelap, but as the brother of a sibling he never came to know; and as the son of a mother, Almira Matayoshi, who had to suffer the horror of giving birth to a jellyfish baby:

> JAMES MATAYOSHI: Today, I stand before you as mayor of Rongelap. But more importantly, I stand before you as a son of Rongelap, a true son of the survivors.
>
> VOICEOVER: It's March the first, a commemoration ceremony of the 50th anniversary of the Castle Bravo hydrogen bomb explosion.
>
> JAMES MATAYOSHI: I wonder if they will tell you about Project 4.1, the study of humans exposed to radiation, drawn in 1953 for the planned 1954 Castle nuclear test series. Project 4.1 contemplated the study of exposed human beings.
>
> MATAYOSHI'S MOTHER: [*translated from Marshallese in subtitles*] My first child born did not look human. It was like a bunch of grapes. The second one came out limp, with no muscles or bones at all. It was like a monster… like a jellyfish. It was all formed with all the body parts but completely limp. It was a jellyfish baby. (*Nuclear Savage*)

It is by mourning for the death of the jellyfish baby, then, that we honor the lives lost in the Pacific, and we witness the horrors of nuclear testing in the Pacific. Yet, here, too, the film insists on not featuring the jellyfish baby only through the eyes of the scientist in whose laboratory the jellyfish baby was born; it refuses to turn the jellyfish baby into a specimen because its short life is witnessed not by the government physician but by its own mother. It is through the eyes of his mother and those of a brother whom he would not live to know that we mourn the death of the jellyfish baby and contemplate the curious detachment of the scientist-physician for whom this jellyfish baby, too, was but a specimen. Insisting on superimposing the wide-angle shot of the scientist looking at the effects of nuclear testing on human bodies and the eye-witness account of the woman owning the body, *Nuclear Savage* addresses the apex of the nuclear horror in the Pacific: It is here, as Graham Huggan and Helen Tiffin have forcefully argued, that it is impossible not to speak, with Barclay, of the "toxic Gothic," (58) a Gothicism triggered by a human being most victimized by nuclear fall-out: the jellyfish baby. As Huggan and Tiffin write,

> The alarming effects of nuclear irradiation are graphically documented, for example, in a powerful section [in *Daughters of the Pacific*] on the Marshall Islands: "I saw a child from Rongelap. Its feet are like clubs . . . . Now we have this problem, what we call "jellyfish babies." These babies are born like jellyfish. They have no eyes. They have no heads. They do not shape [sic] like human beings at all. . . . When they die they are buried right away. They do not allow the mother to see this kind of baby because she will go crazy. . . ." (59)

8.8 No Apology in the "Age of Apology": Genealogies and "Stolen" Generations

What, then, is the ending to this story? And in what context can it end? In return for their suffering, the film makes clear, the human guinea pigs were treated only to a sight-seeing trip of New York. The film ends in a curious void. To this day, there has been no apology issued by the U.S. government to the Rongelapese for the crimes against humanity committed in the Marshall Islands. No-one, Horowitz's film makes clear, has spoken of these tests and the human guinea pigs they involved as crimes against humanity in the first place. What, then, does the absence of an apology mean in the twenty-first century, which has been called the "age of apology" (Gibney et. al.)? In Australia, to be sure, the High Court declared the doctrine of terra nullius to be unconstitutional in its Mabo decision of 1992 (Stephenson, *Mabo*); in 2008, in a historic speech, Australian Prime Minister Rudd apologized to the Aboriginal people of Australia for the trauma inflicted on them, and for the trauma of the "stolen generation":

> Today, we honor the indigenous peoples of this land, the oldest continuing cultures in human history. We reflect on their past mistreatment . . . . We apologize especially for the removal of Aboriginal and Torres Strait Islander children from their families, their communities and their country. For the pain, suffering, and hurt of these Stolen Generations, their descendants and for their families left behind, we say sorry. To the mothers and the fathers, the brothers and the sisters, for the breaking up of families and communities, we say sorry. And for the indig-

> nity and degradation thus inflicted on a proud people and a proud culture, we say sorry. (Parliament of Australia – Department of Parliamentary Services n. pag.)

In this historic apology, to which I will return in more detail in Chapter 9, what is significant is that Rudd can restore a politics of mourning, for mourning the lives which, both psychologically and physically, succeeding Australian governments had destroyed. What is even more important for my purposes here is that he acknowledges the injustice of destroying entire genealogies; he apologizes to the fathers, the mothers, and to the siblings for the trauma and hurt that was afflicted upon them through policies entailing the "stolen generation." Such an apology for the atrocities committed in the Pacific by the U.S. government, Adam Horowitz's film makes clear, has yet to be made. All the film can provide in the place of such an apology is an apology of its own. And yet, it is significant in this context that Horowitz's film itself continues to exist in a void. This fact of an ethical state of limbo is curiously mirrored by the format of the documentary film which was made, by Jewish American filmmaker Adam Horowitz, about Project 4.1: a film which to this day has not found a distributor and can only be streamed from the director's website. The conditions surrounding the distribution of *Nuclear Savage*, then, further substantiate its claim: to this day, the details of Project 4.1 and its implications for the state of U.S. American democracy continue to be classified, even if the archives have been opened. Given the fact that the film does not yet have a distributor; it is as if the horrors of nuclear testing in the Pacific continue to be classified, if only by the fact that a film which reveals the atrocities committed in the South Seas continues to be condemned to a life of virtuality. If Horowitz's film pronounces an apology of its own, then, even this apology is hushed up by a democracy which has not quite owned up to the horrors it committed in the Pacific.

In this chapter, I have been interested in the convergence of four fields of research, and the abolishing of the borders between four different fields or methodologies: postcolonial studies, ecocriticism, indigenous studies and Transpacific studies. At the same time, the film *Nuclear Savage* makes clear that this abolishing of borders is more than academic; in fact, it may be essential to understand the complex constellations of events which made possible the dropping of an atomic bomb on an inhabited island in the Pacific. Life, *Nuclear Savage* implies, precedes our theorizing about it; and the history of the Marshall Islands, and the survivance (Vizenor) of its inhabitants against all odds and in spite of the horrors inflicted upon them by a country which prides itself on being a city upon a hill and a model democracy, gives the lie to assertions that academic schools or approaches should neatly be kept apart.

8.9 Conclusion: The Future Anterior of the South Seas

What, then, about the people of Rongelap? The film ends with a testimony to their survival, against all odds, and of their stubborn refusal to vanish:

> TEACHER: If there was no poison in Rongelap, would you like to stay in Rongelap?
>
> STUDENTS [*in unison*]: Yes.
>
> TEACHER: So do you think you will ever go to Rongelap?
>
> Student 1: Yes.
>
> TEACHER: Yes? One day? And when do you think that will be?
>
> Student 2: When we're old men.
>
> TEACHER: When we're old men and old women. Remember you are a Rongelapese and everyone always loves to go back home.
>
> STUDENT 3: I want to go home.
>
> TEACHER: Right. That song "I Want to Go Home." Right.... (*Nuclear Savage*)

In this as in many instances and struggles for environmental and indigenous rights, not all is well that ends well: In 2011, the Rongelapese were told that their island was now again safe for them to live there. In fact, they were told that they would lose all U.S. government funding unless they agreed to return to their island. Once again, the people of Rongelap saw in this assurance of the alleged decontamination of their island a form of entrapment in the certainties of the life sciences. From the perspective of the Rongelapese, nothing could have been more cynical than for the government to blackmail them, once more, with the power of economics. How could they return to the island that they knew, pace the scientists' alleged assurance, was still contaminated? In this sense, the last scene of the film *Nuclear Savage* is also a testimony to the survivance of the Rongelapese: The people of Rongelap, from their exile in the ghetto of the Pacific, continue to disbelieve Western life sciences, the same life sciences who had for so long turned them into human guinea pigs. For the people of Rongelap, survivance has meant disregarding the predictions, or the alleged certainties, of the life sciences and of the life scientists assuring them that the island was now once again safe for human habitation.

What is at stake here is what I would call the future anterior of indigeneity in the Marshall Islands: Because the half-life of nuclear fallout is 1,400 years, the children now attending school at Rongelap know that when they are seventy, they will have lived out their lives in exile, thinking of the island to which, in their own lifetime, they will not be able to return:

> [*voiceover*] The nuclear weapons tested here by the U.S. government would contaminate these islands and alter the lives of the people beyond their wildest dreams and their worst nightmares. After decades of American weapons testing and military occupation, the traditional life of the Marshall Islanders has largely disappeared. Thousands of Islanders now live in squalid conditions in a tiny island called Ebeye, two miles north of the American missile base. With an estimated 16,000 Islanders crowded onto just 65 acres of land, Ebeye is a slum and it's become known as the ghetto of the Pacific. Many of the Marshallese here are refugees from decades of American nuclear bomb and missile testing and continue to pay a heavy if unseen price for America's defense. (*Nuclear Savage*)

Horowitz's film thus vividly documents a condition of what Huggan and Tiffin have called "nuclear nomadism":

> Other witnesses . . . speak directly from personal memory, recounting their first, confused experiences of nuclear fallout, and their subsequent, unexplained removal to neighboring islands often hopelessly unsuited for human habitation, creating the first wave of "nuclear nomadism" . . . that was to extend for several decades, and the devastating consequences of which can still be felt today. (58)

The last image of the film once again shows the Mayor of Rongelap, the son of survivors and a survivor himself, singing with school children exiled in the ghetto of the Pacific about the desire to finally go home. This scene with its American chorus drives home all the complexity of U.S. involvement in the South Seas. The American flag in Adam Horowitz's film can never again be iconic; it bears witness both to the democratic claims which the U.S. has flaunted and the horrors which it has committed in its name.

If this study investigates the role of medical humanities in American Studies, this chapter has once again been concerned with the relevance of a transnational American Studies. The U.S., I have tried to argue in this chapter, cannot be seen independently of the nuclear horrors it committed, and the violence it continues to commit, in the Pacific. The fruitfulness of a transnational American Studies approach, I would argue, can also be seen in the concept of what I would call a comparative indigenous studies perspective: As I have tried to argue in this chapter, Gerald Vizenor's idea of "survivance" may be powerfully eloquent in describing the resistance, by the Rongelapese, to predictions by American life scientists about the half-life of the nuclear fall-out which had contaminated their island. Even as a comparative indigenous studies perspective must be wary of simply imposing a Native American model on a Pacific context, it may nevertheless be useful in establishing a sense of the striking similarities of programs and policies which resulted in the destruction of indigenous lives and life worlds. This chapter has thus tried to explore the question at whose expense, at the expense of whose lives, medical science progressed in the middle of the twentieth century. The history of science, then, is never neutral, it cannot be seen independently of historical, political and ideological process. Focusing on human lives, on the other hand, and the means we may or may not have on writing and reading these lives, forever calls the bluff of the assertion of the disinterestedness or objectivity of medical science. Rather, what Adam Horowitz's film *Nuclear Savage* makes clear, is that life writing and restoring the testimonies of those whose lives had been written out of medical textbooks except as "human guinea pigs" can be powerful tools in revising medical history.

I would like to end this chapter, then, with a brief discussion of the "politics of recognition" (Taylor, "The Politics of Recognition") as it can be related to both trauma and reconciliation. What would the politics of recognition mean in the context of trauma and in the face of "medical discrimination" (Nelson xi)? First and foremost, it has been argued in trauma studies that the healing of the traumatized individual or collective can emerge only once the perpetrator of the injustice which led to the trauma in the first place admitted to his or her wrongdoing. It is in this sense that in the next chapter, I will discuss the official apologies made by the Prime Ministers of Australia and Canada to the indigenous populations in their respective countries. Moreover, I will read narratives of life writing as forms of evidence, which, arguably, finally resulted in official apologies made by national governments. Yet, recognition – which can then lead to apologies and, perhaps, to forms of healing – can take various shapes. In this context, it may in fact be solace that in 2015, the foreign minister of the Marshall Islands, Tony de Brum, was awarded the "Right Livelihood Award," often termed the "alternative Nobel Peace Prize." This award, even as it cannot replace an official apology on the part of the U.S. government or a formal juridical indictment of the U.S. for the injustice committed in the Marshall Islands, nevertheless constitutes a form of recognition. What is also crucial to note for my purposes here is that the award honored both an individual – Tony e Brum, the Marshall Islands' Minister of Foreign Affairs – and the community he is part of. Significantly, as the website listing the "Right Livelihood" laureates puts it, the 2015 award was given to "Tony de Brum & the People of the Marshall Islands" ("Tony de Brum & the People of the Marshall Islands" n. pag.). The jury describes its reason for this award as follows: The award was given "...in recognition of their vision and courage to take legal action against the nuclear powers for failing to honour their disarmament obligations under the Nuclear Non-Proliferation Treaty and customary international law" ("Tony de Brum & the People of the Marshall Islands" n. pag.). A number of aspects are significant here. In this chapter as well as in the one that follows, I am concerned not just with the relationship between life writing and medicine, but between life writing and the law in the context of what can be termed "medical discrimination" (Nelson xi). Thus, as Adam Horowitz's film *Nuclear Savage* argues, nuclear testing in the Pacific was made possible by a specific form of medical racism targeted against the native inhabitants of the Marshall Islands. Life Writing, I have proposed in this chapter, can be seen as a testimonial in two senses of the term: First, it is a testimonial by a human being whose humanity was direly disregarded by nuclear testing; in this sense, it is an indictment of medical science in a specific historical context. Second, however, it is also a testimonial criticizing the absence of legal frameworks in which such an official indictment could take place. Tony de Brum and the Marshall Islanders are hence honored for "[taking] legal action against the nuclear powers" in the first place, even if this legal action has so far taken place in a void, in the sense that it has not yet succeeded in giving rise to an official court case or an institutional recognition – an institution other, that is, than the committee awarding the "Alternative Nobel Peace Prize." Tony de Brum's work, and his use of his own life narrative in his political activism on behalf of the people of the Marshall Islands, has hence also pointed to a gap in jurisdiction and juridical responsibility: in the void between national legislation and international law, who is to be held responsible for the continuing violations of the rights of the Marshall Islanders? Moreover, the breaches of these rights can be seen both as violations of indigenous rights and of human rights. (This is a distinction, or rather, a misleading distinction, to which I will return in more detail below.) The committee's explanation for giving the Right Livelihood Award to Tony de Brum goes on as follows:

> Tony de Brum has dedicated a lifetime of public service in pursuit of an independent, secure and sustainable Marshall Islands, and he has courageously advanced his peoples' vision of a world free of nuclear weapons. Having witnessed the deleterious effects of U.S. nuclear tests in his country as a young boy, Tony de Brum, as Foreign Minister of the Marshall Islands, took the unprecedented step of filing lawsuits against all nine nuclear weapons states in the International Court of Justice in 2014, seeking to hold them to account for their failure to abide by the provisions of the Nuclear Non-Proliferation Treaty (NPT) and customary international law. As architect of the Majuro Declaration for Climate Leadership, adopted in September 2013, Tony de Brum has also been instrumental in securing the commitment of Pacific Island States to adopt concrete measures to combat climate change. ("Tony de Brum & the People of the Marshall Islands" n. pag.)

Thus, the committee, in its justification of its decision for giving out the 2015 award, links a number of issues which, I argue, must also be addressed from within a framework of medical humanities, even if it has so far been absent from it. The above-quoted passage links the issue of sustainability, environmental justice, and health; it insists on the right to well-being as a human right, a right that must not be infringed upon by the rationale of medical racism. This is an intersection to which I will return in more detail in Chapter 9, which discusses the interface between water rights and indigenous rights in the film *The Cherokee Word for Water* (2013). Moreover, the above-quoted passage also addresses the relationship between illness and health, which must also be central to any discussion of medical humanities. Climate change, of course, is a global issue; in this sense, the measures that Tony de Brum and the Marshall Islanders have adopted to counteract climate change in the Pacific do not only benefit their own community, but may be a model for global environmental action as well. In this study, and especially in the second part of this study, I am thus calling for a framework that links medical humanities to discourses of sustainability and environmental justice. Unless we take this link seriously, I believe, we risk understanding illness only in an individual sense, a sense in which illness affects only a single individual and cannot be seen as a larger picture. If medical humanities are located at the intersection between medicine and the humanities, they must also account for the different ways in which human beings, and communities, are situated differently, in a social, ethnic, or geographical sense. Thus, approaches from the field of environmental justice have stressed that certain communities may be subjected to the "slow violence" (Nixon 45) of environmental damage. Conversely, as documentaries such as *Nuclear Savage* or *Crude: The Real Price of Oil* (2009) make clear, corporations have so far refused to compensate victims or their families on the grounds that, as they argued, no causal connection could be established between entire communities falling ill and the fact that oil was being drilled in the land they lived on.[10] Life writing, as Tony de Brum's work illustrates, is a powerful tool for political activism and for human rights campaigns, a fact which has been explored in Sidonie Smith's and Kay Schaeffer's book *Human Rights and Narrated Lives* (2004). The fact that the Right Livelihood Award was given to Tony de Brum, then, is a step towards the recognition of a struggle in which indigenous rights, human rights, the right to

[10] For a detailed discussion of the film *Crude: The Real Price of Oil* (2009), see Meyer, "Incorporating the Indigenous Subject."

health and well-being, sustainability and environmental justice cannot be separated from one another.

9 Trauma, Repatriation, and Representation: Life Writing as an Alternative Form of Knowledge Production

In the previous chapter on Adam Horowitz's film *Nuclear Savage*, I have discussed issues of trauma with regard to the exposure of the population of the Marshall Islands to nuclear fall-out and the ways in which, through personal testimonies, the Marshallese have had to come to terms with what it meant to be, as Tony de Brum puts it in an interview in *Nuclear Savage*, "human guinea-pigs." The last chapter ended with the question what forms of recognition might ameliorate the effects of trauma and might eventually lead to forms of collective healing. In this chapter, I will be interested in the language of trauma more specifically, as well as in the linguistic form which official apologies may have to take in order to make healing possible.[1] At the same time, I am interested in narratives of life writing as proof or evidence for the reality of trauma. What counts as evidence in both a legal and a medical sense? As I will argue towards the end of this chapter, changes in the life sciences have made it possible to prove the effects of trauma through changes in epigenetics (Elbert and Schauer 64). The evidence of epigenetic results of trauma have, in a sense, supported earlier narratives that attested to the existence of trauma, but which were able to "prove" trauma only in narrative form. If throughout this book, I am interested in a dialogue between life writing and the life sciences, this dialogue has taken a par-

[1] This chapter was first presented as a talk at the "Wissenschaftshistorische Seminar" of the National Academy of the Sciences Leopoldina. I am grateful to Florian Steger and Rainer Godel for inviting me, and for their comments and suggestions, which helped me substantially in revising this chapter.

ticular shape in the context of trauma research and the struggle for human rights and indigenous rights in a variety of contexts.[2]

Quite simply, then, I argue that one justification for including films such as *Nuclear Savage* not only into the field of environmental studies but also of medical humanities, then, is the fact that these narratives can also be seen as narratives of personal and collective trauma. In fact, it may seem problematic to include these narratives only in the framework of indigenous rights; to see these debates only as legal debates, as debates over whether or not to extend specific rights to specific individuals, may run the risk of being cynical. If the breach of individual rights gives rise to illness, the illness of an individual or his or her loss of relatives due to environmental damage or nuclear fall-out, how can the question of rights be separated from narratives of trauma? As I will try to show in Chapter 10, drawing discussions of indigenous performance art, not only have the life sciences and recent discoveries of biomarkers made life writing narratives more powerful, but these scientific developments are themselves reinscribed into life writing performances.

What does it mean or imply to include a chapter such as this one in a book concerned with medical humanities? By including in the framework of medical humanities a discussion of the politics of repatriation, my aim is twofold. First, I want to argue that medical humanities may fall short of their potential if they limit themselves only to individual narratives of illness. What happens, I want to ask, if we inquire not only to cases of illness and ill-health but also to questions of physical and mental well-being? To the extent that narratives of trauma, for instance, are included within a framework of medical humanities, it is impossible to separate questions of medical humanities from aspects of social justice. Traumas are experienced both on an individual level and a communal one. In the histories of indigenous communities throughout the world, moreover, collective trauma has been a direct consequence from centuries of colonial rule. What would it imply, I ask, to exclude these collective indigenous trauma narratives from the framework of medical humanities? At its best, I would suggest, medical humanities can accommodate both individual narratives of illness and collective narratives

[2] For many of the discussions that follow about the relationship between trauma and evidence, I am indebted to Florian Steger.

of trauma and social injustice. In looking at medical humanities from a humanities perspective, then, we may inquire not so much into what medical humanities as a framework for critical inquiry has traditionally included, but also on what it has often excluded. While the first chapters of this book are concerned with life writing narratives about aging and illness which have traditionally been subsumed under medical humanities, then, the second part turns to narratives and concerns which, I argue, have been marginalized by medical humanities discussions. This marginalization, in turn, may have given rise to both a universalist and a color-blind discussion of illness and trauma. Finally, I suggest that the potential of medical humanities may lie in linking questions of illness to concepts of health and well-being. Such an inclusion, in turn, would bridge the gap between medical humanities and frameworks of social and environmental justice. This is a link which I investigate in more detail in Chapter 10.

9.1 The "Museumfication" of Indigenous Lives

I would like to begin this discussion with a life writing narrative. In 1897, an Inuit boy named Minik traveled from Greenland to New York with his father, Qisuk. But what was the reason for their journey? Robert Peary, an American natural scientist, claimed to have literally "discovered" these indigenous inhabitants of the Danish Arctic: Using the familiar and oft-cited language of the imperialist to describe them, Peary saw in these "childlike" Inuit objects of scientific interest, specimen or remnants of a pristine, prehistoric culture seemingly untouched by civilization: "Peary finally saw these untamed natives in 1891. He liked what he saw. For the next eighteen years, they would be 'his' Eskimo" (Harper 2). Not incidentally, these specimen were sold by Peary to the American Museum of Natural History where they could appropriately be exhibited. In New York, the Inuit quickly became curiosities; they were interviewed by renowned anthropologists, especially Franz Boas who had originally commissioned Peary to bring an "Eskimo specimen" back to New York to be studied as live material. Peary, in his turn, reasoned that if one Inuit specimen would bring him fame, how much more fame would the bringing of six native specimen promise? It was for this reason that Peary, on one of his expeditions to Greenland, persuaded six Inuit to accompany him to New York. Eventually, it was decided that

Qisuk, his young son Minik, as well as Nuktaq, his wife Atangana, and their daughter Aviaq come to New York with Peary. Still on board the ship which had landed at the New York harbor, they became instant curiosities: "To the little group of Eskimos, the curiosity of these crowds of New Yorkers was overwhelming. Thirty thousand visitors in two days alone!" (Harper 22). But what happened next?

Soon after their arrival in the new world, Minik's father Qisuk took ill, as did the men who had accompanied them; today, it is known that they must have contracted tuberculosis. Minik had to watch his father get worse and pass away within only a few weeks. Yet, what seems like a tragic accident in retrospective would soon give way to an ethical catastrophe. As Minik would eventually learn, his father's body had been put into a display showcase of the museum which had originally invited them; he had been transformed from a father to a specimen. It is this politics of the "museumfication" of indigenous lives with which this chapter is concerned. For the curators of the museum, Qisuk was not part of a genealogy which was to be honored as such; rather, as the representative of a purportedly primitive species which was allegedly doomed to extinction, he had become a specimen, his body a museum exhibit:

> "[An] upstairs room – at the museum – [became] his father's last resting place. His coffin [was] a showcase, his shroud a piece of plate glass. No quiet of the graveyard is there; the noise of shuffling feet and the tap, tap of the hammers as the workmen fix up other skeletons, is ever present. And when the sunlight fades they turn on the electric lights so that Minik's father may not have even the pall of darkness to hide his naked bones." (Harper 84)

Minik, on the other hand, was deprived of his right to mourn his father's death; the only way for Minik to honor his dead father was to visit the museum which had become his last resting place. As Minik himself would later put it, "'It makes me cry every time I think of his poor bones up there in the museum in a glass case, where everybody can look at them. Just because I am a poor Esquimau boy, why can't I bury my father in a grave the way he would want to be buried?'" (Harper 84).

This moment of forbidden mourning, a form of mourning which has suddenly become impossible, is inextricably intertwined with the politics of the museumfication of indigenous lives. In this context, the display showcase of the museum is the epitome of the disenfranchisement of indigenous groups. Caught up in the vortex of an anthropology which understood indigenous people as demonstration material – from "live exhibits" in the so-called *Völkerschauen* to the display showcase in a museum – indigenous lives were no longer recognized as such.

Minik was denied the right to mourning; a glass case in a museum was to become his father's last resting place, not a burial place which would have been in line with his religion. Today, using the language of the life sciences, we would speak of PTSD (Post-Traumatic Stress Disorder). The young Inuit boy faces the sudden loss of his father; yet, how much greater must that loss be if he can mourn his father not by going to the cemetery, but by visiting him in a museum?

The extent of the museum curators' transgression was even greater than this outline of events suggests. Seeing the boy's despair over his father's death, they were desperately trying to appease him; and they knew that no-one, boy or adult, would react well to their own father's being put on display in the glass case of a museum. It is for this reason that the men resorted to an unusual strategy: Having learned from anthropologist Alfred Kroeber about the Inuit burial rites, they proceeded to stage a mock burial to assure the boy that his father had indeed been properly buried. They had only buried, however, a piece of log:

> [Incredible] as it may seem, the scientists at the American Museum of Natural History had staged a phony funeral for the benefit of little Minik! . . . "At first there seemed no way of appeasing the child son of the dead man. Finally this scheme was hit upon. A fake burial was authorized for the benefit of Minik." . . . The scientists at the American Museum of Natural History decided to duplicate this primitive funeral as best they could on the museum grounds. Years later, William Wallace [one of the museum's curators] would recall the bizarre ceremony . . . . (Harper 86-87)

In this bizarre ceremony which marks one of the darkest chapters of the Western colonization of indigenous peoples, leading to the "museumfication" of indigenous bodies across the world, the American Museum of Natural History and the Bellevue hospital fight for the right to "study" Qisuk's body, the body of an Inuit man who has only seemingly been buried. This, then, is a clash among life science disciplines: both the emerging science of anthropology and medical anatomy stand to benefit from the right to "study" this man's body. And, happily for this sad history of life sciences development, both win: "It was agreed that students at Bellevue should make such use of it as possible in the dissecting-room, and that the skeleton should then be mounted and preserved in the Museum of Natural History" (Harper 85). The dispute had started, moreover, already when Qisuk had lain dying in a New York hospital: "In February of 1898 when Minik's father, Qisuk, lay dying in Bellevue Hospital, that institution had written to Franz Boas at the museum, "I hardly believe Qisuk will survive the night. The body will I suppose belong to the Museum of Natural History of Mr. Peary and they can of course do anything they wish with it. . . " (Harper 85).

It would take another seven years for Minik to find out about this scheme. If the boy had been traumatized before, this recent trauma only exacerbated his situation. As William Wallace, the museum curator with whose family Minik lived after his father's death, recalls:

> The newspapers had found out that the bones of his father were in the museum, and though they never knew of the fake burial or the bone cleaning in Cobleskill, they printed stories about the skeletons. . . . Eventually [the boy] learned that he had not witnessed the burial of his father's remains, but he kept it to himself for a long time. We noticed that there was a change coming over him, and then one day we learned its cause. "He was coming home from school with my son Willie one snowy afternoon, when he suddenly began to cry. "My father is not in his grave," he said, "his bones are in the museum." We questioned him and found out how he had learned the truth. But after that he was never the same boy. He became morbid and restless. Often we would find him sitting crying, and sometimes he would not speak for days. (Harper 96-97)

And why, moreover, was Minik's plea that his father's body be returned to him, never heard, and what was the language in which his plea could not be heard? At the core of this dilemma, quite literally, there seems to be a clash of discourses, one of which – the discourse of life writing – is not recognized as a discourse proper to begin with. Minik's voice and the language of his autobiographical account cannot be heard by museum curators and anthropologists, since as a genre, his account will automatically become subordinated to the scientific account of a vanishing race. Only this clash of discourses – or rather, the discrepancy between what is recognized to be a discourse proper and what is seen merely as an anecdote, a random noise which can never claim to be "scientific" – can account for the fact that what is now exhibited in a glass case of the museum is an item for some and a deceased human being for others. Seen from Minik's perspective, this means that the scientific account about the Inuit as a primitive (and always-already extinct) people is only made possible by placing his father in a display showcase. It is the scientific account, the anthropology of a vanishing race, which makes the museumfication of Qisuk's body possible in the first place, since he is not seen as a father, but a specimen.

9.2 Translating Life Writing into Life Science

Under what circumstances and through what forms of translation, then, could Minik's plea that his father's body may be returned to him, finally be heard? For Minik to be heard, his plea first had to be translated into the language of museum curators and the language of colonialism, and of an anthropology deeply entangled with the logic and the politics of colonialism. In 1986, the historian Kenn Harper, who through marriage had become part of an Inuit community, wrote a biography of the short life of Minik, the young Inuit boy. Harper's biography is not only a biography, but it is also a document of the history of science; and it retells the history of science from the perspective of a young Inuit, who confronts historians of science with a question which is only seemingly simple: "Why am I a scientific experiment?".

Harper's biography of the young Inuit, Minik, hence functions as a missing link between expert discourse and a form of life writing which is only allegedly anecdotal. Seen from Minik's perspective, this means that in order for his story to be heard, two preconditions must be fulfilled: First, the hierarchy between life writing account and scientific treatise must be overcome; and second, the autobiographical or biographical account must be conveyed in a way that it can be understood in the language of science. In this context, it may be useful to revisit the concept of life writing as such. For the concept of "life writing" deliberately blurs the line between biography and autobiography; this blurring of lines, I would suggest, is particularly suitable to the representation of Minik, the "New York Inuit." Throughout this study, I am concerned with the ways – and the media – in which the lives of marginalized individuals or communities can be made visible, and with the question how, through these media, they can leave a mark on the dominant discourses they have been written out of. Where Minik's autobiographical or oral account and his plea that his father's body be returned to him by the museum curators went unheard, it is Harper's biography, written much later, which restores Minik's presence. It is through this biography, in turn, that we are able to re-read the history of science (especially that of anthropology) and of museumfication.

It is in this sense that Harper's biography functions as a missing link. For once the story of Minik's life is turned into a biography written by a historian, it becomes a form of evidence; in the discursive hierarchy with which this chapter is concerned, the biography, if not quite on par with the scientific treatise, is at least located above the "mere" account of someone's life. The historical biography thus highlights the fact that an indigenous life is a life proper, and it sees this life as a form of evidence. Through this form of evidence, moreover, scientific discourse can be exposed for "writing out" this life in the service of scientific disinterest, or rather, of scientific interest in the specimen, not the man. Yet, the question which I would like to ask in this chapter, is this: Under what pressure and under what historical circumstances can the established hierarchy between scientific discourse and life writing account, between life sciences and life writing, be suspended, if only temporarily so?

When Harper first self-published his book in 1986, he was initially faced with outrage; the New York Museum of Natural History, above all, was anything but thrilled about making this dark chapter in its own history public knowledge. As Harper observes in his afterword, "Following the first publication of this book in 1986, the American Museum of Natural History was embarrassed. They had succeeded for many years in covering up the story of Minik and their treatment of the remains of Qisuk and his fellow Eskimos. Now, almost a century after the events in question, the story had come back to haunt them" (224). Only through two newspaper articles which had been written on the basis of Harper's book would the public learn about the men from Greenland, whose bodies had been housed in museum display showcases as items of interest. As Harper goes on to recall, "But public attention waned, and Qisuk's bones continued to lie in a box in the museum under the accession number 99/3610, alongside those of Nuktaq, Atangana, and Aviaq"

(225). At long last, the bodies were returned, and an entire century after the men from Greenland had passed away, they were granted a burial in keeping with their religious belief. Minik himself, who had died at only twenty years of age, would not live to see this happen.

It is thus characteristic of the ironies with which this chapter is concerned, that this form of injustice which had affected Minik in 1897, as it affected ten thousand other members of indigenous communities, would be recognized as a form of legal and historical injustice only in 1993. How did this recognition take place? Minik's petition was finally recognized in 1993, following the publication of two newspaper articles which had been written about Kenn Harper's biography of Minik, the New York Inuit. As Harper recalls in the afterword to his book, justice was restored to the four Inuit whom Peary had once brought to New York almost an entire century later: "On July 28, 1993, the bones of four Polar Eskimos were loaded aboard an American military transport aircraft at Maguire Air Force Base in New Jersey and transported to Thule Air Base in northern Greenland. The journey that had taken over a month in 1897 was accomplished in a few short hours. At Thule, the cargo was transferred to a Greenlandair helicopter for the trip to Qaanaaq, less than an hour away" (227). As Harper goes on to note, today there is a funeral plaque at the grave of the four Inuit, with a sentence whose apparent simplicity belies the complexity of the politics of repatriation, which emerges only from re-reading, and indicting, the entire history of the colonization of indigenous peoples: "A plaque was provided for eventual errection [sic] at the gravesite. It began simply as 'They have come home.' This statement is followed by the names of the four Eskimos with details of their births and deaths and the statement 1897 New York-Imut, 1993 Qaanaamut" (228). It is at this point that Minik's story has come full circle; and it has come full circle through a historical development which at once testifies to the power of biography as life writing. It was through Ken Harper's biography of his life, self-published in 1986, that Minik's voice was finally heard by official discourse. The politics of repatriation, as in the "coming home" of Qisuk and his fellow Inuit, marks the promise of a new beginning in the history of Western nation states. Acknowledging a history of rightlessness for indigenous Greenlanders, the Danish queen finally paid the Inuit men her respects:

> On August 4, 1997, one hundred years after Qisuk, Nuktaq, [his wife] Atangana, and [their daughter] Aviaq left the Thule district for New York aboard [a ship ironically called] *Hope*, and four years after the return of the remains to Greenland and their burial in the graveyard at Qaanaq, the memorial plaque was finally placed over their common grave. Queen Margarethe of Denmark and her husband, Prince Henrik, attended its unveiling in a touching ceremony presided over by the mayor, Lars Jeremiassen, who spoke of the community's wish to honor their forefathers who loved their living and grieved their dead. (Harper 228)[3]

It is in 1997, at long last, that Qisuk's community is given the right to grieve for their dead, of which they had been deprived through a history which strains the limits of belief.

This recognition of injustice and the restoring to indigenous communities of the right to bury their dead, in turn, is part of a change in jurisdiction which would take place only at the beginning of the twenty-first century. In Australia as much as in the U.S. and Canada, the twentieth century ends and the twenty-first century begins with a juridical restoring of justice: This restoring of justice at the same time is inseparably tied to a loss or at least a decline of the power of the museum. The concept of repatriation denotes a number of legislative procedures, owing to which the return of so-called human remains to the indigenous communities from which they originate has finally become mandatory. An

[3] It must be noted here that the men eventually received a Christian burial, not an Inuit mourning ritual. An entire century after the men had been brought to New York, many Inuit in Greenland were Christians. As Harper ironically notes, a fight with the Lutheran church ensued because the Inuit men had been "pagans" "Officialdom almost had one last surprise for the souls of the four returning Eskimos. The Lutheran church, the state church of Greenland and Denmark, had initially decided that, because the Eskimos were pagans and unbaptized, they could not be buried in a Christian ceremony. The decision, however, was reconsidered . . ." (Harper 227). It must also be noted, moreover, that in time Minik, who spent his adolescence fighting for the return of his father's body, asked for a Christian burial, which would be in keeping with the cultural practices of the white American among whom he now lived. Through such a petition, he wanted to appeal to the Christian ethics of anthropologists and museum curators, an attempt, however, which proved to no avail.

entire century later, these laws put into practice what Minik, the "New York Inuit" had once asked for his father. In the U.S., the so-called Native American Grave Protection and Repatriation Act (NAGPRA) is enacted in 1990; in Australia, it would take until 2013 for a comprehensive "Australian Government Indigenous Repatriation Policy" to take effect. As Harper writes at the end of this book, this moment of the enactment, across the globe, of repatriation laws finally marks the convergence of life writing with historical justice. It is hence no historical coincidence that the bodies of Qisuk and his fellow Inuit were finally returned to their community in 1993, three years after the Native American Grave Protection and Repatriation Act had been passed. What emerges here, then, is a global acknowledgment of indigenous rights. It was through the legal success won by Native Americans through NAGPRA that justice could finally be restored to the Inuit from Greenland, who had once been brought to New York in the name of life science. Even if, as Harper outlines, the Inuit from Greenland could benefit from American legislation only through a detour, it was this legislation that had changed the political climate for good. As Harper concludes,

> Then, in 1992, two reporters rediscovered *Give Me My Father's Body*. . . This time the interest in having the bones removed from the museum for burial remained high. Since 1986, things had changed in the conservative world of American museums. Native Americans had made progress in forcing museums to deal appropriately with the remains of their ancestors. In 1990 the Native American Grave and Burial Protection Act was passed. Under this legislation, American museums are required to return skeletal remains to native groups that request them. Qisuk and the other Polar Eskimos, however, were not covered by this legislation. They were Greenlanders, not Americans, and the American Museum of Natural History was under no obligation to send their bones to Greenland or anywhere else for burial. But the museum authorities had had enough. In the summer of 1992, they decided to lay the story to rest once and for all . . . . (226-227)

9.3 The Ceremony of Repatriation

Through this change in jurisdiction, Minik's tragic story seems to have come to a more hopeful end at the beginning of the twenty-first century; yet, as I would like to show in what follows, the discourses which had led to the "museumfication" of his father's body prove to be tenacious and persistent. I would like to discuss a short video depicting a repatriation ceremony from a different national context. In this video, a religious representative of the Ngarrindjeri, Major Sumner, is shown conducting a purification ceremony in front of the National Museum of Scotland:

> NEWSCASTER: The National Museum of Scotland and Edinburgh University have been in possession of Aboriginal remains taken over one hundred years ago. They include the skulls and a woman's ear bone. A delegation from Southern Australia went recently to collect the remains.
>
> VOICEOVER: [*a traditional cleansing ceremony is being shown*]. A traditional Aboriginal ceremony. Major Sumner, an elder from Australia's Ngarrindjeri people, marks the returning of Aboriginal remains. ("Scotland Returns Aboriginal Remains")

Yet, what do we see when we try to describe this historical moment of the present? I would like to argue that our habits of looking are inextricably interwoven with a politics of primitivism; it is in the sense of such primitivism that we may witness in this scene a form of anachronism or asynchronicity. In this tainted vision or vision tainted by the history of the erasure, neglect or disregard of indigenous civilizations, we may come to describe this scene as one of temporal asynchronicity, in which an indigenous past meets a (presumably) modern Western present. It is this reaction, I would argue, which may jumble the emotions with which we may witness this scene, and which accounts for the fact that we may not quite be emotionally moved by the images we see. Rather, we may experience a scene which is part of the ritual of literally "bringing home" the body of an indigenous person unlawfully exhibited in a museum show case with a degree of detachment, precisely because the indigenous traditions at the center of the ritual may seem, to eyes socialized in colonial histories, strangely out of keeping with the (Scottish) setting in which the ritual takes place. Yet, it is the stubborn persistence of this habit of looking – the primitivism ingrained in our habits of seeing – which may serve as an explanation for the fact that Minik's father Qisuk could be exhibited in a museum in the first place. Thus, our own reaction, which emerges from our own cultural and academic socialization, may provide proof for a pernicious anthropological logic which held that Minik's father was not a recently deceased human being, but a find for museum curators to brag about.

This proof, provided by our own eyes against our will, runs as follows: The academic discourse about the so-called indigenous peoples is based on a complex disjunction or differentiation of temporality, which Native American theorist Gerald Vizenor has called "the myth of the vanishing Indian." This warped logic holds that at the beginning of the nineteenth century, indigenous peoples are on the verge of "extinction;" this "extinction," in turn, is due to a Western politics of expansionism. It is in this sense, Vizenor writes in the deliberately polemic style which is one of the hallmarks of his work, that each "Indian" we meet is the last of his tribe. In a bizarre volte-face of imperial thinking, the Western settler community proceeds to mourn the indigenous culture whose destruction it has brought about. At the very moment in which indigenous communities have almost disappeared, the dominant culture sets out to cultivate its memory. This desire for preservation, to be sure, is a well-meaning one, even if it is seriously misguided; it is a desire which takes hold of science and museums, it becomes manifest in sculptures, paintings and novels such as James Fenimore Cooper's *The Last of the Mohicans: A Narrative of 1757* (1826). If, then, each native is the last of his kind, he becomes a specimen or illustrative model at the very moment of this assertion; he becomes the object of anthropological interest. It is at this moment that an ethical short circuit takes place: For looking at Minik and his father Qisuk, the museum's curators see not the human beings that they are but the last "remnants" of a civilization which must be preserved at all cost, and whose erstwhile existence must be documented for future generations. What emerges here is a complex superimposition of two temporal orders. The native is present, but at the same time, he is a remnant from or reminder of a past which must be preserved; in a bizarre volte-face which may be termed the cultural future anterior of indigeneity, this native is said to already be part of the past, not the present.

The aim of a cultural studies or indigenous studies approach, in this context, is to upset our habitual forms of looking, using the repatriation ceremony conducted by Major Sumner as a case in point. The aim of such an alternative politics of looking, then, must be the insistence on seeing Major Sumner as a part of our present, not the past. It is this contemporaneity of indigenous culture, in turn, which Major Sumner himself highlights in an interview in which he reflects on his own role during the ceremony. The body now finally returned to its ancestral community, Sumner notes, was once brought to Scotland on a sailing vessel; it is now returning to Australia in a Boing 747:

> VOICEOVER: Sumner says it's culturally and spiritually important for the remains to be returned to allow the spirits of the dead to rest. And it doesn't matter how they're transported home.
>
> MAJOR SUMNER: They came here on an old sailing ship, and they're going home on a 747 jet, so, you know [LAUGHS], it's a change of times, but they'll get on. ("Scotland Returns Aboriginal Remains")

There is nothing incongruous, then, about Major Sumner's ceremonial dress and the contemporary Australian English coming out of his mouth. To assume these factors as asynchronous with one another, in turn, would be to fall victim to a colonialist politics of looking. In keeping with the religious significance of the event, this form of dress, of course, has been deliberately chosen; the fact that Major Sumner is wearing this form of clothing – as opposed to Western clothing which, once again in a highly imperialist form of thinking, has been associated with "modernity" – is at once part of what Gerald Vizenor has called the "survivance" of indigenous cultures today.

What a habit of looking ingrained in us through the myth of the vanishing native refuses to acknowledge, then, is the fact that, for the duration of the ceremony, Major Sumner slips out of his Western suit and dons traditional dress; a colonialist, primitivist view of Major Sumner in tribal dress would insist, on the other hand, that we are witnessing the last representative of a culture which has long been submerged. Thus, our perception of the repatriation scene, through habitualized forms of looking, may in fact sabotage the ethics of the scene we are witnessing and the emotions which – in spite of the garbled message sent to us by our own eyes which have been habitualized through a colonial gaze – we would like to feel. For at the heart of this scene, there is a righting of past wrongs, of ethical transgressions which led to indigenous bodies being brought into the display cabinets of Western museums in the first place. Our habitualized ways of looking, then, seem to confirm this politics of museumfication rather than resist it. The aim of humanities research in this context, then, is not only to challenge our habits of looking, but to expose the discourses which have conditioned this habitualized gaze. This is also true of our ways of perceiving the museum representatives, whose faces have been painted in the tradition of the Ngarrindjeri: By transforming their own faces and "indigenizing" them, these men are paying tribute to the dead, whose bodies had once unjustly been brought into the glass case of a Scottish museum. The Aboriginal patterns on white Scottish faces will seem incongruous, I would argue, only if we fail to recognize the codes of signification and of recognition at the heart of this repatriation ceremony:

> VOICEOVER: Sumner led a delegation to Scotland to collect the remains including skulls and a woman's ear bone. The skulls have been held in collections belonging to the National Museum of Scotland and Edinburgh University. Sumner burned Eucalyptus leaves as part of a traditional ceremony, which cleanses those who have been in contact with the ancestors' remains.
>
> [*The museum's representatives wearing black suits with their faces painted according to Ngarrindjeri custom, are seen cleansing themselves with smoke from burning Eucalyptus leaves presented to them by Major Sumner*]. ("Scotland Returns Aboriginal Remains")

It is at this very juncture that life writing narratives, whose reach by far exceeds that of mere anecdotes, can help us decode a system of signification through which we will be able to fully understand this ritual of repatriation and the ceremony we are witnessing. Only if we view this narrative and visual ceremony of repatriation through life narratives such as Minik's, we will be able to reverse and to unlearn a colonial politics and the *visual politics* (Mulvey) which gave rise to such colonialist practices, even if in the case of the Scottish museum, the ceremony revolves around the return of indigenous bodies not to Greenland, but to Australia. What is at stake, I want to argue in this chapter, is a transnational, a global politics of repatriation and the restoration of justice to indigenous communities, from the Danish Arctic to Australia.

What would happen, I would like to ask in this chapter, if we were to adapt Laura Mulvey's theory of "visual pleasure" and the gender coding of this pleasure in mainstream film (1975) to a visual politics which has been complicit in erasing from view the contemporaneity of indigenous communities across the globe? To the extent that our eyes insist on seeing Major Sumner's presence against the background of the National

Museum of Scotland as bizarre, we have internalized a visual politics whose pleasure derives from relegating indigenous presences to the past. The act of seeing Major Sumner as bizarre is informed by the very politics which led to the necessity of a repatriation ceremony in the first place: Had it not been for a colonialist imaginary which saw every living native as the last of his tribe, the bodies which are now being repatriated could not have been brought to Western museums in the first place.

Thus, seen through an alternative perspective, the image of an Aboriginal religious representative in front of a Scottish museum of natural history will seem bizarre only as long as we fail to acknowledge a Ngarrindjeri system of signification. What takes place in this ceremony is a burial ritual long overdue; a burial in keeping with an indigenous tradition which had once been denied to Minik, the Inuit boy from Greenland. It is in this context that we may recall the museum curators' staging a "mock burial" of Qisuk, Minik's father. As Kenn Harper emphasizes in his biography of Minik, it was this fake burial rite, mock-native and performed in order to prevent Minik from reclaiming his father's body, which was truly bizarre. What was bizarre, Harper emphasizes, was the museum curators' and anthropologists' blatant disregards of human rights and the ethics of mourning. To speak of Major Sumner's repatriation ritual as bizarre, then, would add oil to a historical fire – the deprivation of indigenous communities of the most fundamental rights imaginable – which has been burning for centuries.

Thus, to speak of the incongruence of Major Sumner's presence in front of a Scottish museum of natural history is nothing less than an entire history of the disenfranchisement of indigenous communities. This history of this deprivation of rights, and the practices of illegitimacy it entailed, started with exhibiting a recently deceased man, Qisuk – who had been invited to a New York museum to speak about his (contemporaneous) culture to begin with – in the display case of the Museum of Natural History. If for this man, a museum glass case is turned into his last resting place, who exactly is bizarre here? Thus, I would like to argue that the presumed bizarreness of the Ngarrindjeri repatriation ceremony in front of the Scottish museum of natural history is not the end, but only the beginning of a debate, a debate which could not be more timely at the beginning of the twenty-first century. It is a debate which revolves around the restoration of justice, and the acknowledgment, long overdue, of an alternative system of cultural signification:

> VOICEOVER: The Aboriginal remains were originally taken from Australia over a hundred years ago. Dr. John Scally from Edinburgh University says it's the right decision to return them.
>
> DR. JOHN SCALLY: So for us today, the small … the tiny ear bone that we've returned today in this beautiful ceremony is the end of the process for us.
>
> VOICEOVER: Although ceremonies like this are cause for celebration, many Aboriginal Australians are still fighting for their ancestors' remains to be returned to their homelands. ("Scotland Returns Aboriginal Remains")

The alleged clash between two different systems of signification, I would like to propose in this chapter, is inextricably tied to the history and the present of indigenous communities. In this ceremony which is only seemingly bizarre, Major Sumner, the religious representative of the Ngarrindjeri, an indigenous community in Southern Australia, reverses historical injustice by restoring to his ancestors a right which they had been denied for centuries: the right of proper burial, and the right of their descendants to mourn the death of their ancestors. The right to mourn, at the same time, is tied to the recognition of a culture which may be different, but which is by no means "primitive."

9.4 Reconciliation and the Politics of Apology

Thus to speak of the bizarreness of this repatriation ceremony could not be more misguided, and it could not be more misleading. Major Sumner is literally a survivor, a survivor of the wrongs and atrocities of Australian colonial policy, a policy which was responsible for the so-called "Stolen Generation." The fact that today, at the beginning of the twenty-first century, Major Sumner can conduct a repatriation ceremony in traditional tribal dress in the first place is a vivid testimony to the "survivance" (Vizenor) of Aboriginal cultures, and the resilience of an indigenous community which, in spite of myriads of political compulsory measures has been able to retain and to continue to develop its cultural tradition. It is in this sense that repatriation is inextricably interwoven with a politics of reconciliation, the reconciliation between white Australians and the Aboriginal communities whose history has been one of disenfranchisement. Major Sumner's very presence in the repatriation ceremony, then, defies the history of this disenfranchisement. The fact that he is able to conduct this ceremony, the fact that at the beginning of the twenty-first century, the bodies of deceased indigenous Australians from museums throughout the world can be returned to the communities from which they had come, is characteristic of an about-face of Australian national policy and a potential new beginning at the outset of the twenty-first century. On February 13, 2008, Australian Prime Minister Kevin Rudd apologized, in a historic speech, to the survivors of the Stolen Generation.

What, then, did it imply, the pernicious policy which led to the "stolen generation"? The Stolen Generation is inextricably tied to the politics of assimilation. It was assumed that in a racialist society, "Aboriginals" would only survive if they assimilated to the dominant society not only culturally, but physically and phenotypically as well. Thus the aim was nothing short of genetic selection. As Henry Reynolds writes in his book *Nowhere People* (2005), referring to the "Protector of Aboriginal Affairs" A.O. Neville, "Neville's solution was biological assimilation . . . . Full bloods should only be allowed to marry other full bloods. In fact, they should be 'rigidly excluded from any association likely to lead to any other union.' And eventually they would die out" (184). In this sense, the politics of assimilation was an allegedly well-meaning one; it is in this sentiment that its perfidiousness lay. The goal of this politics which claimed to be nothing less than a "protection" of indigenous communities was nothing short of an "expunction" of indigenous genetic make-up. Those were seen as worthy of being "civilized" who already possessed "white" genes; it was the aim of subsequent national policies to "generate" from this group of people, who were designated as "half-castes" descendants who would finally be completely white. The extent of psychological trauma resulting from this politics of assimilation could not be more dramatic: Children were literally torn from their parents and brought to boarding schools, where they would have to suffer psychological, physical and sexual abuse. The policy's aim was, as it was often put at the time, "to kill the Aborigine in the child." These children were brought to abhor their own skin color; they were made to simultaneously worship and abhor the whiteness within themselves, thus being literally turned into broken individuals. Most of the children would never see their parents and siblings again. As Neville himself explained, "The child is taken away from the mother and sometimes never sees her again. Thus these children grow up as whites, knowing nothing of their environment" (Reynolds 185).

In 1996, thousands of testimonies of survivors from the Stolen Generation were collected in a report by the Australian Human Rights Commission. These testimonies would later be made public in the documentary *Bringing Them Home* (1997), which is available as a youtube clip:

> *National Inquiry into the Separation of Aboriginal and Torres Strait Islander Children from Their Families.*
>
> MICK DODSON [*Social Justice Commissioner*]: We wish to dedicate this video to those of the Stolen Generation, who had the courage to come forward and tell the inquiry their stories. We also want to dedicate it to the mothers who couldn't come before us and speak of their loss. We also want the video to make the report as broadly accessible as possible to all Australians so that they may know this aspect of our tragic history. ("Bringing them home")

One of the questions which I would like to ask throughout this study is this: In what format are life writing narratives contained? In this chapter, as in the previous chapter on *Nuclear Savage* (Chapter 7), I am concerned with the role of documentary film in collective life writing narratives or rather, oral testimonies. It is in this context that the benefit of "life writing" as a concept for the humanities (and, as I suggest here, also for medical humanities) may lie, as it links oral and written narratives, witness accounts, and documentary film.

Yet, what led to the conducting of the original report by the Australian Human Rights Commission in the first place? What developments, I would like to ask in this chapter, bring about a change in national policy making, the about-face of an entire nation? The report started out from the observation that the vast majority of Aboriginal Australians were suffering from alcoholism and were part of what today is termed "dysfunctional families." Yet, what factors had led up to this dire situation? The Australian Human rights Commission subsequently revealed the devastating consequences, for indigenous communities in Australia, of the history and policies of assimilation. The commission found that the majority of mothers found themselves unable to develop a close relationship to their own children, since they themselves had never known what such a relationship would be like. As the President of the Australian Human Rights Commission, Sir Robert Wilson, puts it:

> SIR RONALD WILSON As one woman said graphically, I'm a rotten mother. I cannot cuddle my children. And that's because I was never cuddled. I never knew what it was to be cuddled. Looking back, I believe perhaps the only time I felt I was being cuddled was when I was being raped. And you would hardly call that a cuddle, would you?" ("Bringing them home")

For the first time in Australia's national history, the blame was cast not on indigenous communities themselves, but on a colonial politics which today's historians have described as a form of cultural genocide. For the first time in the nation's history, the oral narratives and testimonies by survivors of subsequent colonial regimes were being heard; and they were being heard in a political climate that had finally been changed, a climate which investigated Australia's colonial history *in the language of human rights*. It was the discourse of human rights which made the life narratives of the members of the Stolen Generation hearable; many of the children who had once been forced to attend boarding schools, some of them as young as three months old, learned for the first time in their lives that they had had parents in the first place. In the language of human rights, then, and in the psychological language of trauma, the extent of the horrors of the residential schools were revealed for the first time in Australia's history:

> SONG: This story's right
>
> This story's true
>
> I would not tell lies to you
>
> [*Documentary footage shows, in black and white, children who are being brought to a mission school.*]
>
> Like the promises they would not keep

[*An official is shown handing out food to Aboriginal children, all of them perhaps three or four years of age, all dressed in Western clothing.*]

How they fenced us in like sheep

[*Documentary footage shows Aboriginal fathers and mothers are trying to protect their children from being taken away; the next shot shows children in a classroom, their heads bent over their desks.*]

Said to us, come take our hand

Set us up on mission land

Taught us to read

To write and pray

[*A photograph shows two boys dressed in identical shirts and their little sister, stepping off a train, surrounded by police and officials.*]

They took the children away

[*Photograph: A group of boys, all dressed in identical uniforms, their faces sad and unsmiling; a number of other photographs with boys and girls, all dressed in mission school uniforms.]*

Snatched from their mother's breast

Said this is for the best

Took them away.

Taught them that and taught them this

And others taught them prejudice

You took the children away

The children away.

WILSON: The people who were flogged as children and their memory of institutional life is of daily beatings and of periodic sexual abuse. I'll never forget the description of one institution where the children would be in a dormitory, twenty or thirty children, and they would be rigid with terror at night when they heard the steps of an official of the institution coming into their dormitory and wondering if tonight it would be them.

BURNUM BURNUM [*speaking about an Aboriginal Boys' Orphanage*]: They received their job on the negligence of the government, who didn't

> have any important recruiting factors that could allow us to have caring substitute parents. And of course, um, unrepeatable acts were perpetuated upon the boys. This is a tragic chapter in our national history. How can we heal our wounds? How can we really share our pain? There was something like 100,000 children taken away by tricks and force and lies from their mothers. Whole families and communities have been suffering. ("Bringing them home")

Thus it was all the more dramatic and all the more devastating for the survivors who had come forward to testify that nothing followed from the inquiry by the Australian Human Rights Commission. The commission had found that the policies enacted by successive governments with regard to Australia's indigenous populations constituted a form of cultural genocide:

> WILSON: It was genocide. I didn't know it at the beginning but I since have no doubt that it was genocide. One of the definitions of genocide is the fifth clause in the definition of the Genocide Convention and it says, "the removing of children from their communities with a view to extinguishing their culture." Now, you've only got to say that to appreciate that it was genocide. That's exactly what the assimilation policy was all about in its effect. In taking these children, whatever the motives and however good they were, it nevertheless was a necessary part of the practice, the policy to separate them from their families and communities in order to extinguish their culture. And it was not only their culture, their connection with the land, that important connection which is really part of an Aboriginal person's very being – and it was clearly genocide. ("Bringing them home")

Yet, for twelve years, subsequent Australian governments would hush up this conclusion; only in 2008 would Australian Prime Minister Kevin Rudd issue an official apology. In this apology, which I have already discussed in the previous chapter, Rudd apologized for the extent of the trauma which had been inflicted on mothers and fathers, and brothers and sisters, and for the fact that this trauma had been inflicted on the indigenous population in the name of "protection."

The concept of "reconciliation" comprises much more than the formal speech act of the official apology; at its core, there is also a psychological and an ethical dimension. For reconciliation to begin, there needs to be a period of mourning. Mourning, in this context, implies first and foremost the recognition of the life that is being mourned, and that can be legitimately mourned. History, as Judith Butler has argued and as I have elaborated in the previous chapter, goes off track the very moment in which we distinguish between lives that can and that cannot be mourned (*Precarious Life* x). Reconciliation can only begin once this distinction is itself regarded as objectionable and illegitimate. Reconciliation begins with the recognition, on all levels – juridical, political and ethical – that the right to mourn must not be denied to any individual or to any ethnic community.

At the core of an apology, there is what literary studies would term a change of perspective: For the healing of the traumas of the past can only begin once the perpetrator of past wrongs is aware of and recognizes his own guilt. But even more than that: Healing can only begin once the perpetrator of injustice has demonstrated that he is aware of the gravity of his transgression on all levels, physical, psychological and ethical. Only once the perpetrator of injustice, the erstwhile colonializer, can adopt the perspective of the indigenous communities and can describe, from their point of view, the extent of psychological horror which he has inflicted on these communities, can reconciliation begin.[4] It is this change in perspective which is at the center of Prime Minister Rudd's apology: What would have happened, he asks the opponents of the apology, those who had argued against the government's issuing an official apology, if they had had to suffer what the member of the Stolen Generation had to?

Second and as important, there is the necessity of recognizing the life narratives told by the survivors as a form of *evidence*. The most important form of evidence which Rudd relies on in his apology is the evidence provided by life narratives, the life narratives of the survivors of the Stolen Generation; and the traumas conveyed by these life narratives. Rudd's historic speech is thus a direct consequence, I would ar-

[4] Its rhetorical and psychological power notwithstanding, there are many shortcomings of the concepts of "reconciliation." First and foremost, it places the burden of the acknowledgment of the apology on the victims of successive colonial policies. It is the indigenous population of Australia which is now asked to accept the apology, an apology for acts so atrocious that they may in fact be unforgivable. I am indebted to Eva Bösenberg for this aspect.

gue, of the de-hierarchising between scientific discourse – the very discourse which had regarded indigenous men and women as test objects, whose bones could be exhibited in museum display cases or who could be used for a politics of "breeding out" indigenous genes – and life narratives. From the perspective of literary studies and life writing research, this historical moment is so utopian – in the sense of a utopia come true – because it not only puts life narratives on the same level as legislative texts, but because it goes on to reverse this hierarchy: In his apology, Rudd proceeds to read the laws enacted by successive Australian governments through the counter-evidence provided by the life narratives of the survivors of the Stolen Generation. The original hierarchy which saw in a life narrative only a mere anecdote, to whose claims the law was completely oblivious, has completely been reversed in Rudd's historic apology at the beginning of the twenty-first century. In Rudd's apology, it is the life narrative that has become the true point of reference; it is through the life narrative and its power of interpretation that we decide what lives were made possible or rendered impossible by the Australian political and legal systems. For this utopian moment, however temporary, the law has become a mere footnote in the life narrative, whose valence by far exceeds the law.

To an unprecedented extent, Rudd's apology recognizes and acknowledges the life narratives of survivors such Nanna Nungala Fejo, and he recognizes these narratives as what Ottmar Ette, in a different context, has termed "Lebenswissen":

> Some have asked, "Why apologise?" Let me begin to answer by telling the parliament just a little of one person's story—an elegant, eloquent and wonderful woman in her 80s, full of life, full of funny stories, despite what has happened in her life's journey, a woman who has travelled a long way to be with us today, a member of the stolen generation who shared some of her story with me when I called around to see her just a few days ago.
>
> Nanna Nungala Fejo, as she prefers to be called, was born in the late 1920s. She remembers her earliest childhood days living with her family and her community in a bush camp just outside Tennant Creek. She remembers the love and the warmth and the kinship of those days long ago, including traditional dancing around the camp fire at night. She loved the dancing. . . .

> But then, sometime around 1932, when she was about four, she remembers the coming of the welfare men. Her family had feared that day and had dug holes in the creek bank where the children could run and hide. What they had not expected was that the white welfare men did not come alone.
>
> They brought a truck, two white men and an Aboriginal stockman on horseback cracking his stockwhip. The kids were found; they ran for their mothers, screaming, but they could not get away. They were herded and piled onto the back of the truck. Tears flowing, her mum tried clinging to the sides of the truck as her children were taken away to the Bungalow in Alice, all in the name of protection. (The Australian n. pag.)[5]

In the Australian Prime Minister's speech, the distinction between expert knowledge and lay perspective, between the scientific treatise and the "mere" life narrative, has been abolished, if only temporarily so; at the center of his apology, there is the life narrative as the form of an alternative production of knowledge.

The third aspect of the apology, which I would like to discuss here, following the idea of a change in perspective and the recognition of the life narrative as a form of evidence, is an inquiry into the language in which the apology is framed. For the testimonies, the witness accounts by the survivors of the Stolen Generation, are so powerful especially because they convey the extent of the trauma suffered by indigenous Australians due to the pernicious politics of assimilation.

It is at this point that I would like for a moment to return to Minik, the young Inuit. What difference does it make for us to say that Minik mourned his father's death, as opposed to saying that Minik was severely traumatized by the sudden loss of his father and the subsequent museumfication of his body? How does our perception change once we assume that experiences like these often result in forms of PTSD or Post-traumatic Stress Disorder? My claim in this context is this: If we speak of Minik's traumatization in a sense which can be medically diagnosed, this description will seem all the more powerful; there is a sense in which Minik's grief has thus been translated into our language and

[5] For the full transcript of the Prime Minister's speech, see The Australian.

our terminology. His loss, moreover, is not only a cultural one, but it is now recognized to have a psychological and a physical dimension. Our reaction to Minik's loss, as problematic as this may be in a number of senses, may vary to the extent to which we can recognize this loss in the terms of our own inventory of ideas. Minik's own perception, which is only handed down to us through narrative, is thus validated at the very moment in which it becomes measurable through our own methods, our own methodological inventory.

In order to discuss this process of validation, I would like to resort to an example from a field which may at first glance seem unrelated. At the beginning of the twenty-first century, our perspective on indigenous cultures has changed to an unprecedented degree, and it has changed because we now possess the possibility of validating indigenous knowledge through Western methodology. This may be especially pronounced in the field of indigenous medicine. Well into the twentieth century, the indigenous shaman or healer would be derided and dismissed as a remnant of an ancient civilization which had long been extinct. Indigenous medicine was regarded as mere superstition. Yet, to the extent to which the effectiveness of indigenous herbs and medicines can be proven through the methods of Western medicine, a completely different perspective on indigenous systems of knowledge starts to take hold. Such recognition of indigenous forms of knowledge is also true for current climate research. From a humanities perspective, we may be skeptical about such processes of validation: Why should we acknowledge the efficacy of indigenous methods and knowledge systems only once we have measured them by our own yardsticks and validated them on our own terms? These problems and pitfalls notwithstanding, the moment of recognition remains. What arises from this validation is a new form of recognition of indigenous knowledge not as superstition, but as knowledge in its own right.

This validation also relates to the question of the traumatization of indigenous cultures through Western colonial policies which amounted to forms of cultural genocide. Today, we know that traumas can become physically manifest even in a change of an individual's DNA; today, we speak of multi-generational traumas. Thus, Thomas Elbert and Maggie Schauer have referred to the concept of "biological memory" ("*biologisches Gedächtnis*" 66): "Epigenetic modifications constitute molecular correlates of memory formationen. . . . [It has also been emphasized], that long-term epigenetic modifications can be passed on to subsequent generations" (75-76). What is crucial here is that with regard to the proof of epigenetic modifications in the DNA structure, life sciences and life writing can actually work in tandem. As I have outlined above, life writing narratives can provide proof, through narrative evidence and forms of witnessing, of the trauma suffered by individuals in the past. New technologies in the life sciences, on the other hand, can provide material evidence supporting these testimonies. This material evidence, in turn, can also have profound consequences for these individuals and communities finally being granted compensation.

Until the end of the twentieth century, Indigenous Australians as well as Native Americans in the U.S. and First Nations in Canada, were accused of being innately prone to alcoholism, or innately averse to work. Today, on the other hand, there is evidence that alcoholism can directly result from traumatization, as can severe depressions which will render an individual unable to work. To this day, the life expectancy of Australia's indigenous population is seventeen years below that of the majority population. If we take all this into account, how can we begin to see Major Sumner's repatriation ceremony anew and with different eyes? For indigenous Australians, the trauma of the missionary schools lay in the schools' attempts to forcibly "civilize" their students; they were made not only to discontinue, but to abhor their own languages and cultural practices. The fact that today, there are indigenous communities which are able to conduct a repatriation ceremony at once testifies to the survival of an entire culture. Major Sumner's cultural pride and his cultural self-reflexivity, testify to the "survivance" and resilience of indigenous communities in Australia. Once the ceremony is over, we can be assured, Major Sumner will change into his T-shirt and jeans; and he will be living at a time in which indigeneity and Australianness will no longer be regarded as being at odds with one another. It is the promise of such an Australia for which Kevin Rudd vouches in his speech.

9.5 Conclusion: The Twenty-First Century as the "Age of Apology"

It is with the apology, the recognition of trauma and a repatriation ceremony that we have come full circle from a development which had once begun with Minik, the New York Inuit. The beginning of the twenty-first century is marked as a historical moment in which for the first time in history, a global form of reversal seems to have become possible. There is much solace in the idea that the twenty-first century, which has been marked by a resurgence of religious fundamentalism and by global terror, is also the age of apology. A century at the beginning of which an unprecedented number of court decisions have declared previous laws as illegitimate, laws which throughout the world had led to the disenfranchisement of indigenous populations.

Many of these apologies, I have tried to argue in this chapter, proceeded from the life narratives of survivors, life narratives which functioned at one and the same time as testimonies and as an indictment of colonial regimes. Thus, forms of life writing may constitute locations of an alternative production of knowledge; these life narratives oppose the discourse of the life sciences, which regards the bodies of recently deceased human beings as scientific *objets trouvés,* by confronting them with the biographies and autobiographies, which make the lives of these human beings visible as *human* lives.

For the first time in the history of the last five hundred years, the history of Western conquest in North and South America, in Australia and New Zealand, there are formalized and official legal procedures, which are meant to prevent a deprivation of rights for indigenous populations throughout the world, and which set out to make possible the revision of historical injustice. In this new form of legal conception, the United Nations Declaration of the Rights of Indigenous Peoples (UNDRIP, 2007) and the institutionalization of the UN Permanent Forum on Indigenous Issues have certainly been milestones. It is with these measures that the United Nations reacted to the accusation that the Declaration of Human Rights was not sufficient to protect the rights of indigenous populations; that there needed to be another declaration specifically concerned with the rights of indigenous peoples. When we look at the history not only of Australia, this line of argument is certainly conclusive. For as Minik's case vividly demonstrates, the ethical short-circuit in many Western nation-states was precisely the assumption that indigenous groups were *differently* human, if they were human at all. The new, recently enacted laws, in turn, are inextricably connected to the history and the present of compensation, reparation and even reconciliation. These laws, and the apologies which Western governments have finally come around to extending to indigenous communities, at long last enact what had once been denied to Minik, the New York Inuit: The right for recognition of their own genealogy and their own history.

This chapter has assumed the perspective of both transnational American Studies and comparative indigenous studies to investigate what is in fact a global politics of repatriation and (potential) reconciliation. Minik's story, the story with which this chapter began, was one of cultural contact. As Kenn Harper writes in his conclusion, Minik, after he had finally been able to return to Greenland, had never stopped longing for New York; it was in New Hampshire that he would eventually die, still in his twenties:

> Out of place in New York, he felt no more at home when he returned to northern Greenland. The feeling of alienation led him back to the United States in 1916, where he told his old friend, John D. Clark, that the bright lights of Broadway attracted him more than the northern lights. In the fall of 1917, he arrived in northern New Hampshire, and died there one year later. He died among friends . . . . (228-29)

Minik's life narrative, turned into a form of life writing by Kenn Harper, was hence many stories at once: the story of an Inuit boy brought from Greenland to New York's Museum of Natural History by an American explorer, Robert Peary, and the story of an elective New Yorker who would never again feel at home in Greenland even after his return. At the same time, I would argue in this chapter that in the history of U.S. legislation, the passing of NAGPRA can only be fully appreciated as part of a global process and the repositioning of nation states such as Australia and Canada at the beginning of the twenty-first century. It is in this sense, I have proposed in this chapter, that the eventual return of the body of Minik's father Qisuk cannot be separated from the return of the bodies finally reclaimed by the Ngarrindjeri from the National Museum of Scotland. It is Minik's story, and the ceremony conducted by Major Sumner, which give these bodies both a name and a narrative. Life writing is hence an integral part of the politics of repatriation and reconciliation.

Yet why, I would like to ask at the end of this chapter, would a discussion of repatriation and the rights of indigenous communities to mourning and burying their dead be part of a book concerned with medical humanities? I would like to argue that in order for medical humanities to live up to their potential, they must explore not only the current practice of biomedicine, but also its history. The history and present of the life sciences has been important for this chapter, then, on two accounts. First, this chapter has looked into the history of anthropology as a life sciences discipline (avant-la-lettre); second, it has re-read indigenous history through the concept of trauma, which has now been additionally validated through the methods of the life sciences. Minik's story, I have argued in this chapter, is not simply a tragic one; it is a story of trauma, and of trauma inflicted on an indigenous community in the name of science. If indeed we read Minik's narrative as a trauma narrative, then, it can squarely be located within the discourse of medical humanities. To locate Minik's story within medical humanities, then, is to acknowledge his life writing, handed down to us in the form of Kenn Harper's groundbreaking biography, as both a testimony to native survival *and* a patient narrative. The fact that it was denied such status, that it was regarded only as a story or anecdote and not as the patient narrative of a young man severely traumatized by colonial politics, is itself part of an historical amnesia. That the breach of indigenous rights was denied to have a traumatic effect on the members of indigenous communities, was itself a form of violence. As I will elaborate in the next chapter, then, I believe that it is essential to link medical humanities to discussions of social justice. It is in this sense that the process of repatriation, as it sets out to heal centuries of trauma, has everything to do with the framework of medical humanities.

10 Sustainability and Indigenous Life Writing Performances: "Dancing Earth" and *The Cherokee Word for Water*

This chapter takes up an idea which has already been discussed in Chapter 8 with regard to nuclear testing in the Pacific: the link between indigenous rights and environmental justice. Yet, it adds to this nexus the question of sustainability: What, then, does sustainability mean in the context not just of contemporary ecocriticism but also in the context of indigenous rights? What, moreover, would sustainability mean in the context of medical humanities? This paper argues for the inclusion of a variety of topics into the discussion of medical humanities, topics which may so far have been absent from this debate: First, what does it mean to include the notion of sustainability into medical humanities, and how would it change the concept of medical humanities as such? At best, we may argue, medical humanities may be concerned not only with narratives of illness but also with the conditions under which health can be maintained. Can there be a discussion of illness, in other words, without a discussion or awareness of health? In this sense, then, it may not only be useful but essential to include the concept of sustainability into the field of medical humanities. Thus, if my chapter on the film *Nuclear Savage* has been concerned with the consequences of the "slow violence" (Nixon 45) inflicted on the Marshallese, then the antidote to this slow violence of nuclear pollution and other environmentally damaging practices is sustainability. Moreover, sustainability, in the instances I would like to explore in this chapter, is closely related to indigenous rights and the countering of environmental racism.

What, then, about forms of life writing in this context? As I have argued in Chapter 5 with regard to Mikhail Baryshnikov's "HeartBeat: mb" performance, dance, too, can be seen as a form of life writing. Moreover, as in the earlier chapter on the Marshall Islands, I will be concerned here with *collective* forms of life writing. As I will try to show with regard to both the performance art of the Native dance collective "Dancing Earth" and the 2013 feature film, *The Cherokee Word for Water*, both these representations explore the role of indigenous epistemologies and indigenous forms of alternative, communal leadership for developing concepts of sustainability. The performances by the dance company "Dancing Earth" as well as the solo performance by Rosy Simas, and the film *The Cherokee Word for Water* revolve around the nexus of water and sustainability. In both representations, water is linked not only to life itself, but also specifically to human rights and indigenous rights, an intersection which I have already discussed in Chapter 8.[1]

In this chapter, I am interested in the relationship between sustainability on the one hand and, on the other, the sustained presence of the past. While the concept of "sustainability" seems to be future-oriented,

[1] The protests at Standing Rock Reservation against the Dakota Access Pipeline (DAPL) constitute another, recent chapter in the fight for indigenous sovereignty and rights, health and well-being, for clean water and natural resources. The months-long indigenous protests against the 3.8 billion pipeline project that, as the Standing Rock Sioux tribe has been arguing since 2014, cuts through ancestral lands including a sacred tribal burial ground (on land which belongs to Native American communities due to the Treaty of Fort Laramie (1851)) and potentially threatens indigenous water resources on their territory, received international mainstream news media attention throughout 2016 and 2017. Significantly, before being redirected to traverse parts of the Standing Rock Reservation territory, an alternative route of the 1,200 mile pipeline, north of the North Dakota state capital of Bismarck, a predominantly white community, "was proposed but rejected because of its proximity to areas that supply water" (Aisch and Lai n. pag.). After the Obama administration blocked the construction of the segment under dispute in December 2016, President Trump signed executive orders to advance the pipeline's completion a few days after taking office in January 2017. On June 1, 2017, the Dakota Access Pipeline began commercial operations. A few weeks later, a federal D.C. disctrict court judge ruled that the pipeline had not received an adequate environmental review by the U.S. Army Corps of Engineers prior to being put into service. Yet, he did not order the pipeline to cease operations until the requested environmental review is completed, which is not to be expected before the end of 2017. (Aisch and Lai n. pag.; Baker and Davenport n. pag.; Buncombe n. pag.; Hayes n. pag.; Meyer n. pag.; Nicholson n. pag.; Ravitz n. pag.; Wolff n. pag.; Worland n. pag.). I am indebted to Rebecca Schäfer for this point.

the sustained presence of the past evokes the legacy of past injustices and experiences of trauma on both the present and the future. I believe that this deliberate jumbling of tenses is not so much paradoxical as it is imperative. If sustainability is oriented towards the future, the adjective "sustained" is directed towards the past. I will try to propose in this chapter that to understand "sustainability" only with reference to the future is to fall short of a full-scale recognition of Native American pasts and presents. Moreover, the very attempt to separate the future from the present or the past would run counter to indigenous epistemologies, which have insisted on a rejection of temporal linearity and a specific (Western) sense of chronology.

As a performance by Native artist Rosy Simas, to which I will turn in more detail below, vividly demonstrates, there can be no moving into the future without simultaneously reckoning with the impact of the past. What the performance also illustrates, then, is the necessity of countering the "willful" amnesia of settler colonies, willful amnesia that starts with the "terra nullius" doctrine which I have already investigated in the previous chapter. The willful amnesia thus claims a territory that it *wills* to be empty, hence seeking to erase both the presence and the past of indigenous communities and indigenous knowledge systems. Contemporary research projects on sustainability and climate change have embraced indigenous knowledge systems, arguing that what Native American critic Gerald Vizenor has called the effects of a "chemical civilization" will eventually cause the planet to self-destruct.

10.1 The Ecocritical Ventriloquism of "Mother Earth"

I would like to start with an image which, at first glance, may be far from the academic debate on ecocriticism: a poster for the 2012 local election campaign of the German Green Party, *Bündnis 90/Die Grünen*. In its depiction of the vulnerability of our "blue planet," the poster encapsulates the discourse of sustainability. As the image vividly conveys through the wide-angle shot of the earth seen from outer space, our blue planet is vulnerable, endangered, and urgently in need of sustaining, if only for our own sake. Yet, what about the caption which accompanies this image of the small blue planet in the poster? And who, exactly, is speaking here? Who, precisely, is cautioning us to take good care of "Mutter Erde" or "Mother Earth"? This is an instance, I believe, of a particular kind of ventriloquism: it is an ecocritical ventriloquism, I would like to argue in this chapter, of indigeneity, and of an indigeneity which, the poster implies, is ecocritical avant la lettre.

In this chapter, I would like to explore precisely the nexus between indigeneity and ecocriticism, both of which may hinge on the concept of sustainability. In trying to unravel this nexus, I am interested, first, in this recent discovery, by ecocriticism, of a particular concept of indigeneity. The debate on sustainability, I want to suggest in this chapter, led to a particular form of (re)discovery not so much of indigenous rights as of indigenous epistemologies. This (re)discovery, as Julie Rak has recently argued in another context, is far from unproblematic. It is a discovery, above all, of indigeneity in the service of ecocriticism; therefore, it is by no means a discovery or rediscovery of indigeneity for its own sake. It is in this particular context of nostalgia, then, that Western civilization mourns both the environment and a lost form of indigeneity. It is no coincidence, then, that the Indian mouthing "Mutter Erde" in his last dying breath is absent from the picture; we are all the sorrier for the destruction of Mother Earth since the Indian mourning this destruction, the image implies, has already vanished. "We" have destroyed, the image implies, both Native civilizations and the planet which these civilizations had once urged us to safeguard.

There are two pitfalls in the argument inherent in the poster. The first pitfall, as I have already suggested, is the idea of what Gerald Vizenor has called the "myth of the vanishing Indian": Looking at the poster, we mourn not only the small blue planet which we are about to destroy but also the native civilization which, the poster implies through the absence of the speaker mouthing "Mother Earth," we have already destroyed. Sustainability, arguably, is thus closely related to a particular form of nostalgia: the nostalgia for a native civilization which is said to be extinct. Second and related to this is another pitfall: The slogan "Mother Earth," translated, for the purposes of regional campaigning in Rhineland Palatinate into the dialect of "Mudder Erde," also invokes the stereotype of what Krech has called the "ecological Indian." As Greg Garrard has noted, drawing on Krech's concept of environmental primitivism,

> Since the sixteenth century at least, "primitive" people have been represented as dwelling in harmony with nature, sustaining one of the most

> widespread and seductive myths of the non-European "other." The assumption of indigenous environmental virtue is a foundational belief for deep ecologists and many ecocritics. (120)

It is this eco-primitivism of native peoples, which, I believe, recurs in the Green Party poster. This, then, is an appropriation of Native epistemologies minus native peoples.

The question which I would like to explore in this chapter, then, is in what form and through what strategies Native American self-representations can "steal back" the image of themselves as inherently ecocritical. How, in other words, can Native calls for sustainability steer clear of the auto-stereotyping of the eco-Indian? As I will try to suggest in what follows, native self-representations can avoid the trap of the eco-Indian by linking sustainability to indigenous rights. Crucially, the image of the eco-Indian as being an ecocritic avant la lettre hijacks indigenous epistemologies in the service of (Western discourses of) ecocriticism, and in so doing, it *de*contextualizes these indigenous epistemologies from the contexts from which they have emerged. The first step towards re-appropriating indigenous discourses on sustainability, then, is to recontextualize these discourses and to reconnect them to the frameworks – cultural, legal, social and political – from which they arise.

In what follows, I would like to discuss two indigenous representations which can be said to hinge on notions of sustainability: the dance performance "Walking at the Edge of Water" by the inter-tribal dance collective "Dancing Earth" and the feature film *The Cherokee Word for Water*. I believe that it is far from coincidental that both these representations should center on water. In the era of biopiracy and the increasing privatization of natural resources, water and, by implication, health and well-being seem to have become the final frontier.

At the nexus between life sciences and life writing, I am reading Dancing Earth's performance as a form of life writing setting out to combat the power of both the life sciences and recent attempts to privatize nature. Patenting nature – a practice that should be logically impossible in the first place but which unfortunately is not – is hence the first step towards the commodification of nature. Privatization and commodification are sides of the same coin. In this context, too, the future and the past are inextricably connected. Biopiracy, the "plunder of nature and knowledge," as Vandana Shiva puts it (*Biopiracy*), can be countered only through the records form the past which document indigenous knowledge of the power of medicinal effects of these products, *even as* we are aware that they cannot ultimately be *owned*.

10.2 Performing Sustainability in Dancing Earth's "Walking at the Edge of Water"

The performance "Walking at the Edge of Water" by the inter-tribal dance collective "Dancing Earth" begins with an homage, a prayer to water as a life-sustaining force. Dancing Earth's performance "Walking at the Edge of Water" links debates on indigenous rights, environmental justice, indigenous knowledges, and sustainability. It is a plea or petition for the sustaining of water expressed through dance; "Walking at the Edge of Water" is both an ecocritical and an indigenous performance, with neither of these concepts being subsumed by the other. While the first part of the performance celebrates water as a natural force by combining dance elements from a variety of tribal backgrounds, the second act dramatizes the exhausting of natural resources and an environmental destruction the brunt of which has to be borne by native communities. The performance directly points to the destruction of native lands through uranium mining; it links the abuse of water to the environmental destruction of native lands,[2] and implicitly addresses the health risk tied to the mining of uranium. This is a practice, as Joni Adamson has argued, of what has been called "nuclear colonialism" (x). It is this "nuclear colonialism," also, which the performance "Walking at the Edge of Water" contests. As a female voiceover describes in the soundtrack to the performance, "They use 9000 gallons of water every minute mining uranium."

Let me return for a moment to the poster by the German Green party ventriloquizing an imaginary Indian. The small planet in the poster, of course, is a blue planet; and it is blue because the majority of its surface is made up of water, not land mass. It is in this context that the notion of vulnerability which the smallness of the planet conveys may also and

[2] Once again, this is reminiscent of the current debate on Standing Rock Reservation.

especially apply to the contested uses of water. What we need to sustain, above all, is the water which turns the planet blue in the first place. Yet, there is a universality captured in this argument: Mankind, the poster implicitly reminds us, needs water in order to survive. By implication, then, we are all culpable of squandering water as a resource and a life-sustaining force.

It is this universality of culpability which Dancing Earth turns on its head. Who, Dancing Earth asks, has been culpable of squandering water as a natural resource? The performance as an instance of native self-representation, I would like to argue here, zooms in not on the poster or the image of the small blue planet in the poster but *on the hand holding the camera*. Who, the performance asks, flies to outer space just in order to take an image of our small blue planet? And who precisely needs reminding that our earth and its natural resources are too precious to be squandered thoughtlessly? This may well be a form of a reverse of ethnography: Instead of an ethnographic image depicting the Indian as primitive, what we get is an Indian taking a picture of the Western eco-critic taking a picture of the earth from other space. Instead of the Indian primitive, we get a picture of the eco-primitiveness of Western civilization.

It is in this context, the context of the "universality" of an imaginary "mankind," that the reminder not to squander natural resources appears cynical. The context which Dancing Earth invokes is a context in which uranium is being mined on Indian reservations, through the use of millions of gallons of water per minute. Who, precisely, is culpable of squandering water here?

The performance can hence squarely be located in the field of environmental justice, stressing the role of the arts in drawing attention to what Adams has called "environmental racism." A term originally coined by Benjamin Chavis, "environmental racism" can be defined as "racial discrimination in environmental policy-making and the enforcement of regulations and laws, the deliberate targeting of people of color communities for toxic waste facilities, the official sanctioning of the life-threatening presence of poisons and pollutants in our communities, and [the] history of excluding people of color from leadership in the environmental movement" (Adamson 4). Crucially, then, environmental racism can be seen both in the withholding of access to water and in environmental destruction of native lands. It is in this sense that the performance “Walking at the Edge of Water” can be said to be an indictment of environmental colonialism and a performative call for environmental justice. As a review of the performance has noted,

> The second act is about the destruction mankind has wrought over the land. The pollution of the waters. The dancers wear tattered clothing, gas masks and confusion and chaos are prominent themes in this part of the performance. A structured chaos allows you to see how technological advances, making life more connected, have also served to make life disconnected to what the land provides naturally. (“Dance Review: ‘Walking at the Edge of Water” n. pag.)

In blatant irony, the performance stresses the fact that due to environmental damage and environmental racism, the gas mask has become part of contemporary native gear – an aspect that contemporary Native American visual artists such as Bunky Echo Hawk have stressed as well. Bunky Echo Hawk has created a series of paintings called “the gas mask series” which he describes on his website as follows:

> This series came about after learning about toxic, radioactive waste sites popping up in Indian Country. I felt compelled to share the knowledge of their existences, and to tie in the relationship of biological warfare of past years with the construction of these sites, which typically target Indian reservations. I wanted the message to be strong, undeniable, and memorable.
>
> The gas mask is a very formidable image. It conjures up memories of past wars, and perhaps, very tangibly, thoughts of impending wars. The gas mask image bridges the gaps between . . . the present, and the future. Though it is a symbol of war and a targeted nation, it is also one of preparation, organization, and survival.
>
> The gas mask, worn by Native Americans, signifies several other subjects. It is a reference to the Native American demographic collapse, or Holocaust, due largely to primitive colonial means of biological and germ warfare. (Bunky n. pag.)

The gas mask, in both visual art and the dance performance “Walking at the Edge of Water” accomplishes a variety of purposes at once. First, it marks the native subject as a contemporaneous one; not only has the “Indian” not yet vanished, but he is wearing a gas mask, a mask which, in the ancient past which he is said to belong to, had not yet been invented. Moreover, the gas mask shows the native subject's resistance to the environmental destruction of his or her land; wearing the gas mask can hence be seen, in Gerald Vizenor's terms, as an act of "survivance" (vii). At the same time, the necessity of having to wear a gas mask in the first place is a blatant indictment of the economic schemes of Western corporations which mine uranium on native lands.

Finally, the gas mask is the direct opposite of the stereotype of the eco-Indian. What if we were to reinsert the Indian into the Green Party Poster, and if we were to reinsert an Indian wearing a gas mask? What this image would reveal, I would like to argue, is a debunking of the universality implied in the poster: Not only has the Indian mouthing "Mother Earth" not vanished, but he is wearing a gas mask; this gas mask reveals, moreover, that the burden of the destruction of our small blue planet is borne not by white, Western communities but by native peoples and communities of color.

What is central in this context, I believe, is that the dance performance "Walking at the Edge of Water" destroys the temporality implicit in Western discourses on sustainability. Instead of invoking a nostalgia for a lost native civilization – a trope which, the performance implies, is itself part of the logic of Manifest Destiny (Vizenor x) –, the performance, through the image of the gas mask, stresses the contemporaneity of native civilizations. Instead of succumbing to a form of ecocritical cultural nostalgia for the vanishing Indian, it counters the past with the present. Yet, there is one more twist to this argument: The gas mask, as native artist Bunky Echo Hawk has argued, is also a sign of native survival in the face of environmental racism; and it is hence also directed towards the future of native civilizations. The nostalgia of Western ecocriticism is hence countered by native futurism, a futurism which, in this case, is performed through pan-tribal dancers wearing gas masks. As Dancing Earth describes its performance on its website, "This work is motivated by the urgings of Native grandmothers and invokes powerfully relevant water themes of creation, destruction and renewal. *Walking at the Edge of Water* parallels ancestral healing rituals in a dance of inter-disciplinary Native expressions that is both primal and futuristic" ("Walking…Edge of Water" n. pag.; emphasis original).

By referring to elements both "primal and futuristic," then, Dancing Earth stresses the performance of indigeneity, not its "essence." It is in this sense that Dancing Earth refuses to counter the stereotype of the eco-Indian with forms of autoethnography; rather, it revolves around a pan-indigenous (or "inter-tribal," as the website puts it) performance which at the same time resists the relegation of native peoples to the past. By invoking the voices of grandmothers, remembered by their grandchildren, the performance establishes a link to the past; yet at the same time, it stresses the need to redefine and rephrase these voices and their meaning for the present and the future: "[voiceover, female voice] My grandmother she has so much light in her voice when she talks … we rarely drink it, we don't eat fish from it… She talks about it being clear when she was young… you could see to the bottom… and she had such love for the water…" ("DANCING EARTH"). By invoking the voice of the speaker's grandmother, who remembers a time when the water was crystal clear, the voiceover also surveys the damage done to the environment, and the destruction of water: "we do not drink the water …. Rarely do we fish in it" ("DANCING EARTH"). As Joni Adamson has noted, the damage done to native communities through environmental damage is twofold: it poses both a health risk and amounts to the destruction of native ways of life. Adamson notes that indigenous communities, people of color, and rural communities have disproportionately been exposed to environmental justice violations. She writes, "Studies 'found race to be the leading factor in the location of commercial hazardous waste facilities and determined that poor and people of color communities suffer a disproportionate health risk: 60 percent of African American and Latino communities and over 50 percent of Asian/Pacific Islanders and Native Americans live in areas with one or more uncontrolled toxic waste sites'" (Adamson 4). Thus, as Adamson notes, native lands have been bearing the brunt of environmental destruction; even as environmental damage may be ubiquitous, then, native communities as well as people of color have been disproportionately exposed to such damage. What is needed, not only as a deconstruction of the Green Party Poster, is hence an emphasis, as Adamson puts it, on "the crucial intersections between ecological and social justice concerns" (4). It is this linkage, I believe, which the Green Party Poster elides through the universality of mankind and its destruction of "Mother Earth."

10.3 *The Cherokee Word for Water* (2013)

There are a number of overlaps between the performance "Walking at the Edge of Water" and the 2013 feature film *The Cherokee Word for Water*. The question the film asks both implicitly and explicitly is what happens if the "Cherokee word for water" is translated into a Western discourse of rights. The Cherokee word for water, the film emphasizes, does not quite translate into English; and this is a question far beyond either language or linguistic translation, but it is a question of *epistemology:*

> [CHARLIE SOAP, *walking by the river; voiceover*] Long before the United States existed, the Cherokee people had a society based on democratic principles. They were guided by the spirit of balance between the self and community, elders and youth, men and women. One Cherokee community was reminded of that balance in the early 1980s…
>
> The Cherokee word for water is… Ama is how you say it. Ama. [*in Cherokee language, subtitled*] Water is sacred. [*image of a bucket being filled in the river*]. We use water in everything we do. If it wasn't for water, we wouldn't be alive. (*The Cherokee Word for Water*)

If I have argued above that in the context of contemporary native communities in the U.S. the very question of who exactly squanders the natural resources of water is cynical, the film *The Cherokee Word for Water* does this question one better. It is hard to squander water, the film implies, in a rural Cherokee community which does not have access to running water in the first place. It is hard to squander water, the film illustrates, if before squandering it, you have to collect it from a well.

What I am concerned with in this chapter, then, is the ways in which "health," too, may have become a contested signifier and a contested practice at the beginning of the twenty-first century. First, health can be defined as a human right, the right of each and every community to well-being, regardless of the racial or social status of this community. This right, both Barack Obama and the feature film *The Cherokee Word for Water* can be said to argue, has not been extended to minority communities within the U.S., barring African Americans, Native Americans, as well as poor communities from access to health services and non-toxic environments. According to Joni Adamson, "Environmental justice initiatives specifically attempt to redress the disproportionate incidence of environmental contamination in communities of the poor and/or communities of color, to secure for those affected the right to live unthreatened by the risks posed by environmental degradation and contamination, and to afford equal access to natural resources that sustain life and culture" (4).

The film starts, then, with a curiously off-handed depiction of the poverty of both rural Cherokee and rural poor white communities in Bell, Oklahoma:

> [WOMAN]: In this house that we live in, there's no water. There's no inside toilet or anything like that, it's outside. [*The camera shows a girl with her mother, pumping water from a well. Voiceover,* CHARLIE SOAP] If there is no water, many communities begin to scatter, fall apart. That's what was happening by the 1970s. After so many years of broken treaties, empty promises, and deliberate neglect, our Cherokee community stopped thinking about change. They stopped thinking about what we could do together. (*The Cherokee Word for Water*)

The film is curiously pragmatic in the didacticism it elides: Its call for justice, its critique of a form of health discrimination that bars some communities from running water, is never made explicit. Crucially, the WHO guidelines target areas in the developing world which do not have sufficient access to running water and adequate sanitation. What the film invokes, however, is a situation in which this lack of access and the ensuing health risk also pertains to native and rural communities within the U.S.: "Goal 7 . . . of the Millennium Development Goals aims at halving by 2015 the proportion of people without sustainable access to safe drinking water and basic sanitation" ("United Nations Millennium Development Goals" n. pag.).

The film can be seen as both a form of life writing and an indigenous call for environmental justice. It zooms in on the life of a woman who set out to claim the rights of a Cherokee rural community to running water, a woman named Wilma Mankiller. The film begins with Wilma's leaving the city and moving back to the rural village of Bell, Oklahoma:

> Then something happened that no-one expected. It started with the return of one Cherokee woman. Wilma Mankiller. [WILMA MANKILLER *is shown driving back to Mankiller Flats, Oklahoma, her two daughters asleep next to her.*]

> WILMA [*to her daughters*]: We did it! We're home.
>
> FELICIA [*incredulous*]: People live here?
>
> WILMA: Your grandma does. Now we do, too.
>
> [WILMA *and her younger daughter get out of the car. Wilma's mother comes out to greet them, hugs her daughter.*]
>
> WILMA: Hey, ma.
>
> [FELICIA *has stayed in the car, looking on suspiciously. As the scene ends, she puts up the hood of her sweater and huddles more deeply into her seat.*] (*The Cherokee Word for Water*)

As the irony of this scene makes clear, Wilma Mankiller's older daughter Felicia is clearly aware that she seems to have moved to the "Third World," an outlandish time and space where no-one could possibly live. It is this ethnography of primitiveness – a primitiveness both rural and native – which the filmic narrative proceeds to turn on its head:

> *School, Bell, Oklahoma. Women and children are collecting water from an outdoor faucet.*
>
> WOMAN # 1: Do you really think they're gonna close down this place?
>
> WOMAN # 2: No… Sure hate to go to get water every day, though.
>
> WOMAN # 1 [*looking at the school building in front of her*]: This is where my grandma went to school. There's a lot of history here. [*the camera shows the water canister in her hand*]. [*The women and their children turn to carry canisters and buckets of water back home*]. (*The Cherokee Word for Water*)

Crucially, the film zooms in *not* on the alleged primitiveness of the native Bell community which has no access to running water and has to collect water in buckets instead, but on the hand of the administrator barring the Cherokee from having no access to running water. Who, the film asks, is primitive here? The community which does not have access to running water or the social structure withholding the right to running water from some communities while favoring others? What are the color lines, and the lines of poverty, the film asks, which determine the right to water?

Crucially, the film proceeds to claim the right to running water not only for Cherokee or for native communities, but for rural and poor white communities as well; it is a film that insists on linking ecological concerns not, as in the Green Party Poster, to an absent Indian, but to a contemporary Indian with specific indigenous rights. It is a film made by a white, environmental activist director, Tim Kelly in collaboration with the late Wilma Mankiller's husband, Charlie Soap.

Crucially, however, the film does not address the question of what the system denying this rural community access to running water could be; rather, it zooms in not so much on the issue of environmental and structural injustice than on resistance, and communal action. It is in this sense that even though its aesthetics may not be as futuristic as those of Dancing Earth, it is nonetheless future-oriented. There is no nostalgia here, and the eco-Indian is nowhere in sight.

The film centers on the idea of community, and what this community might mean in the twenty-first century. Crucially, the film can be said to revolve around the notion of "gadugi," the solidarity among members of the Cherokee community. Having teamed up with tribal administrator Charlie Soap, Wilma tries to convince the local community to volunteer to build its own water pipeline:

> WILMA [*getting up to greet the people who have come to the community meeting*]: Thank you, Charlie. Good evening everyone. Thank you for coming. As you may know, Charlie and I are here on behalf of the Cherokee Nation. [*In the back of the hall,* DEPUTY CHIEF JACKSON *is seen entering, taking off his hat*]. Now after talking with many you, it's clear that the greatest need here in Bell is water and housing. We have a plan that will bring a water line into Bell so you all can finally get running water. The tribe is gonna provide all the necessary equipment and materials and training but you, the people of Bell, will actually build the water line.
>
> MAN [*raising his hand*]: What if you're not Cherokee?
>
> WILMA: We can build the water line by your house, but you'd have to pay to connect. [*The man averts his gaze, resigned.*] Which brings up another important point: You must be an official member of the Cherokee Nation to get water. Now I know a lot of you are not enrolled with the tribe, but Charlie and I can help you with that paper work. [*looks at* CHARLIE].

> WOMAN [*gets up, speaking in Cherokee, subtitled in English*]: This lady wants me to sign a paper to prove that I'm a Cherokee. Unless I sign, the Tribe won't help me? [*she turns and sits back down*.]
>
> CHARLIE: Flood, we're not that crazy about the policy either. Wouldn't it be worth it? If you can get water?
>
> MAN: So let me get this straight. After we sign all the papers and prove that we're Indian, the Cherokee nation is gonna hire us to dig a water line?
>
> WILMA: No, we're asking you. We're asking all of you, to volunteer.
>
> MAN: The Cherokee Nation's never helped us before. Now they send you out here to ask us to do their work for free? [In the back of the room, the deputy chief is seen, smirking; he is hoping for the plan to fail.] Who do you think you are?
>
> CHARLIE: Wilma's here, not to tell you what to do, but simply to offer her help.
>
> WILMA: And we'll be out there with you, every day.
>
> CHARLIE: Now if we could just come together, like we used to. Gadugi. [In the crowd, people are beginning to nod.] There is no reason why we can't do this. (*The Cherokee Word for Water*)

I believe that the film *The Cherokee Word for Water* is crucial in the context of both indigenous rights and sustainability precisely in its insisting on the multiple meanings of water as a shifting and contested signifier. It is this sense of water as a contested signifier which is evoked in a scene where the volunteers pray over a water pipeline:

> *The volunteers have gathered around a piece of the water pipeline. The men take off their hats.*
>
> CHARLIE'S BROTHER: Creator, maker. Thank you for bringing us together. Thank you for giving us what we already have, and for what you're putting in front of us right now. It is a struggle but we're gonna make it through because you're here with us. [*the camera shows the water line, which has progressed rapidly*.] Again, I thank you for all your blessings. (*The Cherokee Word for Water*)

The act of prayer, insisting on thanking a sublime power for what we already have; water, the film makes clear, precedes the water pipe: It cannot be reduced to a commodity; water will persist long after the water pipe will have corroded and vanished. Instead, the Cherokee community of Bell, Oklahoma, prays both for what is in the water pipe and for what can never ultimately be contained in a water pipe. Even as the water pipe symbolizes access to health and well-being, as well as the simple commodity of tap water, water is never reduced to a commodity.

I believe that the film and this scene in particular could not be more crucial in its appropriation of "water" as what I would call a contested signifier. By insisting that "water" is not a stable but a shifting signifier, the film steers clear of what Ashis Nandy has cautioned against in a different but related context. Nandy, in the context of postcolonial justice movements, has warned us that in the very moment of calling for indigenous or postcolonial justice, the very use of what Mary Lawlor has called "rights language" – a Western language of rights – may corrupt the concepts which lie at the heart of this call for justice. As Lawlor has argued, the minute in which indigenous communities may call for their own rights in a Western language of rights, their project may be doomed:

> [this idea] calls to mind Gayatri Spivak's haunting argument "Can the Subaltern Speak?" in which Spivak wonders whether it is ever possible for an indigenous agent to speak in an indigenous voice and subject position as such in the public spaces and institutions of the dominant societies, given hegemonic representational codes and strategies in representing themselves. In this sense, . . . Nandy's [argument is] that there is something that troubles indigenous subjectivity as such when it attempts to speak in Western public, political forums. (180-81)

What would this mean for the use of "water" in the film *The Cherokee Word for Water*? The pitfall in this call for indigenous rights and an indigenous right to water – or a human right to water which needs to be extended to native communities as well – is the claim of indigenous ownership of water. It is this pitfall, I would like to propose, of which the film steers clear. Since Western rights discourse has hinged on the notion of ownership, any call for access to water on the part of indigenous communities would need to first espouse this idea of ownership. How, then, can rights be claimed without in this very moment jettisoning native epistemologies which do not believe in the possibility of such an ownership of natural resources? This, at first, seems to be an insoluble dilemma; yet, it is a feat which, I want to argue, the film can be said to accomplish.

Crucially, the film *The Cherokee Word for Water* can be seen as *laying claim* to natural elements without, however, simultaneously *claiming ownership*. It is precisely by insisting that water continues to be a shifting and contested signifier that the film resists understanding land solely as real estate, and understanding water solely as a resource. Rather, despite the fact that water can be domesticated through a water pipe, water also has an inherently spiritual quality; it is in this sense that the act of praying over a water pipe is anything but trivial.

Yet, it is equally significant that the title "The Cherokee Word for Water" may actually be a misnomer: In its multiple definitions of "water," the film insists, first, that the Cherokee word for water has multiple signifiers and multiple meanings, and second that the Cherokee word for water includes a form of justice which is extended beyond the Cherokee community to include the poor white community of Bell, Oklahoma. What is key in *The Cherokee Word for Water* is that it addresses the situation of native communities while at the same time referring to the injustices perpetrated against rural (and, implicitly, poor white) communities. It is for this reason, I believe, that the film's call for justice is a highly inclusive one, refusing to cater to what has been termed an "indigenous exceptionalism."

It is thus significant of the film's politics that this form of Cherokee solidarity includes the poor white character, Curly, who helped build the water pipe and for whom the native community of Bell once hosted a bake sale:

> FELICIA [*to Wilma*]: You know, Curly has been out here every day. He loves that backo like a bone and its dog. I don't think he can connect this line. There's not enough money.
>
> WILMA: I wish there was something I could do on my end, but that grant's just for Cherokee families.
>
> FELICIA: He's part of the community, just like the other people here.
>
> GINA [*glad she has come up with an idea*]: Why don't we have a bake sale?

FELICIA: We're gonna need a big cake. And I'm not baking it. [laughs]

A truck is seen approaching. A man in a tan suit is getting out of the car.

JOURNALIST: I'm looking for Wilma Mankiller.

WILMA: I'm Wilma.

JOURNALIST [*shaking her hand*]: Hello, I'm Stan Johnson, CBS news. We'd like to do a piece on your project here, and also, I'd like to interview some principals, like yourself.

WILMA: Well, the people in Bell are the principals. I'll introduce you to them. . . . [*turning around to look at the women*]: Hey ladies, don't you feel like being TV stars today?

In the next scene, the people gather to watch the airing of the feature about Bell on CBS news. They have set up a TV in the community center.

FELICIA: We're having a bake sale Saturday at the community building, to help raise money for the white families to be able to get water, too. And everyone's invited.

There has been a great turn-out at the bake sale.

CURLY [*shyly approaching* WILMA]: Wilma?

WILMA: Curly?

CURLY [*embarrassed*]: I wanna thank you. I wasn't expecting all this.

WILMA: Don't thank me. Thank these ladies over here. (*leading him over to where the women sell the cakes.*)

GINA: Hey, Curly! . . .

CURLY: I don't know what to say. [he has tears in his eyes.] Gina hugs him. (*The Cherokee Word for Water*)

There are a number of aspects implied in a rural Cherokee community hosting a bake-sale for the poor white rural community of Bell, Oklahoma. This is a Cherokee feature film, then, which refuses to engage in Cherokee exceptionalism; even as it is a call for the right to running water as a call for indigenous rights, it is also a call for the rights of indigenous and of poor white communities. Environmental justice, then, cannot be limited in the film to indigenous rights, even as it is closely related to them; rather, the film carefully investigates into the location of social and environmental injustice, showing that a number of disenfranchised communities have been excluded from the right to running water in the U.S. at the beginning of the twenty-first century. It is this coalition, also, which has been invoked by Joni Adamson in her definition of environmental justice:

> In the fall of 1999, delegations of environmental activists, trade unionists, Buddhist monks, indigenous peoples, and "raging grannies," representing many countries of the world, converged in Seattle, Washington, to protest the World Trade Organization's support of multinational corporate objectives and trade agreements that contribute to the building of a global economy where control over local environments, communities, cultures, education, and health care is no longer in the hands of the people but in the hands of big business. (3)

It is this coalition for environmental justice, then, that the film conveys: It is a film made by an "environmental activist" director in collaboration with the Cherokee community of Bell, Oklahoma, and there are a number of "raging grannies," both indigenous and white.

The film ends, then, with the miracle of running water: "Script: The Bell project brought water to 81 families, saved the Bell school, and reignited the spirit of gadugi" *(The Cherokee Word for Water).* At the end of the film, running water is far from being a mere commodity since the film has shown that for some communities, this commodity cannot be taken for granted. The simple act of turning on the faucet thus becomes a meaningful act, and an act significant in the context of both sustainability and environmental justice.

At the same time, the film also ends with documentary footage showing President Clinton awarding Wilma Mankiller the Medal of Freedom in 1998. Bestowed by Congress, the Medal of Freedom is the highest civilian award of the U.S.. It is meant as a recognition of individuals on the basis of "an especially meritorious contribution to the security or national interests of the United States, world peace, cultural or other significant public or private endeavors" (Ray n. pag.). Yet, this recognition, I would argue in light of my previous discussion of *The Cherokee Word for Water*, is far from ambivalent. Even as the film itself refrains from casting blame on any government or "system" denying some communities the right to running water and implicitly, to infrastructures and well-being, such discrimination is nonetheless implicit in the filmic narrative. Thus, the emphasis of Wilma Mankiller's life writing narrative and the film made on the basis of this narrative is on self-help. This politics of self-help, in the context of Native American colonization, is far from ambivalent: In fact, as the film outlines, the rural Cherokee community of Bell, Oklahoma, out of its own initiative sets out to overcome a form of disenfranchisement which should not have existed in the first place. Nonetheless, however, the eventual recognition of Wilma Mankiller's achievement by President Clinton may be a first step, even as this recognition may serve to obfuscate the failure of the political system by which the award is bestowed. As in the bestowal of the Right Livelihood Award to Tony DeBrum and the People of the Marshall Islands, what is at stake is hence a politics of (alternative) recognition, which despite the acknowledgment contained in these awards at the same time may reinscribe a deeper and more ingrained failure of responsibilities on the part of national governments and, to some extent, supra-national organizations.

When Wilma Mankiller passed away in 2010, then, President Obama acknowledged her achievements with the following words:

> I am deeply saddened to hear of the passing of Wilma Mankiller today. As the Cherokee Nation's first female chief, she transformed the Nation-to-Nation relationship between the Cherokee Nation and the Federal Government, and served as an inspiration to women in Indian Country and across America. A recipient of the Presidential Medal of Freedom, she was recognized for her vision and commitment to a brighter future for all Americans. (Vazquez n. pag.)

What is significant here is not only President Obama's recognition of Wilma Mankiller's political achievements, but also her role as a woman activist. Moreover, his recognition that what is at stake here is a "Nation-to-Nation relationship between the Cherokee Nation and the Federal Government" (Vazquez n. pag.) is itself an implicit recognition of the status of Native American communities not as subordinate to the U.S. government but as nations on par with the U.S., at least nominally.[3]

[3] The paradox at the heart of this "nation-to-nation" relationship between Indian nations and the US government has been discussed in detail by Dieter Dörr and

What links Dancing Earth's performance to the film *The Cherokee Word for Water*, then, is more than the simple fact that both should center on water. Rather, both representations point to what may in fact be an epistemological dilemma at the core of the definition of "water" to begin with. As I have tried to argue in this chapter, this convergence in the element and the word for water is anything but coincidental. Rather, the very salience and frequency of water as a natural element, the access to which used to be a human right, points to a specific historical moment in time. At the beginning of the twenty-fist century, these visual performances tell us, the meaning of "water" is no longer clear; rather, what used to be a simple given has ceased to be self-evident. It is in insisting that water has become a complex signifier, and a highly contested one, that the performance by Dancing Earth and the film *The Cherokee Word for Water* converge. Even as both the film and the performance center on indigenous rights, and the indigenous right to water, they steer clear of indigenous exceptionalism, by including, both other communities of color and poor white and rural communities. Both the film and the dance performance insist that there are many words for water. Moreover, it is anything but coincidental that the privatization of water should be at issue in both the performance and the film. The performance explicitly calls for taking arms against the privatization of water; and the film highlights the fact that water is both a commodity and a natural element which can never be commodified, and an element to be prayed over, cherished, and sustained.

One idea that this study seeks to contest, then, is the notion of the "color-blindness" of medical humanities as both a concept and an approach to reading texts about illness, age and disability. Crucially, the framework which seems to be at the heart of medical humanities can be said to be quite similar to that of ecocriticism. As I have tried to outline in this chapter, ecocriticism posits that we are all – "universally," as it were – affected by the increasing destruction of our environment. Yet, as Joni Adamson has stressed, some communities are exposed to ecological damage to an extent that others are not; it is hence crucial to stress, according to Adamson, "ecological and social justice concerns" (4). What

Lindsay Robertson. See Dörr, "The Background of the Theory of Discovery"; Robertson *Conquest by Law.*

would this mean, then, for the framework of medical humanities? What would it mean to speak of medical humanities in a way that is "color-conscious" (Appiah and Gutman, *Color Conscious*)? It would mean a number of aspects which have so far only implicitly been addressed in this chapter. First, a color-conscious medical humanities approach would inquire not only into a given subject's experience of illness, but it would also go on to address the question whether this subject has access to health care, or whether his or her social location bars this person from access to such care. Second, as I have discussed in Chapters 7 and 8, a color-conscious approach to medical humanities would inquire into the potential causes for illness, or rather, into the frameworks from which this illness arose. While there can never be an altogether causal approach to environmental damage and illness, as Adamson has stressed, certain conditions may nonetheless heighten the risk of illness. It is in the sense of a color-conscious medical humanities framework, moreover, that the Bollywood film *My Name Is Khan* may seem especially significant. For as I have tried to outline in Chapter 3, the film not only describes the life of a man with Asperger's, but the social and racial location of a Muslim man with Asperger's in the wake of 9/11. By zooming in only on Khan's disability rather than on the intersection between disability and cultural and social location, the color-blindness of medical humanities as an approach would have been reinforced. It is for this reason, I would like to argue here, that all of the texts that I am discussing in this study can be subsumed under a variety of frameworks, frameworks which I am trying to elaborate on in each of the chapters. It is this multiple contextualization, I believe, which is central to *broadening* medical humanities as a concept. It is for this reason, also, that I have subsumed under a medical humanities frameworks texts which would otherwise not have been discussed from this angle. What may be central to what may be termed a critical medical humanities approach, then, is to inquire into the frameworks under which each of these texts has been subsumed, and into the ways in which an alternative form of canonization may yield altogether different readings of one and the same text.

11 Conclusion

This book has moved from individual autobiographies to collective forms of life writing; from individual stories of illness to collective question of health and well-being. At the same time, it has asked in what form life writing narratives may be accessible to us – in published autobiographies or biographies, in interviews, in documentaries and testimonies, but also as traces in fictional accounts of illness, aging or disability –, and to what extent they are able to influence, leave a mark on or enter a dialogue with constructions of illness, age or disability by the life sciences. Many of the preceding chapters have thus asked under what circumstances scientific knowledge may be decentered, or to what extent it may admit, under certain conditions, the preliminary nature of its own knowledge, even its methodological paradigms. By the same token, I have been interested in the way in which, under particular circumstances, forms of life writing may themselves constitute forms of alternative knowledge, thus pointing to the shortcomings, even obsolescence of a paradigm which assumes a clear-cut distinction between expert knowledge and lay accounts. These latter accounts, I have argued, often center on the notion of lived experience. This notion of experience, in turn, may have been dismissed both by poststructuralist approaches within the humanities which have stressed the aspects of representation and cultural construction and by life science methodologies which, as Marini has argued, have often valued evidence-based medicine at the expense of the narrative dimensions of patient accounts which draw attention to individual experiences of illness or disability (8).

In methodological terms, this study has tried to chart a terrain which can be said to open up spaces between life sciences and the humanities: It has linked life writing research to medical humanities and narrative medicine, both of which already share an interest in (patient) narratives. In this analysis of life writing texts, moreover, I have tried to trace how, in these narratives, definitions of "life" at the beginning of the twenty-first century are subject to redefinitions by biomedical technologies, and what spaces may emerge in the wake of such redefinition. In this vein, I have linked life writing narratives to discussions in bioethics, as well as to the concept of biopolitics. Finally, I have looked at the extent at which new developments in brain research may provide new possibilities of self-articulation for persons with genetic difference.

Thus, I have implicitly tried to argue that investigating life writing texts with regard to new developments in the life sciences and the ensuing redefinition of "life" itself constitutes a form of empirical research. If Lemke suggests, for instance, that empirical research must still be done about how patient groups set out to empower themselves in new forms of collective engagement, I have argued that the role of Michael J. Fox and his advocacy and initiating of Parkinson research may constitute precisely such a case study.

I have thus implied in many of the preceding chapters that opening up a dialogue between the life sciences and the humanities (with their emphasis on life writing) may be crucial in pointing out potential blind spots in each of these disciplines. Thus, the life sciences may have stressed universal concepts of illness, sometimes at the expense of taking into account a patient's individual experience of illness, as well as his or her social and cultural condition. Conversely, the humanities may solely have focused on the narrative dimension of illness or disability, and the notion of individual identity, thus sometimes failing to take into account the fact that, as Marini has emphasized in her recent study of narrative medicine, evidence-based medicine and an attention paid to narrative can in fact coexist (*Narrative Medicine*). I have thus tried to argue throughout these pages that both the humanities and the life sciences may have much to gain from a constructive dialogue bridging scientific explanatory paradigms and (the study of) lived experience.

This book began by inquiring what would be the consequence, for the humanities, of reimporting a product that they had once exported: medical humanities. This question – the question of both outsourcing a particular set of methods and of lines of inquiry and of later "reimporting" them in a changed form – is inextricably connected to the relevance, the scope and the "applicability" of the humanities at the beginning of the twenty-first century. Another way of asking the same question, then, is to wonder about the relevance or obsolescence of the humanities in the age of biomedicine. This question, in turn, is not limited to American Studies as a discipline within the humanities but affects the humanities in general. What is more, recent attacks on the relevance of the humanities have targeted not only the humanities but the social sciences as well. Lacking applicability and a clearly circumscribed set of tools which can then be translated into the job market, both are now said to be obsolete. As a recent article in the German newspaper *DIE ZEIT* observes,

> The professor clearly remembers having the creeping horrors when he collected the "evil letter" from his mailbox. The document exhorted Keiichi Aizawa, Head of German Studies at Tsukuba University, that his institute should offer a "more application-oriented education, which is better attuned to the requirements of society." He found the words "humanities and social sciences," combined in a single phrase, in a sentence using the verb "abolish." (Lill n. pag.; my trans.)

What is ironic in this context is that the "turf wars" between the humanities and the social sciences seem to have backfired in a sense that neither of these sets of disciplines could have anticipated: If the social sciences have long stressed the superiority of their methodologies over the (allegedly) more subjective, more interpretive approach favored by the humanities, both the humanities and the social sciences are now deemed obsolete due to a lack of applicability which, it is argued by the material sciences and the life sciences, they both *share*. As the above-cited article about the situation of the humanities both in Japan and the UK goes on to note, the letter sent to Keiichi Aizawa held that the humanities "always had to have an answer to the question which direct effects its research was to have on the real world. What this implied [Aizawa noted], was the new ideal of measurability" (Lill n. pag.; my trans.).

The claim of the obsolescence of the humanities, then, seems to be widespread, and it appears to be global. As Judith Butler writes in *Precarious Life*, "[A] president of a university made the point that no one is reading humanities books any more, that the humanities have nothing to offer or rather, nothing to offer for our times" (128). The point Butler makes is that the humanities have been faulted for not taking a clear stance, for subscribing, as a clear-cut tenet, only to a clear-cut form of relativism. As she goes on to say, "It was a discussion that turned on the question 'Have the humanities undermined themselves, with all their relativism and questioning and 'critique,' or have the humanities been undermined by all those who oppose that relativism and questioning and 'critique'"? (Butler, *Precarious Life* 129). The answer to this dilemma, of course, cannot be a jettisoning of relativism; as Butler stresses time and again, in the post-9/11 climate of the political hegemony of the "war on terror," such a relativizing of perspectives is needed more than ever. At the same time, the humanities have sometimes been criticized for not engaging with certain forms of critique; critiques which have reproached them with a retreat from the "real." Yet, to argue that any sense of reality is always-already a construction is vastly different from saying that the "real" does not exist.

Such a critique has sometimes arisen in discussions with the life sciences, whose practitioners have at times accused the humanities of not paying sufficient attention to new developments in the life sciences, which may have fundamentally redefined what it means to be human. I believe that engagement and relativism must exist side by side. The humanities, I have tried to argue throughout this book, may have much to win from engaging in discussions with the life sciences; yet, such engagement must not result in the mere proof of the use value or applicability of the humanities. The burden of proof, in other words, should not rest on the humanities alone. What may emerge at this juncture in the history of science, I believe, may be a recognition, by the humanities and the life sciences alike, of what it means to be human at the beginning of the twenty-first century, and how this conceptualization has changed in the era of biomedicine. What if both the humanities and the life sciences set out to redefine their long-cherished concepts of this humanity, through a redefinition informed by the *other* discipline?

This book is hence informed by a sense of pragmatism. At a time when the shutting down of the humanities is almost a foregone conclusion, we have been forced to reconsider the question from which we may have hitherto believe we were aloof. The value of the humanities, arguably, has always been their reflectiveness (Gumbrecht, "Ton der Kontemplation" n. pag.); they have been seen, and have seen themselves, as a moral compass, a seismograph to social, cultural and political changes within a given society. They have sounded moral warnings in the face of changes in which others only saw profitability. As German Studies scholar Aizawa puts it, "The attack on the humanities feels like a hollowing out of society from within. A marginalization of culture, ideals, and values" (Lill n. pag.; my trans.). As a humanities researcher, I cannot not agree with the tenets outlined by Aizawa, ideas and ideals have made the humanities the humanities in the first place. At the same time, I fear that the humanities may sometimes have stopped at this very point, the self-assurance of the relevance of our own field. We may have left it to others, then, to translate our tenets, methods and lines of inquiry into the specifics of their fields. We may not have been interested in breaking down our methods into "tools," which might then be out-sourced to other disciplines. In fact, I believe that we have been skeptical that such a breaking down is even possible. Our love of detail and complexity may have made us reluctant of any short-hand notions or translations of our concepts. Yet, these translations may have been very different from shorthand: they may be eclectic in the concepts they borrow from the humanities, and they may even decontextualize these concepts; but they also *add* to the complexity of both concepts and (humanities) methodologies by fusing them with methods far removed from the humanities. It is thus significant for my purposes here that for instance, the fields of narrative medicine and Critical Race Theory started with scholars and practitioners form other disciplines (medicine and law, respectively), borrowing tools originally based in literary studies. In Critical Race Theory, lawyers and legal scholars re-read the narrative of the law through the tools of literary analysis, thus deconstructing the concept of the supra-narrative quality of the law and reading it only as one narrative among many. It is in this sense that the editors of *Critical Race Theory: The Key Writings that Formed the Movement* (1995) should cite a literary scholar and postcolonial critic, Edward Said, as foundational for the project and impetus of Critical Race Theory's deconstruction of race. As Crenshaw et al. write in their introduction: "The writings in this collaboration may be read as contributions to what Edward Said has called 'antithetical knowledge,' the development of counter-accounts of social reality by subversive and subaltern elements of the reigning order" (xiii). The idea of "counter-accounts" or counter-narratives, so central to literary studies, is hence at the core of Critical Race Theory as a new, interdisciplinary methodology. Similarly, Rita Charon, the founder of narrative medicine,[1] has stressed the complexity of the patient narrative, a narrative which, she argued, could only be

[1] As Marini notes, "Rita Charon at Columbia University in New York was the first to theoretically define narrative medicine and translate it into health care practice" (7).

brought out through the analytical repertoire of literary analysis. As Charon puts it,

> As the physician listens to the patient, he or she follows the narrative thread of the story, imagines the situation of the teller (the biological, familial, cultural, and existential situation) recognizes the multiple and often contradictory meanings of the words used and the events described, and in some way enters into and is moved by the narrative world of the patient. Not unlike acts of reading literature, acts of diagnostic listening enlist the listener's interior resources – memories, associations, curiosities, creativity, interpretive powers, allusions to other stories told by this teller and others – to identify meaning. (qtd. in Marini 8)

How, then, do the humanities react to such borrowing of their methods and approaches in the service of other fields? And are they reluctant to allow for such borrowing? And even more importantly, should they be active or passive in the face of such borrowing? I believe that much can be lost if we see this borrowing, and our being "constrained" to let it happened, only as a more recent attack on the (alleged) lack of the humanities' use value. I believe that the framework in which such borrowing occurs may be immensely fruitful both for the humanities and for the disciplines which borrow from them. As is true of any interdisciplinary project, both disciplines will be altered in the process, and they will be forced to reconsider in the light of a critical interdisciplinary dialogue the concepts they have held most dear and those which they may have jettisoned prematurely. After all, to name but one example, the humanities, changed fundamentally by the tenets of post-structuralism, have been deeply skeptical of the notion of "experience," for a variety of reasons all equally valid. The dialogue with medicine and the natural sciences, on the other hand, may have caused them to discuss different versions of experience, and a potential return to the "real." It is in this sense that I have tried to argue in this book that the genre of life writing may be ideally suited for dialogues between literature and medicine, between life sciences and life writing, since it is situated half-way between fact and fiction.

My belief in this context is this one: First, I believe, following Judith Butler and her discussion of post-9/11 politics and the dire consensus that there are lives which must not be mourned, that the need for the humanities is more urgent than ever; second, however, I am worried that the humanities may make themselves obsolete unless they enter into a dialogue with the disciplines which are now deemed more important or relevant than they are. The value of the humanities has always been their function as a moral compass, for lack of a better concept, which society might follow; a tool for finding direction in an ever more complex social, economic, political, medical and natural world. As Lemke has argued, biomedicine today may provide us with possibilities to change the "nature" of human life to an extent that is unprecedented in human history. From the beginning of life (now changed through reproductive technologies) to the end of life, through forms of enhancement and ways of enabling longevity, we seem to have become masters of our own lives, being able to change adverse conditions which before had seemed unalterable. According to Lemke, "[At the beginning of the twenty-first century] life no longer constitutes a stable ontological and normative reference. With the emergence of biotechnological innovations at the latest, it beomes apparent that processes of life have become malleable to an extent which makes any idea of pristine nature unaffected by human action appear obsolete" (12-13; my trans.). Yet, as Rachel Adams has argued in *Raising Henry* and as Thomas Lemke has stressed from a sociological perspective, we are also faced with decisions which we never before had to take. Which of these options, then, is desirable? And should we desire everything that is made possible through biomedical science?[2] It is this labyrinth of options offered by biomedicine which makes us come face to face with decisions so existential that they seem impossible to make; faced with this inability, where would we turn for direction? As Rachel Adams has argued, it is to forms of life writing (to autobiographies, patient blogs, or self-help groups) that we may turn for guidance. This, I have tried to argued in this book, is the power of life writing and autobiography. As Jason Kingsley and Mitchell Levitz ask in their book evocatively entitled *Count Us In*, might the gynecologists who had once counseled their mothers to have an abortion have acted differently had they read the autobiography of a person with Down Syndrome leading a full life? It is in this sense that life writing can effectively become a counter-narrative to knowledge generated in the life sciences; my aim in this book then, has been to look for instances, in

[2] I am indebted to Norbert Paul for this point.

the history of science and the history of life writing, where a dialogue between these two fields suddenly becomes possible, and to explore the circumstances and conditions in which such a dialogue can occur.

The power of the humanities, I believe, lies precisely in our openness of methodology, the seeming endlessness of the narratives we read as texts. My credo at the end of this book, then, is that the split between the life sciences and the humanities is starting to come to an end. What happens, I have tried to ask in this book, once we believe a genuine dialogue between life sciences and life writing to be possible? One of the most powerful forms of such a dialogue, I have suggested in Chapter 4, is the dialogue between Oliver Sacks and Temple Grandin. This dialogue came about, I have suggested, only through the physician's acknowledging his lack of knowledge about an autistic person's mind; it is this deliberate act of medical humility, in turn, which enabled Temple Grandin, in many different senses of the term, to speak her mind. It is in this sense that *Thinking in Pictures* has changed medical opinions on autism, as Sacks is quick to note. Similarly, Tito Mukhopadhyay's mother Soma, a lay woman, not a practitioner of medicine, developed the rapid prompting method which is now being used in California schools for autistic children; and neuroscientists such as Michael Merzenich have begun to study why this method works. My aim throughout these chapters, then, has been to inquire into the circumstances and conditions in which such a dialogue is possible. Would Oliver Sacks have opened a space for Temple Grandin's narrative to step into if biomedical knowledge of autism had already been advanced at the time? Crucially, approaches such as narrative medicine (which, I have suggested, may have been anticipated by Sacks' decentering of his own medical authority) do *not* argue that the expertise of the medical practitioner be abolished, or that the patient become a biomedical expert of her own condition; they stress, however, the fact that the doctor-patient relationship may be a dynamic one where each can at times admit his own ignorance, and the ensuing need for a co-construction of knowledge.

As the work of Oliver Sacks illustrates, the humanities have thus been crucial for new developments in the practice of biomedicine in the attention they pay to narrative, and to narrative perspective. As Oliver Sacks has put it in his emphasis on the role of narrative in biomedicine, "'Ask not what disease the patient has but rather what person the disease has'" ("Dr Oliver Sacks").[3] What emerges, then is a simultaneous awareness to illness as a universal condition (illness as it affects the human body) and the specific lives which are changed and affected by illness. It is in this sense that I have argued in the preceding chapters that medical humanities as a framework may fall short of its potential if it limits the scope of its inquiry to individual patient narratives, failing to take into account questions of social justice or environmental rights. It is here, I believe, that it is imperative to link accounts from medical humanities to the sociology of medicine. As Alondra Nelson's groundbreaking work about medical racism illustrates, the practice of biomedicine does not emerge from a void; thus, racialist structures may also inform the practice of biomedicine, which in turn has to be aware not only of its medical, but also its social assumptions. It is in this sense that I have proposed in this book that medical humanities, in order to unfold their full potential, need to explore not only narratives of illness, but also stories of health and well-being. These stories, in turn, require that we take into account the social, cultural, political, legal and economic contexts from which they arise; obstacles to the health and well-being of marginalized communities, in turn, must also be the subject of medical humanities.

A number of fields have developed which connect approaches from biomedicine, the humanities, and the social sciences, among them Public Health, Gerontology, Environmental Health Studies, or Environmental Justice Studies, the latter of which I have addressed in my discussion of the contemporary Native American film The *Cherokee Word for Water*. My call at the end of this book may, perhaps, be a utopian one: What would happen if we found reasons not for retrenching and for re-establishing the difference between the life sciences and the humanities, but for assuming that their approaches to human life may in fact be complementary and may hence lend themselves to critical dialogue? To be sure, this would not change, and perhaps must not change, some of the day-to-day practice of either the humanities or the life sciences; as Bettina Schöne-Seifert has argued in an article supporting connections between behavioral psychology and biological psychiatry, there must be,

[3] I am grateful to Angelina Graf for her research assistance, which proved invaluable in the writing of this conclusion.

in everyday life, the strategic reductionism which makes each of these sets of disciplines what they are. According to Schöne-Seifert,

> The main pattern of such "strategies" is to perform deliberate simplifications, through focusing on some aspects and strategically disregarding others, in order to provide an explanation for complex qualities and complex processes of causality. Therefore, a focus on the physical and thus neuropathological aspects of disease seems suitable, in order to detect and to apply the potential of therapeutic forms of influence. . . . (135; my trans.)

Yet, as Schöne-Seifert also implies, each of these fields may stress the shortcomings, the gaps in knowledge, in its current approach. What is crucial about her discussion of biological psychiatry, then, is the fact that Schöne-Seifert stresses the idea that the attention paid to the neurological dimension of illness (which can, for instance, be made visible through brain imaging techniques (Flor 2010) need not result in a dismissal of the level of individual experience, an experience, I would add for my purposes here, which is often conveyed in life writing narratives. As Schöne-Seifert goes on to say, "This is by no means synonymous with negating or neglecting the experiential aspects of illness" (135; my trans.).

Thus, brain research has stressed that while it has come closer to explaining the workings of the human *brain*, it is still at a loss to determine the mechanisms of the human *mind*. As Singer notes,

> The problem with research on the conscious mind is the difficulty of relating these two forms of description to each other, let alone to translate one into the other. I am able to determine when a brain is conscious – this becomes evident through particular qualities in the electrical activity of brain cells –, but I run into problems of representation and thus also of imagination if I am trying to correlate a particular state of the brain with a particular emotion, because I will experience this emotion as private, immaterial, and belonging only to myself. Here, we are confronted with a difficult philosophical problem, a puzzle of cognition theory. (50; my trans.)

The dilemma between mind and brain, as Siri Hustvedt has recently argued and as she has described in detail in *The Shaking Woman* (2011) (which can be read both as memoir and as medical history), is thus far from being resolved (Hustvedt, *The Shaking Woman*). As Onur Güntürkün has suggested, the relationship between mind and brain is a reciprocal one; even as the brain may condition or even to some extent determine the way we think, the brain itself is shaped by our reactions to the society we live in. Güntürkün writes, "Societal structures in their turn influence the way in which individuals think, in the sense that consciousness and society determine one another in a reciprocal manner" (Güntürkün 13; my trans.). What is needed, then, is an interdisciplinary approach which can account both for the biological and the cultural dimension of our lives. As Güntürkün and Hacker go on to observe, "The individual architecture of cognition, affect, [and] action can neither be deduced solely from neurobiology nor from cultural factors alone. Rather, the human mind results from the interplay between brain and society" (7; my trans.).

Given prophecies of doom about their alleged obsolescence and the ascent of the life sciences to *Leitdisziplinen*, the humanities certainly have reasons for fretting; and yet, I believe, much is to be gained from seeking out spaces in which a dialogue with the life sciences may have become possible. What if we were to disregard differences in power, funding and prestige, and enter a dialogue about content, not (economic) context? As I write these chapters, new fields seem to be emerging every day whose hybridity, it seems to me, is less a disadvantage than an intriguing unsettling of the methodological certainties of the fields which they set out to fuse. It is not hard to imagine that these hybrid fields, whose hybridity will come to appear as a difference in degree but not kind, will in time become the rule rather than the exception. Our institutional landscape has already undergone profound changes; as BA programs, many universities across Europe have started offering programs combining different media (literature, theater, film) under the framework of "the arts," with social thought; such combinations, often revolving around a link between social environments, historical developments, ethical concerns and aesthetic expression, are also becoming more common on an MA level. There is a sense in which, many have lamented, such a mixture of fields and perspectives must necessarily occur at the expense of a closer scrutiny of the nuances of literature, or the manifold paradigms of performance known to theater and performance studies; at the same time, the creators of these program have argued that much may also be gained from connecting these different fields. Because of the different methodological frameworks defining the humanities and the life sciences, however, programs linking these two fields are still rare; yet, for instance, the field of biological psychology sets out to connect behavioral psychology and neurosciences. As Onur Güntürkün puts it,

> We have to study thought processes on two levels. I will call them the abstract level, this is the level which we have studied in classical psychology. There is a grammar of thinking, there are mechanisms of thought, there are patterns which tell us much about thinking. And then, thought is generated, created, in the brain, and this is the biological, the "wet" level of thinking. These two levels are tied to one another. The wet level makes the abstract level possible. Yet, how these two levels are interrelated, we have as yet hardly been able to understand. And this is exactly my discipline, biological psychology. I am trying to understand how, in the brain, these patterns are being represented, and how language in its turn has an effect on the brain. ("Onur Güntürkün"; my trans.)

In all these instances, these fields have come into being at a time when before this emergence, no-one thought such combinations were even possible. My point is, then, that just as in the instance of narrative medicine and medical humanities programs, only scientific and scholarly practice can prove the efficacy of these methods. And yet, as I have tried to argue in this study, they may already have transformed the ways we think about our own disciplines.

What, then, would be the role of the humanities in this world of disciplinary unsettling? It has become a truism to say that we live not only by materials, but by metaphors; narratives help us make sense of the world. It is through forms both of fiction (fictional narratives being told in different media, from a film about autism to a book about growing up with Down Syndrome) and of life writing, that we may come to terms with difference, illness, or disability, but also that we may make sense of our own lives, our own way of thinking and of trying to live a full life. The power of life writing, I have tried to suggest in this book, lies in emphasizing that there are many ways to lead a full life. At a time when critics ask about the applicability and the use value of the humanities, what could be of more use than making us see difference differently, making us see difference as socially constructed because we have seen the world through the eyes of a young man with Down Syndrome? What if, through the power of autobiography, we come to see autism not as a disability, but, as Temple Grandin emphasizes in *Thinking in Pictures*, as a difference which in some context, may be an asset? In *Thinking in Pictures*, Temple Grandin describes the working of her own mind from a variety of perspectives: As a psychologist, she describes the workings of her own mind through brain research; as an animal scientist, she compares her own ways of thinking to that of animals, to whom she argues she can relate more than a non-autistic person would, and as a person living with autism, she describes her being in the world and has become a spokesperson for those on the autism spectrum. Grandin writes,

> Since I wrote *Thinking in Pictures*, brain imaging studies have provided more insights into how the brain of a person with autism/Asperger spectrum processes information. Eric Courchesne at the University of California in San Diego states that autism may be a disorder of brain circuit disconnections. This would affect the ability to integrate detailed information from lower parts of the brain where sensory based memories are stored with higher level information processing in the frontal cortex. (*Thinking in Pictures* 26)

What Temple Grandin's groundbreaking autobiography, *Thinking in Pictures*, illustrates, then, is that the dichotomy between the humanities and the life sciences, seen from the perspective of the experience of a life lived with autism, may in fact be counterproductive. Moreover, it is from her perspective both as a person with autism and as a psychologist and animal scientist, that Grandin views this opposition as obsolete. In much the same vein, Nikolas Rose and Joelle Abi-Rached have recently argued that to speak of the "colonization" of our life worlds by the life sciences and by the neurosciences in particular may in fact be both problematic and counterproductive. Instead, they point to what they view as a potential synergy between these different fields. As Rose and Abi-Rached note, "Despite identifying many exaggerated claims and premature promises, Neuro argues that the openness provided by the new style of thought taking shape in neuroscience, with its contemporary conceptions of the neuromolecular, plastic, and social brain, could make possible a new and productive engagement between the social and the brain sciences" (dust jacket n. pag.). To this productiveness, then, the book has sought to add the cultural sciences by looking at the intersection between life sciences and life writing.

It is in this context, also, that we may want to reconsider the idea of "biopolitics" discussed by Nikolas Rose, Paul Rabinow, and Thomas Lemke. If, as Rabinow argues in his conception of "biosociality" (Lemke 125; my trans.), developments at the beginning of the twenty-first century have rendered the division between "culture" and "nature" obsolete, it would seem all the more paradoxical if on the level of academia and with regard to specific sets of disciplines, we were to uphold this distinction. As Lemke notes,

> According to Rabinow, the Human Genome Project and the biotechnological innovations which accompany it result in a redefinition of the two poles identified by Foucault, the poles of the body and of society. What results from this is said to be a post-disciplinary order, which transcends the strict separation between nature and culture and develops a new relationship to processes of life. . . . What we can observe today, it is said, is by no means a biologization of the social, the translation of social projects into biological terms . . ., but a reconfiguration of societal relations through biological categories. (125; my trans.)

If the subject matter which both the humanities and the life sciences set out to study has transcended the nature/culture divide, research must necessarily be transdisciplinary.

The perspectives on human life which have become available to us at the beginning of the twenty-first century, I would argue, cannot be neatly separated into life sciences and humanities; rather, they stress the interrelatedness of these perspectives. It is with the belief that the future, for both the humanities and the life sciences, may be both disciplined *and* undisciplined, and that it may no longer be a future marked by two cultures, that I end this book.

Works Cited

"'My Name is Khan.'" *Manila Times,* Pressreader, 20 Feb. 2010, www.pressreader.com/philippines/manila-times/20100220/282011848514030. Accessed 22 Jan. 2016.

"60 Minutes on Autism." *Dailymotion*, uploaded by meesh, 4 Jan. 2007, www.dailymotion.com/video/xx7ch. Accessed 29 Jun. 2017.

"Alzheimerdemenz: Belastendes Erbe." *Gehirn & Geist*, no. 10, 2016, p. 10.

"Anthropologist on Mars." *OnAol*, uploaded by MAKERS, Apr. 2014, on.aol.com/video/temple-grandin--anthropologist-on-mars.518191675. Accessed 20 Sept. 2014.

"Arnold Schwarzenegger invites 'detained' Bollywood Actor Shah Rukh Khan to Dinner." *The Telegraph*, 19 Aug. 2009, www.telegraph.co.uk/news/celebritynews/6056026/Arnold-Schwarzenegger-invites-detained-Bollywood-actor-Shah-Rukh-Khan-to-dinner.html. Accessed 14 Sept. 2016.

"Baryshnikov Dancing from the Heart H 264 800Kbps Streaming." *YouTube*, uploaded by Bernie Jellig, 20 Feb. 2010, www.youtube.com/watch?v=1CpPPrjjVNI. Accessed 16 Mar. 2016.

"Boston Ballet – Education – Adaptive Dance." *The Boston Ballet*, Inc., www.bostonballet.org/education/adaptive-dance. Accessed 12 May 2016.

"Boy with Down Syndrome Performs 'Nutcracker' with Cincinnati Ballet." *YouTube*, uploaded by ABC News, 15 Dec. 2016, www.youtube.com/watch?v=1H2I_UZFlm8. Accessed 3 Mar. 2017.

"Bringing Them Home: Separation of Aboriginal and Torres Strait Islander Children from Their Families." *YouTube*, uploaded by Australian Human Rights Commission, 11 Jun. 2014, www.youtube.com/watch?v=Sl82VMuuKI0. Accessed 24 Jan. 2017.

"Dance Review: 'Walking at the Edge of Water.'" *Santafe.com,* 22 Oct. 2012, santafe.com/blogs/dance-review-walking-at-the-edge-of-water. Accessed 5 Nov. 2016.

"DANCING EARTH: Walking at the Edge of Water." *YouTube*, uploaded by noreservationspro, 9 Jul. 2013, www.youtube.com/watch?v=MRj_AVAzr_o. Accessed 22 Sept. 2015.

"Dr Oliver Sacks – Narrative and Medicine: The Importance of the Case History." *YouTube*, uploaded by uniwarwick, 20 Mar. 2013, www.youtube.com/watch?v=7PYAnB5Jx-k. Accessed 15 Jan. 2017.

"Janney and Baryshnikov create Electrocardio-Choreography." *MIT News*, 13 May 1998, news.mit.edu/1998/artheart-0513. Accessed 16 Mar. 2016.

"Michael Baryshnikov." *American Ballet Theatre*, n.dat., americanballettheatre.weebly.com/michael-baryshnikov.html. Accessed 15 Apr. 2017.

"Michael J. Fox – Letterman – 2015.04.15." *YouTube*, uploaded by Andrew Lynch, 11 Jul. 2015, www.youtube.com/watch?v=Vnlj-NyiP-Y. Accessed 15 Mar. 2016.

"Michael J. Fox on George Stroumboulopoulos Tonight: Interview." *YouTube*, uploaded by Strombo, 24 Jan. 2013, www.youtube.com/watch?v=DZnixEXIgSo. Accessed 7 Jun. 2016.

"Mikhail Baryshnikov: Biography." *The John F. Kennedy Center for the Performing Arts*, www.kennedy-center.org/artist/A3693. Accessed 16 Mar. 2016.

"Mikhail Baryshnikov: Charity and Art Video for Citizens of Humanity." *YouTube,* uploaded by televisionet, 26 Oct. 2012, https://www.youtube.com/watch?v=srmLI669CAA. Accessed 16 Mar. 2016.

"Mitchell Levitz." *Global Down Syndrome Foundation*, www.globaldownsyndrome.org/mitchell-levitz/. Accessed 26 Jul. 2016.

"New Heights: An A.B.T. Dancer Defies Ballet Convention." *The New Yorker*, 8 Nov. 2004, www.newyorker.com/magazine/2004/11/08/new-heights. Accessed 15 Nov. 2016.

"Onur Güntürkün: Der Natur Fragen stellen." *YouTube*, uploaded by Stifterverband, 26 Jun. 2014, www.youtube.com/watch?v=IXFG57QNzGo. Accessed 25 Sept. 2016.

"Presidential Eligibility." *Constitution Society*, www.constitution.org/abus/pres_elig.htm. Accessed 20 Sept. 2016.

"Scotland Returns Aboriginal Remains." *YouTube*, uploaded by NTDTV, 9 Jun. 2008, www.youtube.com/watch?v=n0s7lkcWJ0g. Accessed 4 Apr. 2016.

"The World Needs all Kinds of Minds Temple Grandin." *YouTube*, uploaded by TED, 24 Feb. 2010, www.ted.com/talks/temple_grandin_the_world_needs_all_kinds_of_minds. Accessed 12 Sept. 2016.

"Tony de Brum & and the People of the Marshall Islands (2015, Marshall Islands)." *The Right Livelihood Award*, www.rightlivelihoodaward.org/laureates/tony-de-brum-the-people-of-the-marshall-islands/. Accessed 4 Dec. 2016.

"Walking…Edge of Water." *Dancing Earth: Indigenous Contemporary Dance Creations*, www.dancingearth.org/walking-edge-of-water-2/. Accessed 21 Apr. 2017.

Adams, Rachel. *Raising Henry: A Memoir of Motherhood, Disability, and Discovery.* Yale UP, 2013.

Adamson, Joni et al., editors. *The Environmental Justice Reader: Politics, Poetics, & Pedagogy.* U of Arizona P, 2002.

Aisch, Gregor and A.A. Rebecca Lai, "The Conflicts Along 1,172 Miles of the Dakota Access Pipeline." *The New York Times*, 20 Mar. 2017, www.nytimes.com/interactive/2016/11/23/us/dakota-access-pipeline-protest-map.html. Accessed 18 Dec. 2017.

Alcoff, Linda. "The Problem of Speaking for Others." *Cultural Critique,* no. 20, 1991, pp. 5-32.

Appiah, K. Anthony, and Amy Gutmann. *Color Conscious: The Political Morality of Race.* Princeton UP, 1996.

Aria, Barbara. "Nonfiction Book Review: Misha: The Mikhail Baryshnikov Story by Barbara Aria." *Publisher's Weekly*, n. dat., www.publishersweekly.com/978-0-312-02610-3. Accessed 16 Mar. 2016.

Back to the Future. Directed by Robert Zemeckis, Universal Pictures, 1985.

Baker, Peter and Coral Davenport. "Trump Revives Keystone Pipeline Rejected by Obama." *The New York Times*, 24 Jan. 2017, www.nytimes.com/2017/01/24/us/politics/keystone-dakota-pipeline-trump.html. Accessed 18 Dec. 2017.

Banerjee, Mita, Anita Wohlmann, and Ralf Dahm. "'Living Autobiographically': Concepts of Aging and Artistic Expression in Painting and Modern Dance." *Journal of Aging Studies*, vol. 40, 2017, pp. 8-15.

Barker, Kristen. "Who Knows: Patient Expertise in the Internet Era." *Medicine and the Other: The Issue of Difference in Medical Knowledge and Practice of the 19th and 20th Centuries*, 6 Oct. 2016, Johannes Gutenberg-Universität, Mainz. Conference Presentation.

Barthes, Roland. "*Death of the Author.*" 1968. *Image-Music-Text*, edited by Farrar Straus & Giroux, 1978.

Bartlett, Jennifer. Preface. *Beauty Is a Verb: The New Poetry of Disability*, edited by Jennifer Barlett, et al., 2011, pp. 15-17.

Bérubé, Michael. *Life As We Know It: A Father, a Family, and an Exceptional Child.* Vintage, 1998.

Blood, Michael R. "People with Disabilities Denied Voting Rights, Group Says." *PBS Newshour*, 10 Jul. 2014, www.pbs.org/newshour/rundown/disabled-people-denied-voting-rights-group-says/. Accessed 20 Mar. 2017.

Blue Hawaii. Directed by Norman Taurog, Paramount Pictures, 1961.

Breckenridge, Janis. Review of *Living Autobiographically: How We Create Identity in Narrative*, by Paul John Eakin. *The Rocky Mountain Review*, vol. 64, no. 1, 2010, pp. 134–136. *JSTOR*, www.jstor.org/stable/25677078. Accessed 22 Feb 2016.

Brown, Lydia X.Z. “Critiquing Temple Grandin.” *Autistic Hoya*, 10 Aug. 2013, www.autistichoya.com/2013/08/critiquing-temple-grandin.html. Accessed 26 Oct. 2016.

Buncombe, Andrew. “North Dakota Pipeline: How It Favours White Community Over Native Neighbours - in One Map.” *Independent*, 30 Nov. 2017, www.independent.co.uk/news/world/americas/north-dakota-access-pipeline-protests-map-white-indigenous-latest-a7448161.html. Accessed 18 Dec. 2017.

Bunky. “About my Gas Mask Paintings….” *The Official Blog of Bunky Echo-Hawk: From Somewhere in Indian Country*, bunkyechohawk.com/gas-mask-paintings/. Accessed 16 Mar. 2017.

Butler, Judith. *Precarious Life: The Powers of Mourning and Violence.* Verso, 2004.

---. *Frames of War: When Is Life Grievable?* Verso, 2009.

Carlson, Marvin. *The Haunted Stage: The Theatre as Memory Machine.* U of Michigan P, 2008.

Charon. Rita. *Narrative Medicine: Honoring the Stories of Illness.* Oxford UP, 2008.

---., and Eric R. Marcus. “A Narrative Transformation of Health and Healthcare.” *The Principles and Practice of Narrative Medicine*, edited by Rita Charon et al., Oxford UP, 2017, pp. 271-91.

Cheng, Anne Anlin. *The Melancholy of Race. Psychoanalysis, Assimilation, and Hidden Grief.* Oxford UP, 2001.

Clifford, James. “On Ethnographic Authority.” *Representations*, no. 2, 1983, pp. 118-46.

---., and George E. Marcus, editors. *Writing Culture: The Poetics and Politics of Ethnography.* U of California P, 2010.

Cohen, David. “Temple Grandin: 'I'm an anthropologist from Mars'.” *The Guardian*, 25 Oct. 2005, www.theguardian.com/education/2005/oct/25/highereducationprofile.academicexperts. Accessed 13 May 2017.

Cooney, Joan Ganz. Foreword. *Count Us In: Growing Up with Down Syndrome*, by Jason Kingsley and Mitchell Levitz, Mariner Books, 2007, pp. vii-x.

Cooper, James Fenimore. *The Last of the Mohicans: A Narrative of 1757 (1826)*. Penguin Classics, 1986.

Couser, G. Thomas. *Vulnerable Subjects: Ethics and Life Writing.* Cornell UP, 2004.

---. *Recovering Bodies: Illness, Disability, and Life Writing*. U of Wisconsin P, 1997.

Crenshaw, Kimberlé, et al. *Critical Race Theory: The Key Writings that Formed the Movement.* The New Press, 1995.

Crenshaw, Kimberlé, et al. Introduction. *Critical Race Theory: The Key Writings that Formed the Movement*. Edited by Kimberlé Crenshaw et al., The New Press, 1995, pp. xiii-xxxii.

Crude: The Real Price of Oil. Directed by Joe Berlinger, Entendre Films, 2009.

Dahm, Ralf. "Berühmte Maler und der Einfluss ihrer Augenleiden auf ihr Kunstschaffen." *Spektrum der Augenheilkunde,* vol. 22, no. 5, 2008, pp. 324-27.

DasGupta, Sayantani. "Being John Doe Malkovitch: Truth, Imagination, and Story in Medicine." *Literature and Medicine*, vol. 25 no.2, 2006, pp. 439-62.

Davis, Lennard. *The End of Normal: Identity in a Biocultural Era*. U of Michigan P, 2014.

DeLoughrey, Elizabeth M. "The Myth of Isolates: Ecosystem Ecologies in the Nuclear Pacific." *Cultural Geographies*, vol. 20, no. 2, 2013, pp. 167-84.

Derrida, Jacques. *Of Grammatology.* Johns Hopkins UP, 1997.

Dörr, Dieter. "The Background of the Theory of Discovery." *American Indian Law Review*, vol. 38, no. 2, 2014, pp. 477-500.

E.T. the Extra-Terrestial. Directed by Steven Spielberg, Universal Pictures, 1982.

Eakin, John Paul. *Living Autobiographically: How We Create Identity in Narrative.* Cornell UP, 2008.

Elbert, Thomas, and Maggie Schauer. "Wenn Gegenwart zur Illusion wird: Spuren belastender Lebenserfahrungen in Genom, Gehirn und Geist." *Geist – Gehirn – Genom – Gesellschaft: Wie wurde ich zu der Person, die ich bin?*, edited by Onur Güntürkün and Jörg Hacker. Nova Acta Leopoldina, no. 405, 2014, pp. 63-79.

Equiano, Olaudah. *The Interesting Narrative of Olaudah Equiano or Gustavus Vassa, Written by Himself.*1789. Lightning Source UK Ltd., 2012.

Fishkin, Shelley Fisher. "Crossroads in Cultures: The Transnational Turn in American Studies – Presidential Address to the American Studies Association, November 12, 2004." *American Quarterly*, vol. 57, no. 1, 2005, pp.17-57.

Flor, Herta. "Bilder für eine gesunde Psyche." *Gehirn & Geist*, no. 1/2, 2010, pp. 50-56.

Fox, Michael J. *Lucky Man: A Memoir.* Ebury Press, 2002.

---. *Always Looking Up: The Adventures of an Incurable Optimist.* Ebury Press, 2009.

Franklin, Benjamin. *Autobiography of Benjamin Franklin.* Millennium Publications, 2015.

Garrard, Greg. *Ecocriticism*. Routledge, 2004.

Gibney, Mark, Rhoda E. Howard-Hassmann, Jean-Marc Coicaud, and Niklaus Steiner, editors. *The Age of Apology: Facing up the Past.* U of Pennsylvania P, 2008.

Gowda, Deepu. "Bearing Witness to Yourself." Narrative Medicine Workshop, 19 Jun. 2016, Johannes Gutenberg-Universität, Mainz. Plenary Address.

Grandin, Temple. *Thinking in Pictures: And other Reports from my Life with Autism. Second ed.*, Bloomsbury, 2006.

Greisel, Beate et. al. *Border Stories: Narratives of Peace, Conflict and Communication in the 20th and 21st Centuries*. Peter Lang, 2017.

Gumbrecht, Hans-Ulrich. "Ton der Kontemplation--Ein Vorschlag zum Überleben der Geisteswissenschaften. " Geisteswissenschaft – Eine Positionsbestimmung, 9 Jun. 2016, Philosophicum P1, Johannes Gutenberg-Universität, Mainz. Keynote Address.

---. "Körper und Technik: Dionysische Faszination der Paralympics." *Frankfurter Allgemeine Zeitung*, 18 Sept. 2012, www.faz.net/aktuell/feuilleton/geisteswissenschaften/koerper-und-technik-dionysische-faszination-der-paralympics-11894760.html. Accessed 10 Aug. 2016.

Gunn, Jeffrey. "Literacy and the Humanizing Project in Olaudah Equiano's *The Interesting Narrative* and Ottobah Cugoano's *Thoughts and Sentiments*." *eSharp*, vol. 10, 2007, pp. 1-19.

Güntürkün, Onur. "Geist – Gehirn – Genom – Gesellschaft: Wie wurde ich zu der Person, die ich bin?" *Geist – Gehirn – Genom – Gesellschaft: Wie wurde ich zu der Person, die ich bin?*, edited by Onur Güntürkün and Jörg Hacker. Nova Acta Leopoldina, no. 405, 2014, pp. 11-35.

---, and Jörg Hacker. Vorwort. *Geist – Gehirn – Genom – Gesellschaft: Wie wurde ich zu der Person, die ich bin?*, edited by Onur Güntürkün and Jörg Hacker. Nova Acta Leopoldina, no. 405, 2014, pp. 7-8.

Hagner, Michael. "Von der Schädellehre zum Neuroimaging." *Gehirn & Geist*, no. 10, 2016, pp. 30-33.

Haker, Hille. "Medizinische Hilfe ist auch soziale Hilfe." *Gehirn & Geist*, no. 10, 2016, p. 77.

Haney-López, Ian F. *White by Law: The Legal Construction of Race*. New York UP, 1996.

Harper, Kenn. *Give Me My Father's Body: The Life of Minik, the New York Eskimo*. San Val, 2001.

Hayes, Kelley. "How To Talk About #NoDAPL: A Native Perspective." *Transformative Spaces*, 26 Oct. 2016, transformativespaces.org/2016/10/27/how-to-talk-about-nodapl-a-native-perspective. Accessed 18 Dec. 2017.

Hess, Christian, and Annina Hess-Cabalzar. *Menschenmedizin: Für eine kluge Heilmedizin.* Suhrkamp, 2006.

Hornung, Alfred, editor. *Auto/Biography and Mediation*. Winter, 2010.

Huggan, Graham, and Helen Tiffin. *Postcolonial Ecocriticism: Literature, Animals, Environment*. Routledge, 2010.

Hustvedt, Siri. *The Shaking Woman, or, A History of My Nerves*. Sceptre, 2011.

Irvine, Craig. "The Ethics of Self-Care in Caring Professions." *Encyclopedia: Journal of Phenomenology and Education*, vol. 18, no. 45-54, 2014, pp. 45-54, doi: 10.6092/issn.1825-8670/4561. Accessed 20 May 2016.

---. "Narrative Ethics: New Clinical Approaches." Narrative Medicine Workshop, 19 Jun. 2016, Johannes Gutenberg-Universität, Mainz. Guest Lecture.

Ishiguro, Kazuo. *Never Let Me Go.* Faber and Faber, 2005.

Ishtar, Zohl dé. *Daughters of the Pacific*. Spinifex Press, 1994.

Jacobson, Matthew Frye. *Whiteness of a Different Color: European Immigrants and the Alchemy of Race.* Harvard UP, 1999.

Jamieson, Alastair. "Airport Denies Body Scanner Photo Claim by Bollywood Star Shahrukh Khan." *The Telegraph*, 10 Feb 2010, www.telegraph.co.uk/culture/film/bollywood/7203872/Airport-denies-body-scanner-photo-claim-by-Bollywood-star-Shahrukh-Khan.html. Accessed 8 Oct. 2016.

Jefferson, Margo. "Revisions; On Having the Grace to Grow Old, Gracefully or Not." *The New York Times*, 23 Aug. 1999, www.nytimes.com/1999/arts/revisions-on-having-the-grace-to-grow-old. Accessed 3 Jan. 2016.

Kadar, Marlene et al., editors. *Tracing the Autobiographical.* Wilfried Laurier UP, 2005.

Kampf, Antje, and Lynn A. Botelho. "Anti-Aging and Biomedicine: Critical Studies on the Pursuit of Maintaining, Revitalizing and Enhancing Aging Bodies." *Medicine Studies: An International Journal for History, Philosophy, and Ethics of Medicine & Allied Sciences*, vol. 1, no. 3, 2009, pp. 187-95. Accessed 3 Dec. 2016.

Kandel, Eric. "A New Intellectual Framework for Psychiatry." *American Journal of Psychiatry*, no. 155, 1998, pp. 457-69. Accessed 26 Jan. 2017.

Kaufman, Sarah. "Heartbeat of a Dancer." *The Washington Post*, 20 May 1998, www.washingtonpost.com/archive/lifestyle/ 1998/05/20/ heartbeat-of-a-dancer/af054e2f-022e-4c35-8185-8fa33b42b7ec/?utm _term=.ddce677b4b4f. Accessed 16 Mar. 2016.

KBR, Upala. "SRK had severe migraines while shooting for MY Name Is Khan-." *Mid-Day.com*, 11 Jan. 2010, www.mid-day.com/ articles/ srk-had-severe-migraines-while-shooting-for-my-name-is-khan/ 69065. Accessed 21 Jun 2017.

Keleman, Stanley. *Taking Charge of Your Life*. Unpublished Manuscript, 2013.

Kern-Stähler, Annette, and Anna Thiemann. "Autism and the American Dream: Progress and Recovery in the American Autie-Biography." *Narrative Matters in Medical Contexts across Disciplines*, edited by Franziska Gygax and Miriam A. Locher, John Benjamins, 2015, pp. 17-31.

Kim, Sabine. *Acoustic Entanglements: Sound and Aesthetic Practice*. Winter, 2017.

Kincaid, Jamaica. *Lucy*. A Plume Book, 1990.

King, Robert, and Michelle King, creators. *The Goodwife*. Scott Free Productions and CBS Television Distributor, 2009.

Kingsley, Emily Perl, and Barbara Gibbs Levitz. Introduction. *Count Us in: Growing Up with Down Syndrome*, by Jason Kingsley and Mitchell Levitz, 2007, pp. 1-9.

Kingsley, Emily Perl. "Welcome to Holland." *Welcome to Holland*, www.our-kids.org/Archives/Holland.html. Accessed 7 Jan. 2017.

Kingsley, Jason, and Mitchell Levitz. *Count Us in: Growing Up with Down Syndrome*. Mariner Books, 2007.

Kisselgoff, Anna. "Dance Review: A Flurry of Dance: Baryshnikov at City Center." *The New York Times*, 23 Jan 1998, www.nytimes.com/1998/01/23/movies/dance-review-a-flurry-of-dance-baryshnikov-at-city-center.html. Accessed 3 May 2016.

Klapper, Bradley. "Feinstein asks White House to Edit Torture Report." *The San Diego Union-Tribune,* 8 Apr. 2014, www.sandiegounion tribune.com/sdut-feinstein-asks-white-house-to-edit-torture-report-2014apr08-story.html. Accessed 24 Jan. 2017.

Knorr-Cetina, Karin. "Jenseits der Aufklärung. Die Entstehung der Kultur des Lebens." *Bios und Zoë: Die menschliche Natur im Zeitalter ihrer technischen Reproduzierbarkeit*, edited by Martin G. Weiß, 2009, pp. 55-71.

Koi... Mil Gaya. Directed by Rakesh Roshan, Filmkraft Productions Pvt. Ltd., 2003.

Kumar, Amitava. *Husband of a Fanatic: A Personal Journey Through India, Pakistan, Love, and Hate.* New Press, 2005.

Lawlor, Mary. *Public Native America: Tribal Self-Representations in Casinos, Museums, and Powwows.* Rutgers UP, 2006.

Lee, Anthony, et al. "I, You, Me, and Autism: An Experimental Study." *Journal of Autism and Developmental Disorders*, vol. 24, no. 2, 1994, pp. 155-76.

Lee, Robert A., editor. *Loosening the Seams: Interpretations of Gerald Vizenor.* Bowling Green State U Popular P, 2000.

Lemke, Thomas, and Peter Wehling. "Bürgerrechte durch Biologie? Kritische Anmerkungen zur Konjunktur des Begriffs »biologische Bürgerschaft«." *Bios und Zoë: Die menschliche Natur im Zeitalter ihrer technischen Reproduzierbarkeit*, edited by Martin G. Weiß, 2009, pp. 72-107.

Lemke, Thomas. *Biopolitik zur Einführung.* Junius, 2007.

Lenoir, Timothy, and Hans-Ulrich Gumbrecht, editors. *Writing Science*, web.stanford.edu/dept/HPST/TimLenoir/WritingScience.htm. Accessed 13 Jan. 2017.

LERU. *Social Sciences and Humanities: Essential Fields for European Research and in Horizon 2020*. Advice Paper, no. 11, 2012, p.7.

Lill, Felix. "Angriff auf die freien Denker: Universitäten in Japan, Großbritannien und den USA verabschieden sich von ihren Geisteswissenschaften. Hält Deutschland dagegen?" *Die Zeit*, no. 15, 14 April 2016, pp. 1-2.

Madsen, Deborah L. *American Exceptionalism*. UP of Mississippi, 1998.

Marcus, Stephen. *The Other Victorians: A Study of Sexuality and Pornography in Mid-Nineteenth-Century England.* Transaction, 2008.

Marini, Maria Giulia. *Narrative Medicine: Bridging the Gap between Evidence-Based Care and Medical Humanities*. Springer, 2016.

Meyer, Robinson." The Standing Rock Sioux Claim 'Victory and Vindication' in Court." *The Atlantic*, 14 June 2017, www.theatlantic.com/science/archive/2017/06/dakota-access-standing-rock-sioux-victory-court/530427. Accessed 18 Dec. 2017.

Meyer, Sabine N. "Incorporating the Indigenous Subject: Environmental Justice, Human Rights, and Independent Film." *Comparative Indigenous Studies,* edited by Mita Banerjee, 2016, pp. 83-112.

Molina, Natalia. *Fit to Be Citizens?: Public Health and Race in Los Angeles 1879-1939.* U of California P, 2006.

Morrison, Toni. *Playing in the Dark: Whiteness and the Literary Imagination.* Vintage, 1992.

---. "Recitatif." *Confirmation: Anthology of African American Women*, edited by Imamu Amiri Baraka, 1983, pp. 243-61.

Mukhopadhyay, Tito Rajarshi. *Beyond the Silence: My Life, the World and Autism.* National Autistic Society, 2000.

---. *The Mind Tree: A Miraculous Child Breaks the Silence of Autism.* Arcade Publishing, 2011.

---. *Der Tag, an dem ich meine Stimme fand: Ein autistischer Junge erzählt.* Rowohlt, 2005.

Mulvey, Laura. *Visual and Other Pleasures*. Palgrave Macmillan, 2009.

My Name is Khan. Dir. Karan Johar. 20th Century Fox, 2010.

National Museum Australia. "The Warburton Ranges Controversy, 1957." *National Museum Australia: Collaborating for Indigenous Rights*, indigenousrights.net.au/civil_rights/the_warburton_ranges_controversy,_1957. Accessed 3 Oct. 2016.

Navarro, Mireya. "Clearly, Frankly, Unabashedly Disabled." *The New York Times*, 13 May 2007, www.nytimes.com/2007/05/13/fashion/13disabled.html. Accessed 11 Aug. 2017.

Nelson, Alondra. *Body and Soul: The Black Panther Party and the Fight Against Medical Discrimination*. U of Minnesota P, 2012.

Nicholson, Blake. "$3.8 Billion Dakota Access Oil Pipeline Begins Service." *The Chicago Tribune*, 1 June 2017, www.chicagotribune.com/news/nationworld/ct-dakota-access-oil-pipeline-20170601-story.html. Accessed 18 Dec. 2017.

Niemeyer, Christof M. "Nanopartikel, Proteine und Nucleinsäuren: Die Biotechnologie begegnet den Materialwissenschaften." *Angewandte Chemie*, vol. 113, no. 22, 2001, pp. 4237-49.

Nixon, Rob. *Slow Violence and the Environmentalism of the Poor*. Harvard UP, 2011.

Nuclear Savage: The Islands of Secret Project 4.1. Directed by Adam Jonas Horowitz, Pacific Islanders in Communications, 2011.

Nussbaum, Martha Craven. *Frontiers of Justice: Disability, Nationality, Species Membership*. Belknap, 2007.

---. *The Clash Within: Democracy, Religious Violence, and India's Future*. Belknap, 2009.

Parliament of Australia – Department of Parliamentary Services. "Prime Minister Kevin Rudd, MP – Apology to Australia's Indigenous Peoples." *Australian Government*, 13 Feb. 2008, www.australia.gov.au/about-australia/our-country/our-people/apology-to-australias-indigenous-peoples. Accessed 2 Aug 2016.

Paul, Norbert, et al. "Captious Certainties: Makings, Meanings and Misreadings of Consumer-Oriented Testing." *Journal of Community Genetics*, vol. 5, no. 1, 2014, pp. 81-87.

Paul, Norbert. "Fundamental Research between Biomedicine and the Humanities." *American Lives*, edited by Alfred Hornung. Winter, 2013, pp. 549-57.

Pratt, Mary Louise. "Arts of the Contact Zone." *Profession*, 1991, pp. 33–40. *JSTOR*, www.jstor.org/stable/25595469. Accessed 24 Jan. 2016.

Prince-Hughes, Dawn. *Songs of the Gorilla Nation: My Journey through Autism*. Harmony, 2004.

Rabinow, Paul, and Nikolas Rose. "Biopower Today." *Biosocieties*, vol. 1, no. 2, 2006, pp. 195–217, doi:10.1017/S1745855206040014. Accessed 15 Mar. 2016.

Rain Man. Directed by Barry Levinson, MGM, 1988.

Randolph, Eleanor. "Heart and Solo." *Los Angeles Times,* 1 Feb. 1998, articles.latimes.com/1998/feb/01/entertainment/ca-14173. Accessed 3 Mar. 2016.

Ravitz, Jessica. "The Sacred Land at the Center of the Dakota Pipeline Dispute." *CNN*, 1 Nov. 2016, edition.cnn.com/2016/11/01/us/standing-rock-sioux-sacred-land-dakota-pipeline/index.html. Accessed 18 Dec. 2017.

Ray, Michael. "Presidential Medal of Freedom." *Encyclopædia Britannica*, 1 Feb. 2017, www.britannica.com/topic/Presidential-Medal-of-Freedom. Accessed 21 Feb. 2017.

Reconciliationproject. "The Doctrine of Discovery is less of a problem than terra nullius." *A Reconciliation Project*, 16 Jul. 2012, reconciliationproject.ca/2012/07/16/the-doctrine-of-discovery-is-less-of-a-problem-than-terra-nullius. Accessed 12 Nov. 2016.

Reynolds, Henry. *Nowhere People: How International Race Thinking Shaped Australia's Identity*. Viking, 2005.

Ring, Trudy. "Oliver Sacks, Famed Gay Neurologist and Author, Dies at 82." *Advocate 50th*, 31 Aug. 2015, www.advocate.com/obituaries/2015/08/31/oliver-sacks-famed-gay-neurologist-and-author-dies-82. Accessed 15 Nov. 2016.

Robertson, Lindsay G. *Conquest by Law: How the Discovery of America Dispossessed Indigenous Peoples of Their Lands.* Oxford UP, 2005.

Robinson, Tom, et al. "The Portrayal of Older Characters in Animated Disney Films." *Journal of Aging Studies*, vol. 21, no. 3, 2007, pp. 203-13.

Rosaldo, Renato. "Cultural Citizenship and Educational Democracy." *Cultural Anthropology*, no. 9, 1994, pp. 402-11, doi:10.1525/can.1994.9.3.02a00110. Accessed 21 Oct. 2017.

Rose, Nikolas S. *The Politics of Life Itself: Biomedicine, Power and Subjectivity in the Twenty-First Century*. Princeton UP, 2007.

---., and Joelle M. Abi-Rached. *Neuro: The New Brain Sciences and the Management of the Mind.* Princeton UP, 2013.

Roy, Arundhati. *The God of Small Things.* Flamingo, 1997.

Sacks, Oliver W. *Awakenings*. Duckworth and Co.,1973.

Sacks, Oliver. Foreword. *Thinking in Pictures: And other Reports from my Life with Autism*, by Temple Grandin, 2006, pp. xiii-vxiii.

Salaam Namaste. Directed by Siddarth Anand, Yash Raj Films, 2005.

Schaffer, Kay, and Sidonie Smith. *Human Rights and Narrated Lives: The Ethics of Recognition*. Palgrave Macmillan, 2004.

Schöne-Seifert, Bettina. "Biologismusvorwürfe gegenüber Neurowissenschaften und Psychiatrie." *Geist – Gehirn – Genom – Gesellschaft: Wie wurde ich zu der Person, die ich bin*?, edited by Onur Güntürkün and Jörg Hacker. Nova Acta Leopoldina, no. 405, 2014, pp. 123-42.

Schroedinger, Erwin. *What is Life? The Physical Aspect of the Living Cell with Mind and Matter and Autobiographical Sketches*. Cambridge UP, 2012.

Scott, Kim. *True Country*. 1993. Freemantle Arts Centre P, 2010.

Sesame Street – Cookie Monster and Jason – LOVE." *YouTube*, uploaded by Tiny Dancer, 6 Dec. 2015, www.youtube.com/watch?v=C-TuLfp3qsw. Accessed 19 Mar. 2016.

Shapiro, Johanna. "Illness Narrative: Reliability, Authenticity, and the Empathic Witness." *Medical Humanities*, vol. 37, no. 2, 2011, pp. 68-72.

Shiva, Vandana. *Biopiracy: The Plunder of Nature and Knowledge*. South End P, 1997.

Singer, Wolf. *Ein neues Menschenbild? Gespräche über Hirnforschung*. Suhrkamp, 2003.

Smith, Zadie. *On Beauty*. Hamish Hamilton, 2005.

Spencer, Danielle R. "The Art of Medicine: All Creatures Great and Small." *The Lancet*, dx.doi.org/10.1016/S0140-6736(15)61192-8, vol. 386, 4 Jul. 2015, pp. 22-3.

Stephenson, Margaret A., editor. *Mabo: The Native Title Legislation.* U of Queensland, 1995.

Spin City. Directed by Michael J. Fox and Garry David Goldberg, Paramount Worldwide, 1996.

Taffe, Sue. "Collaborating for Indigenous Rights 1957–1973." *National Museum Australia*, indigenousrights.net.au/. Accessed 23 Feb. 2017.

Taylor, Charles. "The Politics of Recognition." *Multiculturalism: Examining the Politics of Recognition*, edited by Amy Gutmann, 1994, pp. 25-74.

Temple Grandin. Directed by Mick Jackson, HBO Films, 2010.

The Australian. "Full transcript of PM's speech." *The Australian*, 13 Feb. 2008, www.theaustralian.com.au/news/nation/full-transcript-of-pms-speech/news-story/3143dac870aec0145901e575ae79cc3b19 Sept. 2013. Accessed 15 May 2017.

The Cherokee Word for Water. Directed by Charlie Soap, Mankiller Foundation, 2013.

Thomas, Rachel. "The Male Virtuosos Who Prove that Ballet Isn't Just for Ballerinas." *Royal Opera House*, 7 Feb. 2014, www.roh.org.uk/news/the-male-virtuoso. Accessed 11 Jan. 2017.

Ty, Eleanor, and Christl Verduyn, editors. *Asian Canadian Writing Beyond Autoethnography.* Wilfrid Laurier UP, 2008.

United Nations. "We can end Poverty: Millennium Development Goals and Beyond 2015." *United Nations*, www.un.org/millenniumgoals/environ.shtml. Accessed 28 Mar. 2016.

US Citizenship and Immigration Services. "Citizen Rights and Responsibilities." *Official Website of the Department of Homeland Security*, www.uscis.gov/citizenship/learners/citizenship-rights-and-responsibilities. Accessed 5 Feb. 2016.

---. "The Citizen's Almanac." *Official Website of the Department of Homeland Security*, www.uscis.gov/sites/default/files/USCIS/Office%20of%20Citizenship/Citizenship%20Resource%20Center%20Site/Publications/M-76.pdf. Accessed 24 Jan. 2016.

---. "Civics Questions and Answers for the Naturalization Test." *Official Website of the Department of Homeland Security*, www.uscis.gov/citizenship/see-all-section-items-title/Civics%20Questions%20and%20Answers%20for%20the%20Naturalization%20Test/55254?destination=node/41140. Accessed 5 Feb. 2016.

Vazquez, Michael. "Gale Anne Hurd on The Legacy of Wilma Mankiller (Exclusive Video)." *The Huffington Post*, 5 Apr. 2017, www.huffingtonpost.com/michael-vazquez/post_8525_b_6979656.html. Accessed 20 Nov. 2016.

Vizenor, Gerald Robert. *Manifest Manners: Postindian Warriors and Survivance*. Wesleyan UP, 1999.

Waller, Nicole, and Carl Eduard Scheidt. "Erzählen als (Wieder-) Herstellen von Selbstkohärenz: Überlegungen zur Verarbeitung traumatischer Erfahrungen." *Zeitschrift für Psychosomatische Medizin und Psychotherapie*, vol. 56, no. 1, 2010, pp. 56-73.

Watson, Blake A. "The Doctrine of Discovery and the Elusive Definition of Indian Title." *Lewis and Clark Law Review*, vol. 15, no. 4, 2012, pp. 995- 1024.

Weiß, Martin G., editor. *Bios und Zoë: Die menschliche Natur im Zeitalter ihrer technischen Reproduzierbarkeit.* Suhrkamp, 2009.

---. Einleitung. *Bios und Zoe: Die menschliche Natur im Zeitalter ihrer technischen Reproduzierbarkeit.* Suhrkamp, 2009, pp. 7-10.

Wohlmann, Anita. *Aged Young Adults: Age Readings of Contemporary American Novels and Films*. Transcript, 2014.

Wolf, Christian. "Eine Pille gegen das Anderssein." *Gehirn & Geist*, no. 10, 2016, pp. 70-76.

Wolff. Eric. "Obama Administration Blocks Dakota Pipeline, Angering Trump Allies." *Politico*, 4 Dec. 2016, www.politico.com/story/2016/12/us-army-corps-blocks-dakota-access-pipeline-232172. Accessed 18 Dec. 2017.

Woods, Angela. "The Limits of Narrative: Provocations for the Medical Humanities." *Medical Humanities* vol. 37, no. 2, 2011, p. 73-78.

Woodward, Kathleen. *Figuring Age: Women, Bodies, Generations*. Indiana UP, 1999.

Wortland, Justin. "What to Know About the Dakota Access Pipeline Protests." *Time*, 28 Oct. 2016. time.com/4548566/dakota-access-pipeline-standing-rock-sioux. Accessed 18. Dec. 2017.

Wynne, Brian. "Misunderstood Misunderstanding: Social Identities and Public Uptake of Science." *Public Understanding of Science*, vol. 1, no. 3, July 1992, pp. 281-304, doi.org/10.1088/0963-6625/1/3/004. Accessed 28 Mar. 2017.